Health Care Operations Management

A Quantitative Approach to Business and Logistics

James R. Langabeer II

The University of Texas School of Public Health

Houston, TX

JONES AND BARTLETT PUBLISHERS

Sudbury, Massachusetts

BOSTON   TORONTO   LONDON   SINGAPORE

World Headquarters

Jones and Bartlett Publishers	Jones and Bartlett Publishers	Jones and Bartlett Publishers
40 Tall Pine Drive	Canada	International
Sudbury, MA 01776	6339 Ormindale Way	Barb House, Barb Mews
978-443-5000	Mississauga, Ontario L5V 1J2	London W6 7PA
info@jbpub.com	Canada	United Kingdom
www.jbpub.com		

Jones and Bartlett's books and products are available through most bookstores and online booksellers. To contact Jones and Bartlett Publishers directly, call 800-832-0034, fax 978-443-8000, or visit our website www.jbpub.com.

Substantial discounts on bulk quantities of Jones and Bartlett's publications are available to corporations, professional associations, and other qualified organizations. For details and specific discount information, contact the special sales department at Jones and Bartlett via the above contact information or send an email to specialsales@jbpub.com.

This publication is designed to provide accurate and authoritative information in regard to the Subject Matter covered. It is sold with the understanding that the publisher is not engaged in rendering legal, accounting, or other professional service. If legal advice or other expert assistance is required, the service of a competent professional person should be sought.

Production Credits

Publisher: Michael Brown	Composition: Auburn Associates, Inc.
Associate Editor: Katey Birtcher	Cover Design: Kristin E. Ohlin
Production Director: Amy Rose	Cover Image: © Frank Boellmann/
Production Editor: Tracey Chapman	Shutter Stock, Inc.
Marketing Manager: Sophie Fleck	Printing and Binding: Malloy, Inc.
Manufacturing Buyer: Therese Connell	Cover Printing: Malloy, Inc.

Library of Congress Cataloging-in-Publication Data
Langabeer, James R., 1969-
    Health care operations management : a quantitative approach to business and logistics / James R. Langabeer II.
        p. ; cm.
    Includes bibliographical references and index.
    ISBN-13: 978-0-7637-5051-0
    ISBN-10: 0-7637-5051-4
    1. Hospitals—Business management. 2. Hospitals—Administration. 3. Business logistics. I. Title.
    [DNLM: 1. Hospital Administration—methods. 2. Efficiency, Organizational. WX 157 L271h 2007]
    RA971.3.L338 2007
    362.11068—dc22
                                                        2007007223

6048
Printed in the United States of America
11 10 09 08 07   10 9 8 7 6 5 4 3 2 1

Table of Contents

List of Figures and Tables

Figures

Tables

Preface

While less than 5% of the American population currently works in a healthcare system, the overwhelming majority of adults have been a patient or a guest at a hospital, clinic, or physician's office. Of those, while most remember the quality and care given by nurses and physicians, many have left the facility with an overwhelming feeling of disdain for the inefficient and time-consuming business processes. Excessive wait times, lack of coordination among different departments, duplicate entry of personal information in multiple manual forms, unfriendly facilities, and general lack of customer service are usually attributes assigned to healthcare organizations. While outcome data suggest that the quality of medical care is improving for most types of illness, the attention to detail in day-to-day operational management has not kept pace.

In a time when hospitals' financial situations are increasingly being called into question, hospitals are now starting to get serious about creating operational efficiencies to become more competitive and financially viable. Do hospitals and clinics exist to make profits? Some do; however, most do not. Either way, if hospitals are to survive dismally poor healthcare economics, escalating costs, and increasing competitive pressures, they must apply sound business management. This will ensure that hospitals earn the reasonable return on investment necessary to continue to invest and upgrade buildings, programs, and employees.

A very active debate continues at the national level, primarily focused on health policy research. New programs and policies centered around the concepts of "pay for performance," quality and accreditation, flawed government funding mechanisms, federal and state regulations, publication and sharing of outcome data with the public, and other aspects of the U.S. healthcare system continue to address structural issues that affect the quality and costs of care in general. Additionally, behavioral research into physician judgment and mechanisms to encourage elimination of unnecessary tests and treatments will probably change medical education in the future. All of these can help improve the industry's economics and market structure. But, for now, hospitals and systems must continue to look internally at their own operations and their own management to adapt and thrive in current conditions. Hospitals can't wait for policy to address the structural issues driving healthcare costs—they must apply inspired management to improve organizational performance today.

Principles of operations management, whether they focus on productivity or supply chain management, are common in other industries but have yet to really grab hold in health care. There has been a reluctance to admit the applicability of business optimization techniques to the healthcare industry in general. This, coupled with the lack of sophistication and management education on the part of healthcare managers, limits the ability to fully understand and utilize the concepts, methods, and techniques offered.

Up until about two decades ago, business managers in health care were considered very low level "paper pushers." Senior administrators at most hospitals tended to be clinically trained and apparently didn't see as much value in managing business issues as medical ones. Of course, at that time most hospitals were reimbursed fully for all operational costs and capital costs, plus a small margin. With guaranteed profits there wasn't a big drive for efficiency and productivity management at that time. Times have changed.

Unfortunately, most books on healthcare business management still focus primarily on issues of either governance or finance—both of which are important topics but alone are not comprehensive. Coverage of revenue cycle issues such as reimbursement, patient billing, coding, and collections are well addressed, as are basic accounting and financial reporting topics. Similarly, governance issues such as improving physician relations are well documented. Yet, as important as these topics are, it leaves most of business operations fairly uncovered.

This text focuses on operations management of healthcare organizations, which includes hospitals, clinics, multiple-hospital systems, and other facilities in an integrated delivery network (IDN). For clarity purposes however, the term *hospital* is widely used in this book, and it refers broadly to any large organizational entity—*hospital* is simply easier to use as the unit of measure than saying IDN, healthcare system, clinic, or the like. Hospitals also are the predominant hub of the healthcare system, and they employ the majority of workers, and resources, so they make more lucid examples for most concepts. The tools and techniques used in this text, however, are just as relevant to other healthcare facilities.

This book concerns itself primarily with the topics that haven't been extensively treated in healthcare texts, which are the operational components of business management. These include all areas that help hospitals improve productivity, reduce cycle times, improve cost management, and generally create business value by converting resources into services. Hospital operations and logistics management concerns itself with a few key themes, all of which will be covered in this text: supply chain management, business process and service design, quality management, inventory management, technology and systems, operational planning and scheduling, and performance improvement. All of these are traditional operations research topics that, when applied to hospitals and healthcare organizations, cover the majority of resource consumption.

In other industries, focus on operations and logistics management has existed for several decades. Retail, consumer goods, and manufacturing-intensive industries have made significant progress in applying scientific and mathematic models to management practices. In health care, however, these practices have been slow to be adopted. Only recently have we started to see more of a focus on these topics.

Several organizations—such as the American Hospital Association's Association for Healthcare Resource and Materials Management, the Healthcare Information and Management Systems Society, and the Society for Health Systems of the Institute of Industrial Engineers—have begun focusing on either using technology to drive operational efficiency or using other methods to master operations and logistics management in health care. As with most early stages of development, these organizations have only begun to scratch the surface of operations management in hospitals. The leading organizations that focus on operations management, such as the Institute for Operations Research and Management and the Decision Sciences Institute, have unfortunately concentrated more on industrial organizations than on health care.

This book was written to help practicing executives and administrators, as well as students in undergraduate and graduate healthcare administration programs, understand the importance of sound operational management, using business strategy and logistics to create a competitive advantage for their organization. It presupposes that there will be a growing need for improved cost efficiencies and economics in the coming years, and this mindset is required if hospitals are to survive competitive pressures. The significance and role of business professionals in health care will continue to evolve and improve over time, and therefore it is mandatory that the skills and expertise of hospital business officers continue to improve.

The framework for this book uses an operations management perspective and attempts to set a path for hospitals to pursue a strategy of operational excellence. Therefore, the problems this book addresses are those that are integrated around operations and logistics management, as displayed in **Figure P-1**.

This book will help hospitals address issues such as how to improve processes and reduce costs, how to drive down costs through technology using electronic commerce, and which methods and tools exist to help improve operational performance. This book should be used as a reference guide for those working in hospital logistics, supply

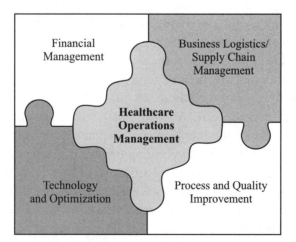

FIGURE P–1 Operations Management in Health Care

chain, and operational management in large hospitals and other facilities in the healthcare industry; ultimately, the book should serve three purposes:

- Present concepts and techniques that many hospitals have not yet adopted, in areas that are not well documented.

- Educate students and administrators on the value of business operations, with a strong focus on quantitative models for decision making.

- Help hospitals become financially successful.

Hopefully, this book will stimulate significantly more research and publication on mastering operations research in health care and using advanced techniques to drive improved competitiveness into health care.

PART I

Operations Management and Financial Health

Part I of this text provides the reader with a foundation of operations management and explains its role in helping to improve health care's financial and business condition. As a service industry, financial outcomes are driven primarily by labor and supply costs, so an understanding of the income statement and the use of key ratios to manage these areas is provided. Understanding the concepts of operations management, and its relationship to financial margins, is also explored.

Chapter 1 offers an overview of the discipline of operations management and that of management in general. Goals of operations management, from cost reduction to network optimization, are described, as well as the key functions and roles performed by operations managers. This chapter sets the stage for the rest of the text.

Chapter 2 is an introduction to health care and hospitals as a business—a business that must generate revenues and sustain itself financially as organizations do in other industries. This chapter defines the hospital, discusses the nature of its goods and services, and provides an overview to healthcare finance. The concept of healthcare production, distinct from operations, is also explored.

Chapter 3 provides an introduction to healthcare finance for the operations manager. An understanding of the drivers of improved financial performance is essential to effective operations management, so this chapter addresses how hospitals earn revenue, and it defines the basic terms used in healthcare finance. Importantly, it defines the key external financial statements that represent the financial condition of the organization, which are used as data sources for a variety of operational analyses in this text. Finally, it discusses the financial distress that is typical in hospitals today.

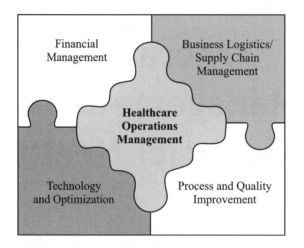

FIGURE P1–1 Operations Management in Health Care

Healthcare Operations Management

Healthcare operations management is a discipline that integrates scientific principles of management to determine the most efficient and optimal methods to support patient care delivery. Most positions today in hospitals are, in fact, roles that involve coordination and execution of operations. This chapter provides the rationale for operations management and describes its evolving role in helping hospitals become more competitive.

THE ROLE OF HEALTHCARE OPERATIONS MANAGEMENT

Most hospitals are nonprofit in nature. Nearly 85% of hospitals are considered not-for-profit and exist solely to serve the community in which they operate. As nonprofits, these organizations are exempt from most federal and state taxation and are *not* expected to show continuous positive growth rates or large profit margins, as most publicly traded firms do. However, if a hospital cannot show some return on the capital or dollars invested, there will be negative consequences. For example, failure to show reasonable margins will likely cause the public bond market (which finances most healthcare growth today) to assign sub-par credit ratings; therefore, the bonds themselves will have poor yields, making hospitals less than stellar investments for bondholders.

Most importantly, the term limited profit margins implies there will be fewer dollars to invest back in the business to ensure that buildings are updated, that equipment is replaced and technology is modern, and that clinical programs will continue to expand and be enhanced. Without these investments, hospitals will probably be unable to attract the most qualified physicians and administrators, which will continue the downward spiral. While some hospitals and healthcare systems wait for changes in the public health policy to save them, the more competitive and successful hospitals are acting now to protect their margins.

In this era of continual pricing pressures affecting the top line of the income statement, and with more than 50% of all hospitals reporting negative profit margins, it is essential that hospitals begin to look toward more sophisticated business strategies to succeed. Differentiated marketing programs and strategies, broader use of advertising, and more careful and precise long-term planning about service lines are all strategies that must be utilized (Rovin, 2001).

Equally as important, there must be a broader adoption of operational and logistical management techniques into hospital business affairs. Monitoring and maximizing labor productivity for all medical support and allied health professionals is critical to maintaining salary expenses. Incorporating queuing theory and scheduling optimization methods helps drive waste and cycle time out of hospitals. Incorporating logistical and supply chain management techniques helps reduce operational expenses, eliminate excess safety stocks, and generally improve working capital management. Most importantly, using technology to further automate and streamline all processes in hospital operations can help reduce costs and maximize efficiencies.

Hospitals and other healthcare organizations cannot rely on the extrinsic factors (such as health policy, federal payer regulation changes, or shifts in managed care market structures) to change their margin potential. That is to say that these are important and probably very significant issues; however, they are covered in other texts and will evolve regardless of the managerial behavior that hospitals employ. These macro-level issues are important, but equally significant are the micro-economic and organization factors that can be affected by operations and logistics management. Operations management can help organizations today.

Think of healthcare profit margins as a balloon, where a variety of extrinsic, or external, factors cause deflationary pressure from the outside. On the inside is the set of decisions and management systems put in place to combat these pressures and essentially inflate the balloon, or expand the margin. In effect, operations management is the set of intrinsic, or internal, processes and decisions that help address costs, process, technology, and productivity. Strategic management, although equally important, is not a focus of this text. **Figure 1–1** shows conceptually the margin-expansion role that operations management plays.

Health care is primarily a service sector, in that the industry provides intangible or nonphysical "goods," as opposed to physical objects that can be seen or touched. Hospital services primarily deliver care through providers to patients and therefore lack a manufacturing or assembling process. These services are unique and somewhat differentiated from

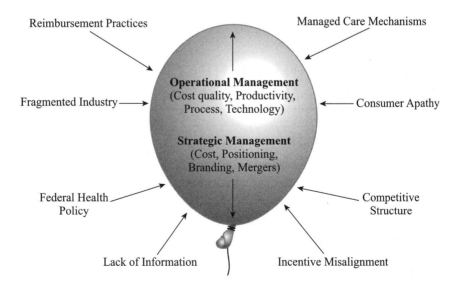

FIGURE 1–1 Operations Management Counters the Extrinsic Pressures Deflating Healthcare Margins

other hospitals, are knowledge-based, and have high levels of customer interaction. Of course, there is a physical good that accompanies the service, which is the focus of supply chain management in hospitals which procures, replenishes, and stores medical supplies and pharmaceuticals as well. In this regard, hospitals have a mix of both tangible and intangible characteristics. All of these attributes make operations management in health care somewhat different than in industries that strictly produce and market physical goods or widgets.

Healthcare operations management can therefore be defined as the quantitative management of the supporting business systems and processes that transform resources (or inputs) into healthcare services (outputs). Inputs are defined as the resources and assets such as labor and capital, including cash, technology, personnel, space, equipment, and information. Outputs include the actual production and delivery of healthcare services. Quantitative management implies a heavy use of analytical and optimization tools, as well as extensive use of process and quality improvement techniques to drive improved results.

Healthcare operations management is a discipline of management that integrates scientific or quantitative principles to determine the most efficient and optimal methods to support patient care delivery. This field is relatively new to health care, but it has existed in other industries for nearly a hundred years.

KEY FUNCTIONS OF HEALTHCARE OPERATIONS MANAGEMENT

The scope of healthcare operations management includes all functions related to the management systems and business processes underlying clinical care. This includes extensive focus on the following: workflow, physical layout, capacity design, physical network optimization, staffing levels, productivity management, supply chain and logistics management, quality management, and process engineering. **Table 1–1** summarizes these key functions and illustrates some of the critical issues and questions that must be addressed for the healthcare enterprise.

Healthcare operations and logistics management include all of these business functions and provide job opportunities for people with titles such as administrator, scheduling manager, operations supervisor, vice

Table 1–1 Key Functions and Issues in Healthcare Operations Management

OM Function	Objective or Issue to Consider
Workflow process	· Are there too many departments or people performing the same task?
	· Do we have an end-to-end map of our major business processes?
	· How many manual processes exist?
	· Are there ways to reduce cycle time, steps, and choke points for key processes?
	· Can we improve speed and patient satisfaction?
Physical layout	· Are our facilities designed with the consideration of speed, capacity, traffic flow, and operational efficiency?
	· Are unit or floor layout designed to eliminate redundancy (e.g., safety stock on all resources)?
Capacity design and planning	· How can we reduce bottlenecks to improve patient through-put for each area?
	· In which cases should we increase the use of technology to improve labor productivity?
Physical network optimization	· Where should we position appropriate par locations, pharmacy satellites, warehouses, and supplies to minimize resources and costs?
	· Do we strategically utilize vendors and their facilities?
	· How can we design and position optimal locations for clinics or resources to ensure lowest total costs?
Staffing levels and productivity management	· How much output can we expect from our staff?
	· Have we maximized the use of automation and electronic commerce to increase productivity?
	· Have we implemented sophisticated analytical models to optimize labor and resource scheduling?
Supply chain and logistics management	· Have we built collaborative planning and forecasting processes to standardize items and reduce total costs?
	· Should we operate "just in time"?
	· Do we use automated, optimized replenishment of medical-surgical supplies to increase turns and asset utilization?
	· How much inventory of each item do we need?
	· Do we use perpetual inventory systems to ensure stringent internal controls and accurate financial reports?
Quality, planning, and process improvement	· Do we use advanced tools for tracking projects?
	· Are we measuring the right performance indicators to bring visibility to trends and exceptions?
	· Do we know how we compare to our key competitors?
	· Have we identified the quality issues that affect goals of customer satisfaction and efficacy, in addition to efficiency, costs, and speed?

president of support services, quality manager, operations analyst, director of patient transportation, procurement manager, management engineer, inventory analyst, facilities manager, supply chain consultant, and so on. Nurses, technicians, and other health providers also play a key role in managing service operations. The advance of operational management positions in hospitals will continue as the need for increased cost efficiency and accountability rises.

THE NEED FOR
OPERATIONS MANAGEMENT

In 2006, the Institute of Medicine of the National Academy of Sciences produced a report called *The Future of Emergency Care*, which is a series of documents that describe the problems facing health care today, especially the emergency care arena. In it, the report outlines a number of recommendations for solving the current crisis. One of the key recommendations called for the following: ". . . hospitals should reduce crowding by improving hospital efficiency and patient flow, and using operational management methods and information technologies" (Institute of Medicine, 2006).

Even others outside of the healthcare industry have identified weaknesses in how healthcare managers manage the processes and systems. IBM has recognized that the service sector needs a greater focus on applying management science to improve process and outcomes and is collaborating with universities to implement what it calls "services science." Irving Wladawsky-Berger, IBM's Vice President for Technical Strategy and Innovation, was quoted recently in the *New York Times* as saying, "All those processes [in a hospital] get done in a relatively ad hoc way. If we want to apply information technology and engineering discipline to improve the quality of the service to reduce errors and to improve productivity, you need people who know how to design a hospital system" (Holstein, 2006). Clearly, even those on the periphery of the healthcare system understand the complexity and the lack of sophistication that currently exist in the industry.

Many other researchers and associations have called for operations management to help drive improvements and efficiencies into the healthcare system (Herzlinger, 1999). Hopefully, the rest of this book will help students and practitioners do just that.

GOALS OF THE OPERATIONS MANAGER

The operations manager may hold any number of job titles discussed earlier, but generically I will refer to the role "operations manager" to describe all such positions in this text. So, what do operations managers do? They have multiple broad goals and functions in the hospital, including all of the following: reduce costs, reduce variability and improve logistics flow, improve productivity, improve quality of customer service, and continuously improve business processes. These are outlined in more detail in the following sections.

Reduce Costs

Operations managers' primary role is to take costs out of the healthcare system. Finding waste, improving utilization, and generally stabilizing and reducing the overall cost of delivering services are essential functions. A hospital with appropriate tracking and management systems—that can isolate all personnel, material, and other resources utilized for delivery of care—will be much more likely to reduce costs because it understands the underlying cost structure. Identifying costs and eliminating unnecessary waste and effort is at the forefront of an operations manager's priority list.

Reduce Variability and Improve Logistics Flow

Operations managers continuously look for the most efficient and optimal paths for movement of resources, whether those resources are physical or information flows. Similarly, there is a continuous focus on reducing variability. **Variability** is the inconsistency or dispersion of inputs and outputs. Variability threatens processes because it results in uncertainty, too many or too few resources, and generally inconsistent results. If there are 10 patients typically seeking care in a specific clinic within a certain time period, and then 20 appear the following period, it will be difficult to staff, to control waiting times, and to manage patient flows.

Improving flow means seeking higher throughput or yields for the same level of resource input. **Throughput** is the rate or velocity at which services are performed or goods are delivered. If a hospital typically sees four patients an hour and can increase throughput to six per hour, this is a

50% improvement in logistical flow and throughput. Similarly, if patient volumes double but a hospital maintains the same historical inventory levels of pharmaceutical supplies, this represents significant improvements in material flow, because assets have higher utilization and turns.

Staffing and resource consumption should be tied directly with patient volumes and workload: if patient volume increase, so too should resources. Unfortunately, many healthcare facilities do not understand patient volumes and the variability that exists from hour to hour and day to day. Managing this variability allows a change in staffing mix and scheduling to accommodate the changes, without staffing at the peaks (which causes excessive costs), staffing for the valleys or low points (which will cause long lines periodically due to limited resources and therefore service quality issues), or staffing for the average (which is the most common suboptimal approach). **Figure 1–2** shows how variability changes over time, which necessitates both capacity and demand analyses.

Logistics is defined as the efficient coordination and control of the flow of all operations—including patients, personnel, and other resources. The role of operations managers is to facilitate improved logistics and throughput by using streamlined process and facility designs to increase capacity, workflow, and throughput.

FIGURE 1–2 Variability Creates Chaos and Inefficiency

Improve Productivity

Hospitals have a tendency to hire additional staff faster than in other industries. This is partly driven by the highly structured organizations that are common in health care and partly because of the historical lack of focus on costs. In years past, hospitals were reimbursed from government and other payers on a "cost-plus" basis—meaning that whatever the cost to deliver, hospitals would be reimbursed fully plus a small profit margin. When pricing is guaranteed to cover costs, there is not a tendency to be overly cost conscious. Even though the industry moved away from this nearly two decades ago, the mentality and behavior of many hospitals have been slow to adapt. **Productivity** is defined as the ratio of outputs to inputs. Improving productivity implies a search for higher levels of output from all employees and other assets. This is one of the most vital roles of an operations manager.

Improve Quality of Customer Service

Health care cannot become so focused on cost and efficiency that quality starts to diminish. Improved quality implies reduced medical errors and improved patient safety, in addition to higher levels of patient satisfaction. Maintenance and improvement of high quality and service levels, both from patient care and other business services (such as the cafeteria or admissions), are expected from an operations manager. Across all industries, higher quality services lead to the ability to secure higher prices, which drives increased market shares and operating margins (Buzzell & Gale, 1987).

Ensuring that services continue to improve patient satisfaction levels, and simultaneously reduce response and waiting times, are key deliverables to providing higher quality services. The **cost-quality continuum** refers to a theoretical trade-off in which a focus on one side of the equation leads to diminishing returns on the other. A focus on costs might lead a hospital to reduce services provided, which might affect overall quality. Operations professionals must balance both and help make optimal decisions on many fronts.

Continuously Improve Business Processes

In highly structured organizations, business processes tend to be unique to each department and are not highly cross-functional or integrated. The operating room in one hospital may handle procurement of goods one way, while the same hospital's gynecology department handles it another. There is typically no sharing of best practices internally, standardization of processes that can lead to improved learning and economies of scale, and very little multidepartment workflow automation. Each department in large hospitals today operates as an independent business, which creates multiple efficiency problems. The role of operations management is to find ways to carry out business processes while improving process efficiency and effectiveness. **Figure 1–3** shows the operations management process of converting inputs into outputs.

COMPETITIVE ADVANTAGE OF OPERATIONS

Overall, if a hospital is successful at delivering on each of these goals throughout the facility, it will deliver improved operational effectiveness. **Operations effectiveness** is a measure of how well the organization is run. It considers both the efficiency of resource inputs and usage and the effectiveness of overall management in achieving desired goals and outcomes (Kilmann & Kilmann, 1991). **Operational excellence** is a term often used to describe a business strategy that focuses exclusively on maximizing operational effectiveness.

A hospital that is operationally effective is heading toward increased competitiveness. **Competitiveness** is management's ability to respond to

Creating value by converting inputs (resources) into efficient and effective outputs (services)

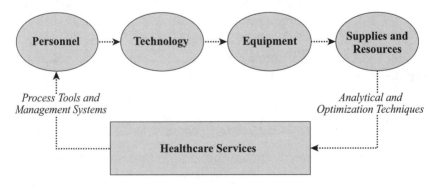

FIGURE 1–3 The Operations Management Process

environmental changes (such as changes in reimbursement practices) as well as competitor's actions (such as adding new facilities or expanding existing service lines). If a hospital can achieve a competitive edge or advantage over other hospitals, and can sustain this position, it will have higher operating margins and will be able to continue improving, expanding, and surviving. Operations management is critical to this outcome.

Competitiveness is often driven by innovation. **Innovation** is the continuous search for a way to do new things or just do current things better. Organizations innovate by using new technologies or finding ways to change the playing field so that processes that once were considered essential are no longer necessary. The electronics industry is an example in which firms continuously innovate. A firm that was competitive based on analog technology had its perspective of the world shaken up considerably when digital technology was created, and the products that the firm once made were completely irrelevant. In addition, continuous innovation often results in hypercompetition, which ultimately is characterized by economics wherein both prices and costs decline (D'Aveni, 2006). For example, when digital video disc players were first introduced, prices were nearly $1,000. Today they can be purchased for as little as $30 in discount stores. The prices of cell phones, televisions, computers, fax machines, and many other electronics all follow the same pattern. In healthcare, innovation also helps to improve competitiveness.

FACTORS DRIVING INCREASED HEALTHCARE COSTS

Imagine that rather than a healthcare organization's annual budget increasing between 5% and 15% (the range of industry average annual changes), expenses could be maintained and even show signs of deflation, or negative price/cost growth. This would be very beneficial to a hospital's financial condition if it could reduce costs and maintain similar pricing levels.

The historical argument justifying continuously growing healthcare inflation rates typically focuses on five points:

1. Consumers are aging and living longer and are increasingly consuming or utilizing a greater number of services than in prior years.

2. The costs of medical technology and equipment continue to rise, and this represents a growing percentage of capital budgets for most organizations.

3.   The labor costs of key resources (such as physicians and nurses) are governed by market shortages for these positions, which have increased steadily the past few decades.

4.   Prices of pharmaceuticals, which represent a sizable portion of medical treatment plans, continue to escalate to cover high costs of research and development, long U.S. Food and Drug Administration approval cycles, and generally high industry margins for pharmaceuticals.

5.   Emphasis on strict managed care, which appeared to be the predominant model a decade ago, is slowly shifting and diminishing in practice.

The result has been a steadily increasing cost of care. Using the Department of Labor, Bureau of Labor Statistics (BLS) data highlights this fact. The BLS tracks inflation growth through its consumer price index (CPI). The CPI is a mathematical calculation of the average pricing changes over time, using a market basket approach. The general CPI for all items in years 1999 through 2005 showed an increase of less than 14% over 7 years, or around 2% per year (Bureau of Labor Statistics, 2006). Compare that with the cost of medical care, which rose nearly 30% in that same time period—nearly double that of the rest of all other goods tracked. **Figure 1–4** shows this growth over time.

Overall spending for health care in the United States has risen steadily between 13% of the national gross domestic product (GDP) in 1993 to

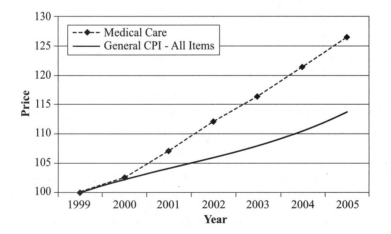

FIGURE 1–4 Controlling Exponential Price Increases in Health Care
Source: US Department of Labor, Bureau of Labor Statistics, 2006.

more than 16.5% of the GDP in 2006, and economists project that this will double again in the next decade and likely reach 20% by 2015 (Heffler et al., 2005). While some hospitals wait for the national debate to continue, it is important to first look at the intrinsic factors in the organization that are driving excessive costs: redundancy, inefficiency, bureaucracy, waste, paper, limited productivity, lack of performance monitoring, poor deployment of information technology, and generally unsophisticated levels of management.

LEARNING FROM OTHER INDUSTRIES

Although health care is unique and has its own set of challenges, hospitals can learn a great deal from other industries that have evolved faster due to technology or process innovation, industry economics, more aggressive competition, reduced barriers to entry and exit, or just better trained business managers. For example, if managers looked at a hospital as being similar to the retail industry, they could better understand how to lay out floors, design configurations to achieve more efficient movement and handling, and use analytical forecasts to drive all aspects of the business. There is a lot to learn from the more operationally effective industries. The tools and techniques that are most similar should be borrowed and applied to health care where appropriate.

For example, in the airline industry, thousands of planes move through the sky fairly seamlessly. A plane lands every few seconds at major airports throughout the world, and yet there are very few accidents (as a percentage of total flights), very high levels of on-time rates (given numerous factors such as weather and security), and very little lost baggage. Nearly 67 million passengers boarded planes in August 2006 in the United States alone (Bureau of Transportation Statistics, 2006). Airlines have learned to operate using speed and volume as an advantage. When an airplane lands, it has very little time before it must be turned around and take off to another destination. This changeover process allows less than 30 minutes, on average, to completely refuel, check maintenance and mechanical conditions, validate aviation systems, restock food and supplies, change over personnel, and unload and reload hundreds of passengers. Think of this changeover as it relates to the process a hospital goes through when changing out beds after a patient is discharged (i.e., admitting and bed management process). A lot can be learned from how another industry approaches a somewhat similar problem. **Table 1–2** summarizes what operations managers in health care can learn from other industries.

PRINCIPLES OF MANAGEMENT

Operations management is one of the disciplines of the broader field of management. According to most theorists, management concerns itself with four key functions: planning, organizing, leading, and controlling. **Planning** involves the establishment of goals and a strategy to achieve these goals. In health care, planning can be strategic (such as deciding which geographic region to invest in a new facility), or it can be operational (such as how many employees to have on staff for each shift). **Organizing** includes making decisions about what tasks will be done, where, when, and by whom. Organizing uses a variety of tools, such as an organization chart to manage people's roles and reporting relationships, process flow charts for improving activities, and Gantt charts for managing projects. **Leading** includes motivating employees, building support for ideas, and generally getting things done through people. Providing direction and clarification to expectations, as well as the role of change management, or preparing the organization for changes to come, are instrumental to providing leadership in hospital operations management. **Controlling** includes all tasks to monitor and track progress toward goals, ensure performance improvement, and make corrective changes in strategy where necessary. The use of status reports, budgets, procedures, and a multitude of other tracking tools is useful in helping enhance management control.

Managers wear many hats and play many roles. They might serve as a figurehead, they make decisions, they reward employees, and they handle

Table 1–2 Teachings from Other Industries

Retail	Building layout and configuration, customer flows, use of forecasts and planning, electronic commerce
Airlines	Scheduling, logistics, strategic pricing (yield management)
Chemicals	Efficiencies, economies of scale, extensive use of linear programming and quantitative modeling
Electronics	Technology innovation, product life-cycle management, pricing strategy
Telecommunications	Command and control center

conflicts and solve problems. Managers help plan tasks, organize them, direct them, and continually adjust and control. Henry Mintzberg, one of the earliest researchers on management processes, described the nature of manager's work as grouped around three key themes: informational, decisional, and interpersonal (1973). *Informational* roles refer to collecting, monitoring, and disseminating information from the external and internal environments to work teams. *Decisional* roles refer to making key decisions for the organization, such as allocation of scarce resources, rewards and penalties for employees, and negotiations with employees and others. *Interpersonal* roles include training and motivating employees, serving as spokesperson, facilitating communication exchanges among various groups, and serving as a liaison.

The study of management continues to evolve. It has moved through a variety of schools of thought: from scientific management, to process-focused, to human behavior, to decision or management sciences theory, to social and open systems (Certo & Certo, 2005). These schools of thought represent different contexts or perspectives upon which a manager's role and tasks should be based. For example, the systems theory schools emphasize that a manager views the organization as a living organism, which is changing and adapting and which operates by an integrated network of open processes. Behavioral schools tend to focus on viewing management from a psychological aspect, highlighting the importance of understanding what motivates employees and how human and cognitive factors influence work environments.

For purposes of operations management and looking for ways to improve operational effectiveness, the school of thought that is the most relevant is that of scientific management.

THE SCIENTIFIC AND MATHEMATICAL SCHOOLS OF MANAGEMENT

Operations management seeks to apply quantitative and analytical techniques to achieve the goals of reduced costs, higher quality, higher productivity, improved processes, and improved logistical flows. The role of mathematics started to drive concepts of industrial efficiency in what is now known as the scientific management era, which began prior to the turn of the 20th century.

Scientific schools of thought historically focused on use of concepts such as "time and motion" studies, which measured how long business processes took, seeking ways to reduce the variability of the results and continuously shrinking the times and associated costs. Early work by Frank and Lillian Gilbreth helped drive a focus on continual improvements—finding ways to do things faster and with fewer resources. In fact, the Gilbreths' research has had a profound impact on health care as well (Gilbreth & Carey, 1966). In the early 1900s they were credited as observing the productivity of surgeons and found that the introduction of changes in both staffing and work flow could significantly alter physician productivity. The introduction of a surgical nurse—to help provide surgical instruments and supplies when needed to free up the surgeon, thereby improving overall productivity—was one of the key recommendations made. In addition, the Gilbreths recommended other hospital improvements, such as a tray to hold common surgical instruments. These are just two of the contributions made by scientific management to health care.

Frederick Taylor, one of the original management researchers and the "father of scientific management," was often quoted as saying that scientific management is a great "mental revolution" (Matteson & Ivancevich, 1996). By this, he meant that a scientific approach encourages a different perspective or outlook that can change management behaviors and results. This revolution led to some key concepts, such as specialization, division of labor, and mass production. The concept of **specialization** suggests that if a person repeatedly performs just one task, he or she will be able to perform that task faster and with higher quality than others, because he or she has repeated exposure to the process and has learned from his or her experiences. Specialization, in many regards, is what leads hospitals to structure their organization around units such as nursing or materials management. Continued specialization helps to produce well defined roles and tasks, concentrated work efforts, and higher efficiencies. This is also known as **division of labor**. **Mass production** is the concept of the creation of rapid production processes through the use of assembly-line techniques. Mass production has been embraced by most other industries, but, in many respects, it is not relevant in health care.

The scientific era has been shown to have a number of failings and issues, which led to several other schools of thought. The lack of focus on human behavior, on alignment of rewards of employees with those of the organization, and on understanding the need for job rotations and expansion all are major issues that well-rounded managers have to consider. Thus, many of the analytical concepts of scientific management remain vital to healthcare operations management. First, scientific management suggests the need for a strong understanding of processes, their costs and resource utilizations, constraints, and cycle times. Second, scientific management encourages an initial focus on understanding expected outcomes and subsequently designing management systems and business processes around this operational strategy. Third, the variability of processes has to be smoothed out and consistently managed. Finally, scientific management shows that in many cases, quantitative approaches can help create mathematically optimal results for common management decisions and problems. These four fundamental concepts are the foundation of the operations management discipline.

POWER AND DECISION MAKING IN HEALTH CARE

Decisions in health care do not follow the traditional, logical processes used in industrial organizations. In other industries, where profit maximization and shareholder wealth are the primary motives, decisions are primarily driven by goal alignment for both managers (those that run the business) and owners (shareholders who invest in equity or debt and have a claim on the profits and assets). Decision making tends to follow cost-benefit models and focus on risk minimization, cash flows, and return on investment. Although disputes and conflicts may arise because of incomplete or imperfect information (as described in the agency theory of economics), these disputes can typically be minimized by changing incentives, behaviors, and structural mechanisms.

In health care, however, there is incomplete alignment of goals between different agents, or managers, in the organization because of three issues:

1. *Goals are unclear.* There are clinical goals, financial goals, educational or academic goals in some cases, societal goals, community goals, and so on. The ambiguity that exists in terms of priorities and focus makes goals much less acute than in other industries.

2. *Organizations are complex.* In industrial organizations, the organization is focused clearly on the key aspects of buying, making, sell-

ing, and moving products to the marketplace. In health care, reporting relationships often involve complex matrices and dual-reporting structures. This is definitely not the "command and control" structure, focused on speed and efficiency of decision making, that might work in other places.

3. *Relationships are ambiguous.* Many business units in health care are interconnected, but they often behave as if they were not. Independence of departments and providers helps create an environment that is less team focused than in other industries, making relationships important for purposes of mutual support as allies. Also there are continuous power struggles in the healthcare arena between different factions of employees. This creates ambiguity in decision making.

Physicians are typically the most dominant players and have a very substantial role in most major organizational decisions (Young & Saltman, 1985). Power conflicts with nurses and other providers are frequent and have developed (for structural reasons) in the struggle for control over patients, their care, and overall patient management processes (Coombs, 2004). As such, several formal power bases have emerged: business managers, who increasingly are becoming more professional and sophisticated; physician leadership, which historically dominates the power pendulum; and nursing leadership, which probably has the most intimate knowledge of patients and their needs.

Those who control the "production" process in most industries tend to have the most influence and can control decision making for many things. In the production of health care (i.e., delivery of treatments and provision of care) physicians are by far the dominant players, yet their role in most operational management processes in most hospitals is waning as professional business managers evolve.

Decision making in teaching hospitals and academic medical centers is even more complicated—through the introduction of another dominant party: academic faculty and researchers (Choi, Allison, & Munson, 1986). In the largest hospitals, this complexity in decision making is complicated by large business infrastructures, which may employ hundreds or thousands of individuals in all types of support functions, from admissions to patient finance to facilities.

Three characteristics define this complexity of decision processes: problematic preferences, unclear technology, and fluid participation (Cohen,

March, & Olsen, 1972). These characteristics, together with "streams" of both problems and choices, can be combined in unclear decision processes in a "garbage can," where they can often address the wrong problems at the wrong time. This garbage can tends to allow issues and solutions to resurface in strange ways, which often results in a lack of clarity and focus.

With all of these dominant players and complexities, many hospitals have become large bureaucracies. These bureaucracies make it difficult to make important decisions, address financial and business issues, change behaviors and business processes, and implement new technology.

Sophistication in operations and logistics management requires not only understanding concepts and their application to health care, but also understanding the persuasive and leadership characteristics necessary to navigate the bureaucracy, influence dominant power groups, engage support for ideas, and ultimately gain approval and acceptance of changes. These changes will come only if business executives achieve more dominant power positions, which can evolve only as operations and logistics executives are recognized for their contributions, specialized education, professional expertise, and leadership skills. Collaboration within these multidisciplined organizations is just one way to retain more control in the decision-making process.

THE ROLE OF TECHNOLOGY

With its focus on improvements, OM rests highly on the use of technology and automation. Decisions about capital investment in new information and management systems are always at the forefront of the modern operations manager's mind. Technology should be considered whenever quality and efficiency is low. Processes that are repetitive in nature and that can be replaced by less expensive automation are also suitable for a technology investment.

Technology often serves one of three roles:

1. Automate manual processes.
2. Improve transaction processing capabilities.
3. Improve the quality of analysis, reports, and decisions.

Technology has the ability to substantially alter the economics of a process. Processes that can be mechanized allow for faster production or delivery, with less resource usage—two keys to improving operational effectiveness. The decision to substitute capital, or technology, for labor—especially in areas of business support services—is the only way to reduce processing and transactional costs over the long run. For this reason, several other chapters in this text address the issue of technology and its role in productivity enhancements.

TRENDS IN OPERATIONS MANAGEMENT

There are several trends that are being widely considered and adopted in hospitals. These are depicted in **Table 1–3**, and the trends correspond to the role or function of operations management most closely related to it. Some of these will be highlighted in this section, while others will be discussed in other parts of this book.

Outsourcing is the contracting of an outside firm to perform services that were once handled internally. Outsourcing is quite common in many industries, and in health care it has been used successfully for cafeteria operations, bookstore management, investments, and even nursing and other clinical care areas. Outsourcing is not a new concept, but it has a slow adoption rate in health care, where decisions such as these are often quite difficult to make, especially when they result in the dismissal of employees from hospital payrolls. However, outsourcing, when used

Table 1–3 Roles and Trends in Healthcare Operations Management

Primary Role of Operations Managers	Evolving Trends
1. Reduce costs	Standardization
	Optimization
	Resource tracking systems
2. Reduce variability and improve logistical flow	Integrated service delivery
	Analytics
	Supply chain management
3. Improve productivity	Information technology
	Return on investment
4. Provide higher quality services	Evidence-based health care
	Six Sigma
5. Improve business processes	Outsourcing
	Globalization

selectively to target the right areas, can be quite beneficial from a cost perspective.

Outsourcing relies on the notion that a hospital should focus on its core competencies—delivering clinical care—and not on some of the less mission-centric functions, such as housekeeping, materials management, finance, and information technology. When analyzing pre- and post-performance improvement, the evaluation of internally performed or selective outsourcing costs needs to be undertaken to ensure all options are explored and the most operationally effective process remains.

Integrated service delivery is another trend that has been developing over the past few years. Many researchers have pointed to the excessive cost of care as being driven by the medical community's continued desire for specialization and concentration on discrete diseases and treatments, rather than integrative, comprehensive care (Porter & Teisberg, 2006). In response to this, hospitals are looking for ways to push care toward more integrative medicine, including higher sharing of information, resources, and collaboration. The impact on operations management will include redesign of business processes and changes in the number and frequency of logistics networks.

Supply chain management is the integrated management of all products, information, and financial flows in a network designed to pull products from manufacturers to consumers. In health care, there has been widespread adoption of improved sourcing and inventory techniques, designed to lower overall supply expense ratios (which typically account for 25% to 50% of all hospital costs). Significantly more detail about the use of supply chain and logistics management will be covered in Part III.

Another trend in healthcare operations management is globalization. The world is becoming smaller, and vendors from all around the globe are competing for business in retail and other industries. Health care has only recently felt the effects, but this trend will continue. When firms look for outsourcing opportunities (e.g., in information technology), they are now able to turn to vendors as far away as Ireland and India to help manage their information technology operations infrastructure. Medical care that might once have required specialists on site is now only a television away, allowing physicians to practice medicine without even setting foot in the hospital. Vendors for certain medical supplies, pharmaceuticals, and equipment are emerging and starting to compete for business as potential suppliers, requiring hospital managers to understand global logistics. As more and more hospital services become automated, the location of the technology does not matter. This is the true impact of globalization, and it will require adjustments by hospital management.

Investments in a hospital's information technology infrastructure are quite common today. Electronic medical records, computerized physician order entry, enterprise resource planning, picture archival communication systems, supply chain management, and many other systems are much more prevalent today than in years past. Investments in a number of lesser-known technologies for admissions, cashiering, inventory management, and even bed management are also becoming more common.

The basic premise of most technologies is that they provide some return that, when quantified, is greater than the costs associated with it. In some cases, this is simple to calculate, as when a system creates known financial value and has well-defined costs. In others, when the information technology produces vague benefits (such as extending a system's end of life or improving clinical quality), the returns are more difficult to measure and quantify and thus are more complex if creating a cost-benefit comparison. Regardless, the trend in leading hospitals is to conduct thorough return on investment analyses that clearly define the pre- and post-environment and then make comparisons of the delivered or earned value for the project. Significantly more about this will be discussed later in this text.

The growth in deployment of resource tracking systems is also quite interesting. Information systems and technology are being developed specific to health care to allow for tracking of patients, equipment, supplies, pharmaceuticals, bed occupancy, and much more. Microprocessor chips, bar coding technology, global positioning systems, and radio frequency identification systems are all technologies that are being slowly adopted in larger hospitals. Many of these use existing wireless frequencies and infrastructure, so they are becoming easier to implement at lower costs. These tracking systems allow for closer monitoring of utilization patterns, location analysis, stationary or down times, and logistical flows, which thus helps better manage the number, type, and mix of resources required. Improved operational effectiveness results from improved utilization and higher asset productivities. Many of these technologies will be described later.

Another trend that is being followed closely in operations management is that of standardization. **Standardization** is the use of consistent procedures, resources, and services to achieve consistent results across multiple departments. In a system or network, standardization suggests that two hospitals could use the same basic medical supplies for multiple procedures, rather than a wide variety of them, which helps reduce inventory and purchasing costs and creates some economies of scale. Standardization also refers to the use of common standards for information systems, as well as personnel and operational processes. Standardization helps ensure alignment among departments, helps promote familiarization and learning curves, and helps reduce the number of transactions processed—which all result in lower costs and higher productivity.

Finally, many hospitals practice what is called evidence-based health care. **Evidence-based medicine** applies the scientific method to medical practice and seeks to quantify the true outcomes associated with certain medical practices by applying statistical and research methods (CEBM.net, 2006). Evidence-based health care, as it applies to logistics or operations, emphasizes that prior to decisions being made, the options are conscientiously analyzed for the effects each would have on operations. For example, if a certain piece of equipment needs to be replaced, evidence-based medicine suggests that the true costs and outcomes associated with this item be carefully analyzed over time; a replacement piece of equipment undergoes the exact same controls to guarantee and quantify the total impacts of this change on the system. Evidence-based health care, in its use of quantitative methods and in seeking to comprehensively analyze operations, is completely in alignment with operations management theory. The use of quality management processes such as Six Sigma, which attempts to improve process and outputs through continuous improvement techniques, is beginning to gain a solid foundation in the healthcare industry.

CHAPTER SUMMARY

Operations management is the quantitative management of the supporting business systems and processes that transform resources into healthcare outputs. It is focused on achieving operational effectiveness—defined as lower costs, higher productivity, and continuous process improvement. There are five key goals of the operations manager: reduce costs, reduce variability and improve logistics flows, improve productivity, improve quality of customer service, and continuously improve business processes. Operations management is a field within the discipline of management, and it evolved initially from the scientific management school of thought.

It has progressed into a much broader and comprehensive discipline. There are many trends evolving that are changing healthcare operations, and many of these are discussed in later chapters.

KEY TERMS

competitiveness, controlling, cost-quality continuum, division of labor, evidence-based medicine, healthcare operations management, innovation, leading, logistics, mass production, operational excellence, operations effectiveness, organizing, outsourcing, planning, productivity, specialization, standardization, throughput, variability

DISCUSSION QUESTIONS

1. What is operations management in health care?
2. What are the five key goals of operations managers?
3. Does operations management affect a hospital's competitive advantage?
4. What are three of the key trends affecting hospital operations?
5. Who is considered the "father" of scientific management?
6. What are the common sources of cost increases in health care?
7. How does the medical care CPI relate to cost increases for other items?
8. What four things can be learned from scientific management?
9. What are the three reasons decision-making processes in health care are more ambiguous than in other places?
10. How does evidence-based medicine support operations management techniques?

EXERCISE PROBLEM

1. Royal Hospital currently receives more than 10,000 boxes of pharmaceutical supplies per month. All of these items are manually inspected and logged to ensure adequate receipt prior to payment. Eight employees manage receipts and deliveries, while four em-

ployees manually record and track them. A new software package that allows automated scanning of bar codes will replace all or some of the employees used for manual tracking, or at least allow redeployment to other areas of the hospital. What are some of the key questions that must be explored to fully understand the impacts of technology and whether a capital investment should be made to substitute capital for labor?

REFERENCES

Bureau of Labor Statistics. (2006). U.S. Department of Labor. CPI Tables accessed from www.bls.gov.

Bureau of Transportation Statistics. (2006). *U.S. Air Carrier Traffic Statistics—August 2006.* Washington, D.C.: Department of Transportation.

Buzzell, Robert D., and Buzzell T. Gale. (1987). *The PIMS Principles: Linking Strategy to Performance.* New York: The Free Press.

CEBM.net. Centre for Evidence-Based Medicine, University of Oxford Institute of Health Sciences. Website accessed October 2006.

Certo, Samuel C., and S. T. Certo. (2005). *Modern Management.* 10th ed. New York: Prentice Hall Publishing.

Choi, Thomas, Robert F. Allison, and F. Munson. (1986). *Governing University Hospitals in a Changing Environment.* Ann Arbor, MI: Health Administration Press.

Cohen, Michael D., James G. March, and Jonah P. Olsen. (1972). Garbage Can Model of Organizational Choice. *Administrative Science Quarterly, 17*(1): 1–25.

Coombs, Maureen A. (2004). *Power and Conflict between Doctors and Nurses: Breaking through the Inner Circle.* New York: Routledge Publishing.

D'Aveni, Richard A. (2006). *Hyper-Competition.* New York: Free Press.

Gilbreth, Frank B., and Ernestine G. Carey. (1966). *Cheaper by the Dozen.* New York: Cromwell.

Heffler, Stephen, Sheila Smith, Sean Keehan, Christine Borger, M. Kent Clemens, and Christopher Truffer. (2005). Trends: U.S. Health Spending Projections For 2004–2014. *Health Affairs, 10*:79–93.

Herzlinger, Regina E. (1999). *Market-Driven Healthcare: Who Wins, Who Loses in the Transformation of America's Largest Service Industry.* New York: Perseus Books Group.

Holstein, William J. (2006). And Now a Syllabus for the Service Economy. *The New York Times,* December 3, Business Section, p. 10.

Institute of Medicine. (2006). *The Future of Emergency Care: Key Findings and Recommendations.* Washington, D.C.: National Academy of Sciences.

Kilmann, Ralph H., and Ines Kilmann. (1991). *Making Organizations Competitive: Enhancing Networks and Relationships Across Traditional Boundaries.* San Francisco: Jossey-Bass Publishers.

Matteson, Michael T., and John M. Ivancevich. (1996). *Management and Organizational Behavior Classics*. 6th ed. Chicago: Irwin Publishing.

Mintzberg, Henry. (1973). *Nature of Managerial Work*. Reading, MA: Addison-Wesley.

Porter, Michael E., and Elizabeth O. Teisberg. (2006). *Redefining Health Care: Creating Value-Based Competition on Results*. Boston: Harvard Business School Press.

Rovin, Sheldon. (2001). *Medicine and Business: Bridging the Gap*. Gaithersburg, MD: Aspen Publishers.

Young, David W., and Richard B. Saltman. (1985). *The Hospital Power Equilibrium: Physician Behavior and Cost Control*. Baltimore: Johns Hopkins University Press.

Health Care as a Business

Goals of This Chapter
1. Define *hospital*
2. Describe the roles of a business operations manager in health care
3. Explain the different classifications of hospitals
4. Describe what makes a teaching hospital unique
5. Describe the sources of reimbursement from payers

Those of you who find yourselves working as business professionals in a healthcare setting for the first time will undoubtedly be overwhelmed on the first day of employment. The first thing to notice is that there is a much greater focus on medical activities than business activities in most facilities. Another first impression is that the layout and design of workflow and facilities are often extremely inefficient, cluttered, and almost an afterthought. The information systems in all but the most advanced hospitals have not yet discovered or adopted electronic commerce, process automation, and real-time operational reporting, as you would expect to find in retail or manufacturing industries. In additions, hospitals have not yet begun to focus on key business issues as have almost all other industries over the past few decades. This is good news for those just joining the industry, because it promises significant change and opportunities for improvement.

Before operations management can help make a difference in health care, using quantitative tools and techniques to drive improvements across all areas of the business, it is important to understand the context of the modern hospital—what it is, how it started, and where it is going.

HOSPITALS ARE BIG BUSINESS

Hospitals are large and complex organizations and differ from most traditional organizations in many ways. First, hospital missions focus on the more abstract goals of improving community health or curing and eliminating disease. Meanwhile, other types of companies typically have a two-prong mission of maximizing profits and satisfying stakeholders, which helps to clearly focus employees and others on efficiencies, revenues, and cost reductions.

Hospitals also offer an intangible product, unlike a widget that can be easily packaged and sold. This service, which is somewhat unique and not widely available, distinguishes the production of health care from the production of other goods.

Typically, hospitals are not profit-maximizing entities, and historically, most have not been overly concerned about negative margins or break-even income statements. Most other organizations focus solely on maximizing the wealth of the owners or shareholders and to a lesser degree on the social or public benefits that are derived from the production of their goods or services.

Additionally, the primary performance outcome of a hospital is measured in terms of "quality," abstractly measured by a wide range of mortality and morbidity indicators, and not business metrics such as economic value, return on investment, or net income. This lack of focus on the more common financial metrics separates health care from most other industries, which use indexes that daily monitor the efficient flow of information about the organization and communicate the value generated, as in a stock exchange. As a byproduct, there is very little free flow of information about most healthcare organizations, and this lack of perfect information further distinguishes the healthcare industry.

Very importantly, hospitals are governed to a large degree by professionals who lack formal training in business management, unlike other firms where those educated and professionally trained in business disciplines clearly govern all aspects of the business. This is one of the primary reasons financial and business implications of key decisions might be secondary to the more relevant medical issues that dominate most physicians' mindsets. The business managers who are recruited are often not trained as well in business or financial acumen as those graduates who tend to migrate toward the traditional profit industries, such as energy or banking.

Healthcare facilities also commonly work on a 24-hour-per-day basis, creating obvious labor and scheduling inefficiencies. Some industrial organizations do this as well, but they do so only to the extent that the decision to remain opens generates positive cash flow. Decisions about hours in health care are driven largely by societal needs and expectations for round-the-clock medical service and availability of care at all times.

Finally, hospitals have community and other stakeholder interests that create goal ambiguity. In most towns, hospitals are as sacred as a church or civic building and are not admired as much for their economic engine as for their healing powers.

Nonetheless, hospitals have to manage the same set of business resources as any other type of organization, whether talking about financial resources, personnel, equipment, supplies, technology, facilities, etc. Hospitals employ hundreds or even thousands of people, with payrolls that can reach several hundred million dollars. They serve as a marketplace and are suppliers of valuable services to hundreds of customers daily. They are buyers, procuring a vast array of supplies, pharmaceuticals, and technology. To function efficiently, hospitals have to manage people, money, time, and business processes. They are economic engines that generate significant cash flows and provide economic value for their organization and their community. In short, hospitals are a business. Managing these business affairs then is a difficult challenge, and historically there has not been much focus in this area.

Nearly 5,800 hospitals operate today, employing nearly 5,500,000 people and managing gross revenues of over $500 billion (Bureau of Labor Statistics [BLS], 2004; American Hospital Association [AHA], 2006a). These are significant resources, requiring dedicated and trained business managers who can help ensure appropriate fiscal responsibility, maintain overall costs, improve productivity, and ensure positive operating margins. Yet, business and management professionals in hospitals represent less than 5% of all employment (BLS, 2004).

While the size of hospitals varies—anywhere from 10 beds to more than 1,000 beds—the administrative organizations and operational managements are quite similar. Some have a large network of outpatient clinics, while others focus exclusively on inpatient surgeries and treatments. There may also be differences in funding sources, types of services offered, or mix of patients served, but the overall aim of business operational management should be similar. Finding methods and means for improving business operations should be the primary goal of business officers in hospitals.

WHAT IS A HOSPITAL?

A hospital is an organization devoted to delivering patient care, and it serves as the central hub for the entire healthcare industry. There is at least one hospital in nearly every city, and larger cities might have several dozen. Historically, hospitals were viewed as a "facility" placed to serve those who need overnight stays (i.e., primarily inpatient) or surgery, or who were otherwise extremely sick. The very early definition of hospitals was as a place people went to die, but as the quality of care has improved, so too have the national health outcomes, measured primarily in terms of morbidity and mortality rates. Consequently, fewer people go to hospitals to die than to get well or to prevent illness.

The basic definition of a **hospital** typically involves providing services clustered around three key terms: observation, diagnosis, and treatment (Samour, 2006). **Observation** involves analyzing or studying patients and running tests and checks—all of which ultimately lead to a diagnosis. The **diagnosis** is the physician's or medical provider's explanation for the cause or source of the problem or symptoms. **Treatment** is the course of action that the hospital will take to make the patient better, lessen the symptoms, or otherwise care for the patient. All of the services that a hospital provides are typically organized around at least one of these areas.

The healthcare industry has become somewhat more integrated, or consolidated, in recent years. **Horizontal integration** refers to consolidation, mergers, acquisitions, or alliances among several competitive or cooperative hospitals. Horizontal integration has resulted in a large number of *multihospital systems,* defined as an organized system of hospitals that share central services, common ownership of assets, and/or centralized governance and management. **Vertical integration** refers to the acquisition or alliances of other parties involved in other phases of the healthcare value chain, such as payers, clinics, or physicians. Physician-hospital alliances and hospital-sponsored health maintenance organizations (HMOs) are common structures within vertically integrated systems. Whether vertically or horizontally integrated, an **integrated delivery network** refers to any combination or integration between a hospital and other providers or partners in the healthcare industry that works together collaboratively across a spectrum of care to provide more competitive and comprehensive services.

In economic terms, the "production" capabilities (i.e., the conversion of supplies, labor, and other resources into medical services) of health care are performed by physicians, nurses, technicians, and a host of other allied health professionals. Physicians of course have traditionally retained most of the power in health care because they have long played the dominant and central role. They are the most academically qualified, spend the longest time in training programs, and have the most systematic view of disease and anatomy. A physician is also called a "medical doctor" or simply a "doctor" in most places.

The new role of the hospital is evolving, as hospitals have extended their ownership and influence from a "facility" to a "system," which might include multiple buildings, offices, or practices distributed throughout a large geographic area. Hospitals now often include ambulatory or outpatient clinics, physician offices, treatment centers, and other services that are not necessarily housed in the primary hospital. Hospitals have come a long way since the construction of the first hospital, the Pennsylvania Hospital in Philadelphia, in the mid 1700s.

From a business perspective, it is important to understand the type of hospital in order to understand its mission, background, and orientation. There are several ways to classify hospitals, but the most common is by ownership type, type of service or specialty offered, and length of stay.

Most hospitals in the United States are primarily considered **community hospitals**, in that they are available for use by an entire community. Community hospitals represent the significant majority of all hospital-based care and include all nonfederal, short-term hospitals, whether they are for-profit, not-for-profit, or public. When people think of the "typical" hospital, they are thinking of the community hospital. Community hospitals focus on short-term stays, usually less than 30 days, and **acute care**, defined as being focused on a specific episode or event requiring care. Sometimes both for-profit and not-for-profit community hospitals are grouped together and called private hospitals, to distinguish them from public and government-owned facilities. In addition, churches control some of these private nonprofit hospitals. Well-known healthcare systems are controlled by the Baptist, Catholic, Protestant, and Seventh Day Adventist religions. Besides community, there are federally owned hospitals, such as the Veterans Administration, which manages a network of more than 150 hospitals and nearly 1,000 clinics and other facilities (Department of Veterans Affairs, 2006).

Hospitals listed with the AHA fall into one of four classifications (AHA, 2006b):

1. General (providing a broad range of services for multiple conditions).

2. Specialty (services for a specific medical condition, such as oncology).

3. Rehabilitation (focused on restoring health).

4. Psychiatric (providing care for behavioral and mental disorders).

Historically hospitals have been owned by either nonprofit, church, or government agencies and have been considered organizations offering public or social goods. This mix has been changing over the past three decades. In 1976, approximately 13% of community hospitals were for-profit or investor owned. In 1986 there were nearly 15%, and in 2006 there are 17% investor owned (AHA, 2006b). As this mix shifts, a higher level of competitiveness and financial focus will continue. The largest for-profit hospitals systems are HCA Inc., Tenet, HMA, Triad, and Community Health. Of these, the most prominent, HCA, had annual revenues exceeding $25 billion in 2005 with nearly 190,000 employees in 182 hospitals (Hoovers, 2006). **Figure 2–1** shows the hospital breakdown by type in 2005.

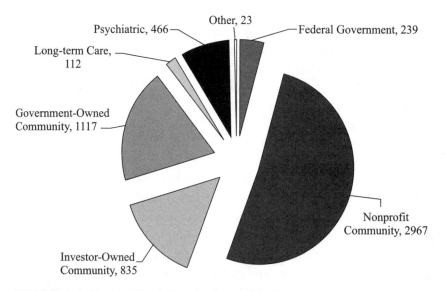

FIGURE 2–1 Hospital Breakdown by Ownership Type
Source: Data from American Hospital Association.

TEACHING HOSPITALS

The largest major hospitals tend to fit into another classification called **teaching hospitals**, which suggests that a fairly large percentage of resources are devoted to academic and research missions, in addition to patient care.

Teaching hospitals were once thought of as the "cornerstone" of the American healthcare system (Iglehart, 1993). As the healthcare industry continues to evolve, this leadership role might be in jeopardy, as teaching facilities struggle to gain a competitive position with all the other entities in the healthcare industry, including group practices, independent primary care clinics, and ambulatory surgery centers.

Teaching facilities are usually the largest, most sophisticated hospitals in the predominantly urban markets they serve (Langabeer & Napiewocki, 2000). They are almost always significantly larger than their non-teaching-hospital competitors, in terms of number of employees, types of service lines offered, number of beds, number of admissions and discharges, size of financial budget, and most other measures of scale. Teaching hospitals have significantly more resources invested in facilities and technologies to provide advanced treatments for the unusually complex cases that they serve.

Teaching hospitals are committed to the principles of higher education. This means that the medical doctor-practitioners are primarily teachers and research faculty members who are affiliated with an accredited school of medicine, whose goal is to educate and formally train licensed medical doctors. Currently, there are more than 126 university medical schools accredited by the Association of American Medical Colleges (AAMC) in the United States and another 16 in Canada. Teaching hospitals offer *medical residencies*—training programs specially designed to instruct graduate medical trainees in clinical settings before they are legally licensed to practice medicine. Most major teaching hospitals have at least four residency programs. The Council of Teaching Hospitals (COTH) of the AAMC maintains a list of more than 400 major hospitals and many more "minor" ones (i.e., those with less than four residency programs). COTH membership requirements include a documented affiliation agreement with a medical school accredited by the Liaison Committee on Medical Education. For a complete listing of all of the major teaching hospitals, see Appendix A.

The other core component of academic medicine is a focus on applied clinical and even basic biomedical research that can help improve the ability to observe, diagnose, and treat patients in the future. Advancing knowledge for new treatments, practices, and techniques will help improve the state of practice in the future and is a critical academic concern for teaching hospitals.

Many factors distinguish a teaching hospital from other community hospitals. First, they are the largest and have the broadest scale and scope (as discussed earlier). Second, they train physicians and provide research, which are not always well reimbursed and funded. Third, they have complex organizations because they are typically partnered with medical schools and academic health centers, which have collaborative arrangements. Fourth, they have more stakeholders than most community hospitals, given the broader mission that they serve. Fifth, given the three-pronged mission (research, education, and patient care), they tend to have a more financially difficult time balancing all three needs than most single-focused community hospitals.

PAYERS AND HOSPITAL REVENUES

Hospitals fund their operations by collecting for services offered to patients through a variety of payers. A **payer** is a party to a transaction that will provide reimbursement through specific mechanisms and protocols, typically based on negotiated or settled pricing. In a small percentage of hospitals, self-pay (i.e., fee-for-service) or private payments directly by the patient are collected, but the overwhelming majority of hospital reimbursement is based on principles of insurance and risk management, where money is collected in advance for probable future claims. **Insurance** refers to reimbursement calculated by probabilities of loss or incidence of other risks, and it is administered typically by what is called a third party. A **third-party payer** is a middleman between the hospital and the patient, typically shares the financial risk, and is responsible for understanding the costs and outcomes of all types of procedures and services they cover. Third parties also negotiate with the hospital to establish reimbursement guidelines and acceptable pricing.

The largest payer in the United States is the federal government, through the Centers for Medicare and Medicaid Services (CMS) in the Department of Health and Human Services. Medicare and Medicaid represent somewhere between 30% and 60% of an average hospital's gross revenues, depending on the hospital classification. **Medicare** is the federal government health insurance plan that offers care to more than 40 million patients who are elderly, disabled, or have end-stage renal disease. The U.S. Congress created Medicare in 1965 under Title XVIII of the Social Security Act to improve access to medical care by providing for health insurance that covers a portion of medical expenditures. Medicare has three primary components: Parts A, B, and D. Part A provides inpatient hospital coverage for participants, as well as some posthospital treatment and hospice care. Part A is paid for by a required payroll tax deduction from the entire American population. Part B is a supplemental insurance program that requires monthly premium contributions by the participant; it covers physician services, emergency room services, and outpatient visits. Part D is Medicare's prescription drug benefit program, which offers discounts on outpatient drugs to lower income seniors and disabled individuals. Medicare Part A funds the largest portion of hospital reimbursements of the three parts.

The federal government also administers Medicaid. **Medicaid** is designed to meet the healthcare needs of certain individuals with low incomes who otherwise might not be afforded quality patient care. Medicaid was established under Title XIX of the 1965 Social Security Act, at the same time Medicare was formed. Medicaid is financed by a federal/state matching formula, where the federal government is fiscally responsible for the majority of the finances, somewhere between 50% and 83%, depending on the state. The federal portion of the match is inversely related to per capita state income. Therefore, wealthier states have increased fiscal responsibility for health care, and the U.S. government plays a smaller role. States are able to control their own policies, so reimbursement for direct and indirect medical education costs vary from state to state.

In 1997, the U.S. Congress passed the Balanced Budget Act (BBA), designed to balance the federal budget by the end of 2002. Although it was not successful in that endeavor, the BBA stands as a landmark piece of legislation for health care because of its goals and its outcome on reimbursement practices and rates. Although the BBA had several goals, including creating options for senior citizens and reducing fraud and abuse, the primary goal of the BBA was to reduce Medicare costs and extend the life of the Medicare Trust Fund; in 2005, the trust fund balance stood at around $295 billion (CMS, 2005). To achieve this, CMS continues to find ways to specifically reduce hospital inpatient and outpatient reimbursements in both Medicare and Medicaid.

In 2005, Medicare provided healthcare reimbursement of $330 billion. Based on trends, the CMS estimates that in the next 10 years the trust fund will be exhausted, which suggests that both Medicare and Medicaid will continue to look for ways to drive down costs and cut reimbursement rates.

The other large nongovernmental payers are commercial insurers. Two of the largest and most well-known insurers are Blue Cross Blue Shield and Kaiser Permanente. Nongovernment payers represent the remaining 30% to 40% of hospital reimbursement in a typical hospital. These types of payers have significant influence: they are paid for by company labor benefits and have the market power to require significant deductions in pricing in return for allowing their insurers to seek medical care at the hospital.

Private managed-care companies can have a number of different structural arrangements, which determine how they are organized, the level of access to care that they allow, and the extent to which services are reimbursed. There are three primary arrangements that describe most managed-care companies: health maintenance organizations, preferred provider organizations, and point-of-service plans.

Health maintenance organizations, or **HMOs**, are managed-care arrangements in which physicians and providers develop contractual relationships to supply specific services (most of which emphasize preventive care) at negotiated reimbursement levels. The plans typically provide coverage for providers or facilities inside their networks at a fixed price per visit, with policies that cover deductibles, co-pays, and out-of-pocket expenses. There is a strong financial incentive for HMO members to seek care inside the network, because a significantly lower percentage of expenses are covered outside of the network that the managed care company has defined. HMOs almost always require a referral from a primary care physician inside the network to access another provider or specialist. HMOs also usually offer some form of drug benefits for outpatients and inpatients.

Preferred provider organizations are loosely organized networks of providers and physicians that have contractually negotiated to offer discounts on certain services. Unlike HMOs, however, they encourage members to seek care from specific providers (i.e., preferred) in return for lower costs and higher benefits. Members seeking care from nonpreferred, or out-of-network providers, will have higher costs and reduced benefits.

Point-of-service plans also offer a network of preferred providers, like HMOs, but they provide the member with flexibility to seek care outside of the network, albeit at a higher cost and with higher out-of-pocket expenses. There will be reduced benefits for providers or facilities outside the network, and they typically require a referral from a primary care physician, similar to the HMO arrangement.

Each of these managed-care plans for private payers, as well as the government payers described earlier, are the parties responsible for ultimately reimbursing hospitals for services offered to the patients they cover. Each of these different types of payers has a certain degree of leverage, based on the size of their network, the number of enrollees or members in the plan, and the number and type of patients they cover. Therefore, each payer has varying level of ability to influence and establish hospital reimbursements. The same services and supplies provided to two different patients may have the same prices billed on the hospital invoice for both patients, but the ability for a hospital to collect the entire amount is entirely based on the individual payer that is reimbursing the hospital. One payer might cover 60% of all costs billed, while another might reimburse the entire amount. Negotiations, settlements, and pre-established reimbursement programs for all payers govern the extent to which costs will be reimbursed. In general, Medicaid is considered to be the payer that reimburses the lowest for all services—in most cases not even fully reimbursing providers for the total cost to deliver care. Other payers might reimburse at cost for specific services that might be specialized or hard to find but reimburse significantly less for services that are very competitive and general.

A hospital's revenue is therefore dependent on the **payer mix**. An individual hospital's payer mix is determined by a number of extrinsic factors, including geographic region, type of patients served, number and type of service lines offered, socioeconomic demographics of the surrounding community, and even market share. In addition, a firm's business strategy and ability to tailor services toward specific payers help determine payer mix. **Figure 2–2** shows the percentage of funding that hospitals received industrywide in 2004.

What does all this mean for hospitals? It means that hospitals have to become focused on all aspects of the profit margin. We are entering an era of competitiveness in health care, where efficiency and margins have to become primary performance indicators. Hospitals will have to continue to squeeze all possible revenue from each procedure delivered and negotiate using competitive and analytical data on costs and outcomes to max-

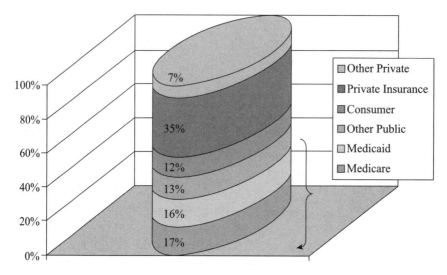

FIGURE 2–2 Funding Sources for U.S. Hospitals
Source: Data from Centers for Medicare and Medicaid, Office of the Actuary, 2004.

imize pricing rates in the **Charge Description Master**, which lists all prices for all services and supplies the hospital provides. On the cost side, hospitals have to reduce total cycle time and service delivery time; automate as much of the business process as possible; reduce labor costs associated with service lines that have low reimbursements; and, by using the most sophisticated budgeting and financial tools, continually drive improvements to the bottom line.

Together, reimbursement rates represent gross patient revenues for a hospital, but deductions are nearly always taken by payers for volume, exclusions, and pricing discounts to reflect the payer's contractual terms. In addition to gross patient revenues, a significant source of revenue for hospitals comes from donations and fundraising efforts, parking and cafeteria operations, gift shops, and especially interest and investment income. According to the CMS' National Health Statistics Group, 7% of all healthcare reimbursement was from other private sources such as these. The typical hospital has significant working capital: large amounts of cash are constantly moving in and out of accounts. Investing these dollars wisely often means the difference between a hospital that makes money and one that does not. Without all these sources of nonoperating revenues, most of the U.S. hospitals would have significantly negative overall profit margins annually.

While many thought that the BBA and the advent of managed care created devastating turbulence in hospitals, managing the hospital business will only become more difficult.

HOSPITAL BUSINESS OPERATIONS

The management of hospital business operations can be broken down into a few major roles and responsibilities, including finance and accounting, business logistics and supply chain management, physical plant or facilities, human resources, information technology, and business planning and performance improvement. There are a number of job opportunities in each of these areas for a typical hospital.

Finance and Accounting

Finance and accounting represents a large and growing portion of health care. Finance professionals are responsible for managing a wide variety of functions, including accounting, billing, collections, financial reporting, payroll, treasury and cash management, investment management, records management, budgeting, and accounts payable. While some of these focus on transaction processing, such as accounting, payables, and payroll, others are more focused on analysis and reporting, such as investments and budgeting. Financial analysts, accountants, and other professionals can find many challenges in this area of health care.

Logistics and Supply Chain Management

Supply chain management is one of the fastest growing sectors in health care. The search for cost savings of key resources and supplies and for better management of goods and services in the physical supply chain is responsible for creating job opportunities for analysts and professionals interested in a wide number of fields, including purchasing, receiving, inventory, transportation, distribution, logistics, and laundry and linen.

Physical Plant or Facilities

As hospitals continue to expand beyond just single, multifloor buildings, the need for additional resources and different types of facilities' expertise keeps growing. Many hospitals are part of systems or networks with several facilities, each of which has a need for design, planning, construction, maintenance, housekeeping, and security operations. Roles for architects, engineers, and general business managers to help manage these business support services keep increasing.

Human Resources

The average hospital employs about 1,000 employees, although that number can range from 50 to more than 10,000. As large employers, there is continued need for business skills focused on providing general personnel management, as well as specialized services such as recruitment, compensation, and benefits. Organizational development and training are also common in larger hospitals.

Information Technology

Information needs require management of telecommunications, data services, information reporting, systems project management, and infrastructure support. Significant improvements in labor productivity can be gained by investing appropriately and wisely in technology to automate manual processes, as well as other technologies to improve access to information and work flow.

Business Planning and Performance Improvement

Although not typically a department in smaller hospitals, there is a much stronger focus on continuous improvement today given the financial condition and competitive environments most hospitals face. As this occurs, there has been a strong rise in demand for professionals who can help provide internal analyses and decision support in areas such as strategic planning, business process reengineering, process improvement, competitive intelligence, performance benchmarking, accreditation preparation, and quality management. This area is a small but growing opportunity for students and other professionals with keen analytical, people, and facilitation skills.

Each of these areas involves substantial level of resources and commitment. By no means are these all of the opportunities for people interested in business careers in hospitals, but they are some of the most common. Many of these areas will be discussed in significantly more detail in subsequent chapters.

CHAPTER SUMMARY

Hospitals represent society and community interests, but they are also a business. They consume significant resources and require extensive management over a variety of functions. Managing these resources and functions require employees new to the industry, and those currently employed, to upgrade their knowledge of finance, management, and business operations management to help the industry continue to thrive, as well as weather the turbulence that threatens a hospital's ability to survive. There are a number of different types of payers and managed-care organizations that reimburse hospitals for their services. Only by using all available advanced tools, methods, and techniques will hospitals be able to use business operations management to improve competitiveness and financial position in health care.

KEY TERMS

acute care, Charge Description Master, community hospital, diagnosis, health maintenance organization (HMO), horizontal integration, hospital, insurance, integrated delivery network, Medicare, Medicaid, observation, payer, payer mix, point-of-service plan, preferred provider organization, teaching hospital, third-party payer, treatment, vertical integration.

DISCUSSION QUESTIONS

1. Is health care a "business?"
2. What are five of the key factors that distinguish a hospital from other industrial organizations?
3. Define an "average" hospital in terms of size (employees, revenue, beds).
4. What is the difference between Medicare and Medicaid?
5. What is a payer? What impact do payers have on a hospital's revenue?

6. What is the role of a teaching hospital in the healthcare industry?

7. What makes governance of academic hospitals more complex than community hospitals?

8. What are the different types of managed-care plans?

REFERENCES

American Hospital Association (AHA). (2006a). *Hospital Statistics.* Chicago: AHA.

American Hospital Association (AHA). (2006b). *Guide to the Healthcare Field.* Chicago: AHA.

Bureau of Labor Statistics. (2004). *2004 Career Guide.* Washington, D.C.: U.S. Department of Labor.

Centers for Medicare and Medicaid Services. (2005). *Monthly Trend Report for Medicare, Medicaid, and SCHIP.* Washington D.C.: U.S. Department of Health and Human Services.

Department of Veterans Affairs. (May 2006). *Organizational Briefing Book.* Washington, D.C.: U.S. Department of Veteran Affairs.

Hoovers. (2006). Website research.

Iglehart, J. K. (1993). The American Health Care System: Teaching Hospitals. *The New England Journal of Medicine, 329*(14):1052–1056.

Langabeer, James R., and John Napiewocki. (2000). *Competitive Business Strategy for Teaching Hospitals.* Westport, CT: Greenwood Publishing.

Samour, Patricia Q. (2006). *Hospitals: What They Are and How They Work.* Boston: Jones and Bartlett Publishers.

CHAPTER 3

Healthcare Finance for the Operations Manager

To understand how operations management can benefit hospitals, it is important to understand the financial condition and environment that hospitals work in. To improve productivity and operating efficiencies in processes—and to understand how such a reduction also saves money—it is necessary to isolate those costs, identify them on the financial statement or general ledger, and incorporate them in financial analyses. Yet, too many operations managers do not know where to turn to find financial data, even though these data are necessary to achieve operational efficiency by analyzing process costs, staffing levels, and productivity. While business and operations managers might not need to record journal entries or explain all the intricacies of accounting, it is important to conceptually understand the impact that operations has on the bottom line. This chapter lays the foundation for interpreting financial statements.

FROM RETROSPECTIVE TO PROSPECTIVE

Since the introduction of the prospective payment system in 1983, there have been continued financial pressures placed on hospitals. Prior to this legislation, enacted to preserve the Social Security and Medicare trust funds that are projected to have deficit balances in the near term, most hospitals were on a retrospective or cost-plus reimbursement system. In this context, **retrospective** literally means to look backward at all costs incurred. This means that regardless of the total cost to deliver services, including both operational and capital components, insurers would fully compensate actual costs, plus a component to represent a small profit margin. In an era where revenue was unconstrained, there was no need for cost efficiencies or fiscal discipline in spending or utilization patterns.

Then, in 1982 and 1983, several pieces of legislation were passed to introduce prospective payment systems. One of these was the Tax Equity and Fiscal Responsibility Act, which made several major changes in Medicare reimbursement practices. This became the stimulus for prospective payments, which became even further adopted in 1997 with the Balanced Budget Act. **Prospective payment** represents a methodology in which fee schedules are calculated based on treatment type or illness classification and are paid in advance of the treatment without regard to actual costs incurred. These are reimbursement or payment programs, not rate regulations, and the result was an end to cost-plus pricing.

Since this time, hospitals have endured a variety of reimbursement practices, all aimed at reducing costs and improving financial stewardship. One such practice is capitation. **Capitation** is a method of physician or provider reimbursement that transfers financial risk of care to physicians and away from health plans or insurers, by limiting payments to a fixed-dollar amount. Standard primary care capitation would reimburse the provider on a per-member per-month basis, such that a flat payment is made per capita to a defined population over a certain period of time. Capitation is generally not used by payers as much today as in the early 1990s.

Fee-for-services (FFS) is now relatively unused, but it was the original reimbursement method where hospitals are paid directly for every service performed. FFS now represents only a small percentage of an average hospital's total revenue. Similarly, discounted FFS reduces the fees by a specific discount rate. From the payer or reimbursement prospective, there are problems with both of these methods. For example, hospitals see them as incentives to perform more services—the greater the utilization or number of procedures or resources utilized, the greater the potential reimbursement. Most payers are not in favor of these approaches, since there is not an alignment around incentives.

Per diems are fixed daily payments to cover all services and procedures performed. They are essentially daily rates that limit the exposure for a payer but provide revenue caps for the hospital. They are effective in some cases, but they might cause a hospital to treat patients longer, generating higher average lengths of stay, in order to maximize revenue.

The most popular payment method in use today, which is favored by both payers and providers, is the use of diagnosis-related groups. A **diagnosis-related group (DRG)** is a classification scheme, primarily used for inpatient treatment that categorizes all patients through principal and secondary diagnosis, procedures provided, age, sex, and other factors. Although DRGs are required under Medicare, they are also used by a number of commercial insurers and payers because of their comprehensive classification schema. Under the DRG system, hospital rates are set based on the patient's illness and the length of time required to treat that illness in an inpatient setting. Many private insurers prefer fixed per diems for inpatients, where a fixed daily "allowance" is provided for all services performed and supplies consumed. Private insurers tend to use negotiating and contract management processes to establish pricing; they use contracts where negotiated discount provisions are based on market coverage, type of service, and volume of activity. In general, the use of a standard fixed rate reimbursement for each type of service performed, adjusted for case complexity, is the standard for most hospitals.

The financial implications from these changes in hospital reimbursement mechanisms are enormous. The risk and pressure of holding costs down below the aggregate net revenue collected is being transferred from the payer to the provider. This change calls for a different type of administrator and the need for managing costs, maximizing staff productivity, and limiting unnecessary processes.

PROFIT MARGINS

Profit margins are found by subtracting expenses from revenues, and they represent the residual value to fund the future. Since the 1980s, the average profit margins for community hospitals have been extremely unsatisfactory. Economics suggest that with long-term industry profit margins near 0% on average, hospitals exit the market because it is unattractive to both new entrants and current organizations. Hospitals exit through bankruptcy, acquisition by another competitor, or simply dissolution. According to the American Hospital Association (AHA), more than one-third of all hospitals have negative profit margins.

That is exactly what continues to happen over time to U.S. hospitals. Significant consolidation of both beds and hospitals continues each year. In 1991 there were more than 5,300 community hospitals and more than 920,000 beds. In 2001, that number had dropped to nearly 4,900 hospitals and 840,000 beds (AHA, 2006). Meanwhile, demand continues to rise. The number of admissions rose from 31,000,000 in 1997 across all community hospitals to nearly 35,000,000 in 2004 (AHA, 2006). The rise in outpatient volumes has grown even more quickly. The chart in **Figure 3–1** shows the change in hospital demand and supply over the last eight years.

When supply is consolidated yet demand remains strong, pricing and margins typically rebound. That is exactly what we have seen in hospitals recently. Profit margins shrank from around 7% to 4% in 2001. Now, as supply is starting to stabilize (the number of community hospitals has re-

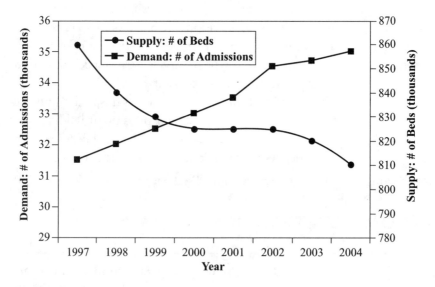

FIGURE 3–1 Hospital Industry Economics: Supply Falling and Demand Rising
Source: Data from American Hospital Association.

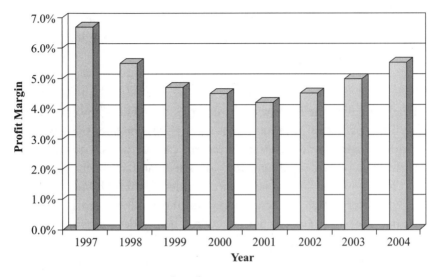

FIGURE 3–2 Average Hospital Profit Margins
Source: Data from Modern Healthcare, 2005.

mained around 4,900 for the last three years), the industry is seeing a rebounding of profit margins. The last few years' margins have climbed from 4% to nearly 5.5% (see **Figure 3–2**). Hopefully this trend will continue, but many of the remaining hospitals are continuing to expand and add additional capacity (e.g., beds, clinics); in the long run, this additional capacity will influence margins.

Yet this tells only half of the story. Some research suggests that nearly 50% of large hospitals have negative operating margins (Langabeer, 2006). Investment income and ancillary sources of revenue can typically contribute between 20% and 50% of total margins for an average hospital. Therefore, real operating income margins are usually between 1% and 3% across the board. With the continued rising cost of medical technologies, equipment, and other capital costs, sustaining an organization for the long term at single digit margins is nearly impossible.

INCOME STATEMENTS

It is important to understand all components of a hospital's financials. This includes being able to look at all of the key statements—income statement, balance sheet, and cash flow—and be able to utilize metrics and line items to fully understand a hospital's operation. The **income**

statement is one of the most important ones, because it measures a hospital's profitability by tracking revenues, expenses, and margins. It works off the basic accounting principle:

$$\text{Revenues} - \text{Expenses} = \text{Profit Margin}$$

Beginning with the top line of the income statement, a hospital reports gross revenues. Gross revenues represent the gross or total billings to all government and private insurers for patient care activities. Gross revenue is typically reported separately for outpatient and inpatient activities. Gross revenue is the sum of all services rendered, through bills issued to payers for every DRG, current procedural terminology, and Healthcare Common Procedure Coding System code. These codes represent the hospital, professional, and technical services provided, and they are billed based on the pricing maintained in each hospital's Charge Description Master (CDM). This CDM is a listing of all services and prices that the hospital delivers; it is essentially a price list, based on gross charges to be billed to payers. An assumption for private payments or for co-pays or other out-of-pockets costs is that all billings that are the patient's responsibility will be paid in full.

A hospital's gross billings, however, do not represent what will be realized, given that sizable discounts are taken based on contract negotiations (i.e., for private insurers) and for other rate caps, allowances, exclusions, or limitations. A discount or **deductions** category appears that reflects an allowance for payments that will probably not be collected. This could be because of exclusions, contractual adjustments, discounts, or other deductions for the difference between what is billed and what the insurer will pay. Deductions for many hospitals can average between 20% and 60%, depending on the payer mix and types of services offered. For example, if a hospital's CDM shows a price for a specific service, such as a chest X-ray for $2,500, that is the gross revenue expected and would be consolidated with all other services performed to calculate the top line on the income statement. Based on the payer mix represented in the services offered in a specific period, there would be an adjustment to discount this based on the reality of what the payer will reimburse. For instance, if the $2,500 service was capped by a payer at $1,000, then $1,500 would appear in the deductions line accumulated with all other deductions, and $1,000 would be added to net patient revenue.

The difference between gross revenues and discounts and deductions is what is called net patient revenues. **Net patient revenues** are the actual expected revenues (gross revenues less deductions and allowances) for a hospital system and are more commonly used for hospital comparisons than gross revenues. Net patient revenue is the same as operating revenue.

Under the expense side of the income statement, hospitals typically place their highest expenses first, followed by lesser categories. For instance, if personnel expense was $15,000,000 and supply expense was $17,000,000, then supply expense would be the first expense category reported.

Depending on the level of detail that a hospital reports internally and externally, all expense categories can be hidden or aggregated to "total operating expense". Typically, the major categories that should be itemized include medical supply and drug expense, personnel or labor expense, administrative expense, general service expense, teaching expense, nursing, depreciation, and other operating expense. In other statements, the separate major divisions are detailed separately, such as intensive care unit, emergency, or obstetrics/gynecology. The two largest operating expenses in most hospitals are typically personnel and supply expenses. Labor expenses can account for nearly 60% of all costs, while supply and pharmaceutical expenses typically average around 20% to 30%. More detail about supply expenses will be provided later in this text.

The difference between net patient revenue and total operating expense is operating income or operating margin. Operating margin reflects the profits cleared in the course of normal business or operations and is one of the most important metrics for determining a hospital's financial health. As stated earlier, almost one-third of all hospitals had negative operating margins in the most recent year of publicly available financial data. An average operating margin of between 1% and 3% is very common for most hospitals, especially larger urban ones. Smaller, rural hospitals tend to have even lower margins.

Most hospitals are able to improve their financial performance by maximizing the non-operating- or non-patient-related activities. These activities are commonly referred to as "below the line" because they are not operating activities and are not reported in operating income. They include fundraising and donations, which can total between 5% and 10% of net income for a hospital or, based on industry-average calculations, between $250,000 for a community hospital and $10 million for a larger teaching hospital. In addition, investment and interest income is a major source of nonoperating revenue. Many hospitals have an in-house treasury or investment management professional to help direct the movement of cash, manage working capital, support bond and debt offerings, and invest in various equity markets. The role of treasury professionals in hospitals is a fairly small field, but its impact can be quite significant, adding as much as 20% to operating income.

A sample hospital income statement is shown in **Table 3–1**.

INCOME STATEMENT RATIO ANALYSIS

Ratio analyses are important management control activities to ensure that operations are headed in the right direction and that they are competitive with other organizations. Ratios allow the details from statements to be put into common formulas that help track financial health and condition. There are several key ratios that should be monitored to assess an organization's financial condition, including profitability, liquidity, and efficiency. Specifically, ratios that measure profit margins, return on capital

Table 3–1 Hospital Income Statement

ABC Hospital Income Statement	August 31, 2006
Inpatient revenue	$1,500,300,000
Outpatient revenue	$430,320,200
Total patient revenue	$1,930,620,200
Deductions, discounts, and allowances	($1,000,000,000)
Net patient revenues	$930,620,200
Total operating expenses	($830,220,200)
Operating income	$100,400,000
Other income (donations, contributions, gifts)	$5,200,500
Income from investments	$15,000,500
Governmental appropriations	$0
Auxiliary and nonpatient revenue	$3,000,000
Total nonpatient revenue	$23,201,000
Total other expenses	($124,400,000)
Net income or (loss)	($799,000)

(ROC), labor productivity, and supply expense are vital in healthcare operations management.

Profit Margin Ratios

One of the most common ratios examines operating margin and total margin percentages. Operating margin is defined as:

$$\text{Operating margin} = (\text{Operating revenue} - \text{Operating cost}) \div \text{Operating revenue}$$

In the sample income statement shown in Table 3–1, total operating or net patient revenue was $930.6 million, and total operating expenses were $830.2 million. The margin was $100,400,000, or 10.8% of the operating margin percentage—which, if this were a real hospital, would be an excellent margin percentage.

Total margin percentage is very similar. It is calculated as:

$$\text{Total margin percentage} = (\text{Total revenue} - \text{Total cost}) \div \text{Total revenue}$$

Again using the data in Table 3–1, where total revenues were $953,821,000 and total costs were $954,620,200, the total margin in dollars was a loss of $799,000. Dividing this by the total revenue yields a −0.1% total margin percentage.

This is why it is important to understand the difference between total and operating margins. It is possible for a hospital to lose money in operations and still have positive total margins, or vice versa. Understanding this is essential to knowing which area to focus on and how cost conscious the hospital will have to be to reduce operating costs.

Return on Capital

ROC is a measure of the level of financial return generated by a hospital's operations in a specific accounting period. This return produces a ratio that can be compared with all hospitals and across other industries. The higher a hospital's return on capital, the better that hospital performed relative to the competition (although it is impossible to determine if a true economic profit—not accounting profit—has been earned without analyzing the cost of capital).

ROC is measured by multiplying a hospital's operating margin, expressed as a percentage, by the total asset turnover ratio. Although a more direct method of calculating ROC would be to simply divide invested capital by net income, the effects of accounting changes, depreciation methods, and financing policies tend to distort the ratio, thereby reducing reliability and accuracy. Return on capital combines both income statement and balance sheet variables and produces a reasonably optimal estimate of financial viability. Operating margin is calculated by subtracting operating expenses from the total operating revenue and dividing this figure by the total revenue generated. Total asset turnover is calculated by dividing total revenues by total assets, which will be discussed in the balance sheet section.

$$\text{Return on capital} = [(\text{EBIT} \div \text{Revenues}) \times (\text{Revenues} \div \text{Invested capital})]$$

or

$$= [\text{ Operating margin} \times \text{Asset turnover }]$$

Labor Productivity Ratios

Other key analyses using income statement data involve analyzing the labor and nursing costs. Using a combination of the personnel expense labor line plus hospital volume and activity indicators (e.g., number of discharges, number of beds, number of adjusted patient days), key staffing and productivity analyses can be conducted to see if the hospital is improving over time or relative to competition.

Consider this example. A hospital with 10,000 annual discharges incurred a labor expense of $15,000,000. The labor cost per discharge (or labor cost) would then be $1,500 per discharge. If the same figures were $14,700,000 and 8,200 discharges a year earlier, then the ratio would be $1,793. This means that the hospital did get more efficient or otherwise had lower labor intensity from one year to the next. If, however, the neighboring hospital across the street, which offers the same set of services and is relatively the same size, has a labor cost per discharge of $1,200, then there is still significantly more work that would need to be done to reduce costs and improve overall competitiveness. Obviously, the lower the figure, the better, assuming that lower-paid employees does not translate into lower-quality care or other service outcomes. Other similar ways to analyze personnel expense are to use net patient revenue divided by the number of full-time equivalent employees (FTEs) to get revenue per employee. An FTE is a measure of the total number of hours that an employee should work (e.g., an employee that works 40 hours is considered 1.0 FTE, while a part time 10-hour-per-week employee is considered .25). Most hospitals typically average between $80,000 and $120,000. The higher the figure, the better the ratio and the more competitive the hospital.

Supply Expense Ratios

Because medical supplies and pharmaceutical expenses contribute so significantly to overall cost behaviors in hospitals, it is essential to analyze these expense categories separately (Healthcare Financial Management Association, 2005). A key metric that should be analyzed is supply cost per unit of patient activity. Typically, if a hospital were primarily inpatient based, the best denominators for all ratios would be inpatient days, number of admissions, or number of discharges. If a hospital has a higher mix of outpatient visits, it would be best to use a denominator such as number of clinic visits or number of outpatient treatments performed. If a hospital has a fairly even split between inpatient and outpatient volumes, the only metric that accommodates for a mix of both inpatients and outpatients properly is "adjusted patient day." An **adjusted patient day** can be calculated based on the relationship between inpatient and total revenue multiplied by the inpatient days. The specific formula is defined as:

$$\text{Adjusted patient days} = (\text{Total gross revenue} \div \text{Total inpatient revenue}) \times \text{Number of patient days}$$

Supply costs include the sum of all purchases of surgical supplies, general medical supplies, laboratory supplies, oxygen and gases, linens, dietary products, radiology supplies, and office supplies (AHRMM, 2005). The added costs of freight and tax, less rebates and discounts, are also included in this supply expense category.

Because supply expenses can account for 15% to 50% of a hospital's operating expenses, depending on the type of specialty and patient acuity, it is important to focus on this area. Later chapters of this text will help to focus efforts around:

- Reducing supply acquisition costs.
- Reducing costs of holding inventory and storing materials.

- Speeding up the turn rates for supplies to improve working capital and have overall higher asset efficiencies.

To calculate supply ratios, there are several common options for the denominator, such as supply expense per discharge, supply expense per bed, supply expense as a percentage of total operating expense, and supply expense per adjusted patient discharge. Alternatively, pharmaceutical or drug expense could be divided by the same denominators.

If a hospital has total medical supplies and drug expense of $15,000,000, total operating revenues of $100,000,000, and 15,000 annual discharges, they would have a 15% cost-to-revenue ratio and a $1,000 cost per discharge ratio. Compared with a similar hospital in the same geographic region with an $800 supply cost per discharge, the competing hospital would be seen as more efficient and probably has greater profitability.

This all assumes, of course, that the complexity or intensity of the types of patients the hospital serves is relatively the same. An adjustment is necessary to make these figures relative so that they can be compared across institutions. In theory, the greater the intensity, the more medical supplies that will be consumed, and the lower the intensity, the fewer the supplies. A common way to adjust for patient mix differences between hospitals is to calculate a **case mix index (CMI)**. Case mix index is calculated by averaging the DRG weighting for all patients served over the course of an accounting period. All patients are coded with a DRG (representing the resource consumption requirements based on a patients diagnosis, treatment, age, gender, and procedures performed), so the DRG weights are the best-known indexes to adjust for case mix. They typically are used only for Medicare reimbursement, but the calculations can be applied to all costs.

If the CMI turns out to be less than 1.0, then the supply cost per discharge would be greater than the original calculation. The formula is

$$\text{Supply cost per discharge} = (\text{Supply expense} \div \text{Number of discharges}) \div \text{CMI}$$

For example, if supply expense per discharge was $800, as in the previous example, and the CMI for all DRGs performed was 0.77, then the total supply cost per discharge would be $1,038. If another hospital had a supply cost per discharge of $1,200 but a CMI of 1.4, then the adjusted cost would be $857. The second hospital would be considered to be more efficient in supply utilization.

BALANCE SHEET

Users of hospital financial statements cannot make informed decisions about the organization's financial condition without examining the balance sheet in addition to the income statement (Finkler & Ward, 2006). A **balance sheet** is a representation of the accounting propriety equation:

$$\text{Assets} = \text{Liabilities} + \text{Equity}$$

Equity is often called net assets in government organizations. There are simply too many interrelationships among revenues, expenses, assets, and liabilities to ignore either of these statements. For example, assume that supply expenses reported on the income statement were low one month, but looking at the balance sheet you see an unusually high accounts payable balance. Accounting entries commonly balance figures between both statements. For instance, purchasing expenses can be accrued and put on the balance sheet, and supplies or pharmaceutical expenses can be held in inventory on the balance sheet. These temporary differences require users to understand and interact with both statements simultaneously.

The purpose of financial statements is to maintain a historical perspective of financial performance over time, using standards to allow for comparison purposes, which will allow one to diagnose the strengths and weaknesses of a firm. A balance sheet, as one of the key statements, is designed to show how the assets, liabilities, and equity of the hospital are distributed at a specific point in time. It is often called the **statement of financial position**. It is usually prepared at regular intervals, such as each quarter, the end of each month, and especially at the end of an accounting year. Most hospitals are either on an academic-year (i.e., September 1 through August 31) or calendar-year basis (i.e., January 1 through December 31).

When looking at the balance sheets, assets are listed first and they are arranged based on categories in decreasing order of liquidity, based on how quickly they can be turned into cash. Cash, therefore, is the first asset that appears under the asset section. Liabilities are listed second and are arranged in order of how soon they must be repaid or are due. Equity, or net assets, is listed third on the balance sheet. A sample balance sheet appears in **Table 3–2**.

Table 3–2 Hospital Balance Sheet

ASSETS		2006
Current Assets:		
Cash and equivalents	$	325
Short-term investments		175
Accounts Receivable, net		550
Inventories		250
Prepaid Expenses		50
Total Current Assets		1,350
Long-term Assets:		
Land and Buildings, net	$	750
Property and Equipment, net		500
Investments		200
Total Long-term Assets		1,450
TOTAL ASSETS		**$ 2,800**
LIABILITIES AND EQUITY/NET ASSETS		
Current Liabilities:		
Accounts payable	$	360
Taxes and other payables		40
Accrued Liabilities		80
Other ST Liabilities		10
Total Current Liabilities	$	490
Long-term Liabilities:		
Long-term Debt		180
Other LT Obligations		20
TOTAL LIABILITIES	$	690
Equity/Net Assets		$ 2,110
TOTAL LIABILITIES AND NET ASSETS		**$ 2,800**

An **asset** is anything the hospital owns that has immediate or long-term monetary value. Examples of assets are cash, marketable securities and investments, prepaid expenses, accounts receivable, inventories, fixed assets (also called plant, property, and equipment), and other assets. Assets can be further divided into current and long-term, or long-lived, assets. Current assets are those that will be converted into cash within 12 months or the current operating cycle, whichever is longer. Long-term assets are all those that are longer than one year or the current operating cycle.

Liabilities are the claims of all vendors and creditors against the assets of the business and represent all debts owed by the hospital. Current liabilities are debts that must be paid within one year, such as accounts payable, short-term notes payable, accrued expenses, taxes payable, and the current payment on long-term debt. Long-term liabilities are amounts owed with a maturity of more than one year, such as mortgages payable and long-term bank notes.

The difference between an organization's assets and its liabilities is the net assets, equity, or net worth of the business. It represents the investment of the owners, plus any profits retained, minus any losses incurred.

WORKING CAPITAL

Let's define working capital, because that is an important concept for operations. **Working capital** can be calculated by subtracting current liabilities from current assets. The excess of what we will soon be converting to cash, minus the liabilities that will consume cash, is working capital. Conceptually, it is the funds necessary to finance the conversion operating cycle for a hospital—from delivering services to receiving funds to paying invoices for materials used. The higher the figure, the more liquid a business is considered and the higher its ability to pay its debts.

Working capital represents the levels of inventory, cash, and accounts receivable on the books at any point in time. The current liabilities primarily represent payments to be made for accounts payable, such as supplies, materials, or services. From a supply chain perspective, both sides of the working capital equation are important because they reflect how efficiently the hospital is ordering, storing, and paying for goods and services. From a financial perspective, the amount of money in cash should be held to as little as possible, while still being able to make all required payments; the rest of the funds are held in marketable securities or accounts that have higher yielding interest and investment income. The key with working capital management is to match the amount of money needed in the short term with the amount of funds available and keep all other assets in assets with higher returns, such as investing in a new building that will produce clinical revenue or in an equity fund.

One common working capital indicator used to measure efficiency is the number of days of working capital that a hospital holds. If a hospital has $22 million in current assets, $15 million in current liabilities, and has average monthly operating expense of about $26 million, then the calculation would be:

$$
\begin{aligned}
\text{Days of working capital} &= \Big[(\text{Current assets} - \text{Current liabilities}) \\
&\div \left(\frac{\text{Operating expense}}{360} \right) \Big] \\
&= (\$22,000,000 - \$15,000,000) \\
&\div (\$26,000,000 \div 30) \\
&= \$7,000,000 \div \$866,667 = 8.07
\end{aligned}
$$

Alternatively, working capital can be measured by its separate components, such as number of days of cash on hand or number of days of inventory. Understanding which component of working capital is increasing or decreasing over a period of time, or relative to competitor hospitals, will help determine the drivers of changes to working capital and focus operational management efforts.

OTHER FINANCIAL RATIOS

Common analyses performed on the balance sheet for operations management purposes include working capital indicators, debt ratio, inventory utilization, and asset management, among others.

An important measure for healthcare operations examines the percentage of debt that the organization maintains to sustain operations. The debt ratio examines the percentage of total assets financed by debt, and is calculated as follows:

$$
\text{Debt ratio} = \frac{\text{Total liabilities}}{\text{Total assets}}
$$

For example, the balance sheet in Table 3–2 showed $690 in total liabilities and $2,800 in total assets, which gives a 25% debt ratio. The lower the figure, the more equity is used to finance operations, which could suggest inefficient use of debt. On the other hand, too high a ratio suggests greater debt exposure, which tends to exaggerate earnings artificially.

Another important balance sheet ratio is the inventory turnover ratio. The simplest way to calculate inventory turns is:

$$
\text{Inventory turnover ratio} = \frac{\text{COGS}}{\text{Average inventory}}
$$

Cost of goods sold (COGS) is the term used to represent the cost of the materials or supplies that are stored in inventory, and average inventory is the mean value reported between two financial reports. For example, on the balance sheet in Table 3–2 the inventory was reported at $250. The previous year it was also $250, so the mean inventory is $250. Assuming that total cost of goods sold was $2,500, the inventory turnover ratio would be 10 ($2,500 ÷ $250).

Accounts receivable (AR) is an important component to analyze, because it represents future revenue to be recognized. The faster that this can be converted into cash, the better. The most common AR calculation is called "days sales outstanding" (DSO) or average collection period, which defines how long on average the hospital has to wait to convert the receivables into cash. It is calculated as:

$$DSO = \frac{\text{Accounts receivable}}{(\text{Revenue}/360)}$$

Using the earlier figure, total accounts receivable is $550 (in millions) and daily revenue averages are $2,585,056 ($930,620,200 ÷ 360). Therefore, the DSO calculation is 212 days. In most modern hospitals, an average of days of AR outstanding is somewhere between 30 days and 75 days.

The last balance sheet ratio that is quite common focuses on the relationship between current assets and current liabilities because it suggests how solvent or liquid the hospital is. The current ratio is calculated as:

$$\text{Current ratio} = \frac{\text{Current assets}}{\text{Current liabilities}}$$

Using the data in Table 3–2, current assets are $1,350 and current liabilities are $490. Therefore, the current ratio is 2.75 times. In general, a higher ratio indicates a larger safety margin, but it might also suggest inefficient use of assets, since the higher returning assets typically are long-term investments.

FINANCIAL DISTRESS IN HEALTH CARE

Small and rural hospitals on average have lower financial performance than their large urban counterparts. While urban hospitals have significantly more competition (e.g., there are approximately 20 hospitals in San

Diego and more than 60 in Houston), they also have higher market share and a larger population of potential demand. A study conducted to specifically look at the largest, most advanced, most highly respected urban hospitals found that they too have deep financial pressures (Langabeer, 2006).

Analyzing severe financial distress, especially bankruptcy, in hospitals is more difficult than in other industries. There has been virtually no research to classify and predict business failure in hospitals. In other industries, businesses are considered to have failed when they enter formal bankruptcy proceedings, but with most large hospitals, it typically never reaches this point. Being primarily nonprofit, hospitals manage to find alternative ways of turning around the business prior to filing formal bankruptcy proceedings for liquidation or re-organization with the Internal Revenue Service and the Securities and Exchange Commission, as most publicly traded firms do. Instead, financial distress and formal filings would be immediately preceded by a number of other strategies to avoid bankruptcy. These financial strategies include a spin-off or divestiture of assets or service lines, a merger or acquisition with another hospital, a bailout or subsidy from the hospital's stakeholders, a request for additional funds from a government or parent structure, an organizational turnaround or change in management control, or significant increases in debt offerings. All of these are more common outcomes of hospitals in severe financial distress.

To foresee severe financial distress, a bankruptcy prediction model could be used to help understand the near-term future of hospitals and help these hospitals create strategies in advance. The most widely followed models are those of Dr. Edward Altman, who developed a multiple discriminate analysis based on business failures in the manufacturing sector. It has since been revisited and amended for other types of industries as well (Altman, 1993). The Altman Z-score model has been used to detect bankruptcy early by many analysts, bond rating agencies, investment firms, traders, and academics. The success of predicting near-term financial distress is quite impressive, but it has rarely been applied to health care.

The Altman Z-score model for service and retail firms is calculated using the following equation (Morris, 1997):

$$Z = 6.56X_1 + 3.26X_2 + 6.72X_3 + 1.05X_4$$

where:

X_1 = Net working capital (Current assets – Current liabilities) / Total assets

X_2 = Retained earnings / Total assets

X_3 = Earnings before income taxes / Total assets

X_4 = Book value of equity / Book value of debt

This Z-score model builds on the interrelationships of many different financial aspects, similar to that of a balanced financial scorecard, and calculates an index or score for each firm based on all of the independent variables shown earlier (i.e., working capital, total assets, retained earnings, fund balances, book value of liabilities, and net patient revenue).

In using this model, a score is generated for each hospital. A score of less than 1.1 indicates an organization is in imminent danger of bankruptcy. A score greater than 1.1 but less than 2.6 indicates a neutral zone and requires special care and focus on improving financial health. The last group, those greater than 2.6, indicates hospitals in very good financial condition.

When this model was applied to 50 of the largest hospitals in the United States, the mean Z-score decreased from 4.67 in 2002 to 4.08 in 2004, indicating that across these hospitals the probability of bankruptcy or financial distress has increased (Langabeer, 2006). While the average for the entire sample is greater than 2.6, there are two problems with the scores. First, they are trending the wrong direction for the sample across the time frame examined, and second, the distribution of hospitals within the population is skewed toward the lower ends. In other words, the highest performing hospitals are artificially skewing the means, which suggests that the wide variability and dispersion of results artificially makes this sample's financial performance better than it is.

Using 2004 data, 14% of the hospitals studied had a very likely probability of short-term bankruptcy or failure. The overwhelming majority, nearly 50%, was in the cautionary zone. In total, 64% of the hospitals studied were in a crisis situation, despite the fact that this same group of hospitals had a mean operating margin of nearly $30 million and only four had sustained losses from operations that year.

Looking at this, the higher-performing group had a Z-score nearly 4 times higher than that of the low-performing group. One of the key differences that stands out is that the total dollars of debt load per bed is nearly double in the lower-performing group, while the average cash on hand is more than 75% greater. This suggests that those hospitals closer to bankruptcy tend to hold on to cash longer, possibly as a defensive mechanism, and have significantly greater debt loads. Additionally, the higher-performing group has nearly 13 times more net working capital than those in financial distress. This would indicate the importance of good working capital management and optimal financial leverage.

Based on the statistical findings of this research, some suggestions can be offered to enhance the probability of avoiding financial failure for hospital management:

1. Carefully understand the degree of financial leverage utilized. In some hospitals, it appears debt financing is used excessively, creating financial issues over the long run. While cash is obviously important, a proper mix of cash versus debt financing needs to be used. The best performing hospitals had high levels of working capital, lower days of cash on hand, and significantly less debt service.

2. Focus on multiple financial metrics and build a financial scorecard. Operating margins and Z-scores are not significantly correlated, nor are days of cash on hand, so it is important that these traditional accounting metrics are not used as sole indicators of long-term viability. It takes a comprehensive integration of all financial metrics to accurately predict financial distress, so building a performance scorecard that integrates the key metrics of leverage, operating efficiency, profitability, asset turnover, and working capital is critical to fully understanding the financial health of a hospital.

3. Adjust business strategies. Based on this sample, the business strategy could be focused on consolidating service lines around those that are the most profitable and maximizing number of beds available to seek higher inpatient volumes instead of outpatient visits. Of course, each local market condition will help determine the right business strategy, but hospital administrators need to focus closely on those variables that drive financial health.

Despite the prestige and reputation of major hospitals, as a group even they are in financial distress. If this trend continues, expect to see a higher incidence of mergers and acquisitions or divestitures of assets and services, as well as other strategies designed to combat failing businesses. Nearly one out of every six hospitals sampled was predicted to be near immediate bankruptcy, and the overwhelming majority are not far behind. It will take a significant effort for these hospitals to continue to treat their operations as a clinical and research "business," but they must do just that if they are to survive in the current climate.

CASH FLOW STATEMENT

The third and most common financial statement is the statement of cash flows. Cash is required to pay short-term bills, to fund payroll, and to finance daily operations. But monitoring the cash balance sitting in bank accounts is not sufficient to fully understand how it is being earned, and how it is being used.

For public companies traded on stock exchange markets, the Securities and Exchange Commission requires disclosure and reporting of a company's cash flows. In the healthcare industry, which is primarily nonprofit, there is significantly less use of the statement of cash flows; even if it is not required, it should be utilized.

The **statement of cash flows** represents all of the cash inflows a hospital receives from its ongoing business activities and investments, as well as its cash outflows for expenditures, labor, and other activities. The cash flow statement shows both sources and uses of funds and reconciles both the income statement and the balance sheet back to changes in cash flow.

The cash flow statement is very useful to help analyze whether business activities are positively or negatively affecting a hospital's cash position. With most hospitals maintaining cash reserves of several days to several weeks of operations, it is important that business managers closely examine their efforts to ensure they are positively contributing to cash flows over time.

This statement helps a hospital better manage its cash position, which is a critical component of working capital. It is a critical metric that hospital administrators must focus on to ensure that more cash is being "earned than burned." Knowing whether a change in cash position is due to *operations* (i.e., inflows and outflows related directly to services provided in the normal course of observing, diagnosing, and treating patients) or whether they come from *investments* or *financing* activities is essential to understanding a hospital's true financial position. A sample statement of cash flows is provided in **Table 3–3**.

Table 3–3 Statement of Cash Flows

Cash Flow from Operations	$1,500,000
Net Earnings	
Depreciation	$ 45,000
Decrease in Accounts Receivable	$ 15,000
Increase in Taxes Payable	$ 2,000
Less Decrease in Accounts Payable	$ (25,000)
Less Increase in Inventory	$ (15,000)
Net Cash From Operations	$1,522,000
Cash Flow from Investing	
Equipment	$ (400,000)
Cash Flow from Financing	
Notes Payable	$ 15,000
Cash Flow from FY2006, Net	**$1,137,000**

Cash flow statements can be produced in two formats: direct and indirect. The indirect method appears to be most commonly used, probably because of its simplicity. The indirect method reconciles net income as the top line and makes adjustments for all entries that do not affect cash. Depreciation, for example, reduces net income, but because it is a noncash activity, it will be added back to reconcile to the cash flow position. The direct method reports cash outflows and inflows only, without attempting to make reconciling adjustments back to net income. Both methods produce the same results, which is net cash used or provided by all types of operating, investing, and financing activities.

Under the operating activities, the indirect method sums all cash inflows and outflows primarily from the income statement items (e.g., net income, adjustments), but it also looks at changes in current assets and liabilities. The calculation of cash flows for operating activities formula looks at the beginning and ending income statement and balance sheet and performs the following computation:

+ Net income
+ Decrease in current assets (if any)
+ Increase in current liabilities (if any)
+ Depreciation
+ Amortization of any intangible assets

+ Amortization of bond discounts
+ Any operating losses
− Increase in current assets (if any)
− Decrease in current liabilities (if any)
− Amortization of bond premiums
− Operating gains

= **Net cash provided (used) by operating activities**

Similarly, a calculation for investing activities looks at both long-term assets bought or sold, as well as short and long-term investments. Finally, a net cash flow from financing activities explores the changes in long-term liabilities; any dividends payable; and any issuing stock, treasury stock, and debt (although these are less common in most nonprofit hospitals). The net cash flow sums all three of the components to see the changes in net cash flow used or provided by operating, investing, and financing activities, and it gives a very clear picture of whether the organization generated or burned cash during the period.

AUDITED FINANCIAL STATEMENTS

All of the three financial statements described in this chapter—income statement, balance sheet, and statement of cash flows—help show the overall financial health and condition of a hospital. However, obtaining these statements for benchmark comparisons with other hospitals is very difficult. For-profit, or publicly traded, firms are required to disclose their statements to the public as a condition of being listed on a stock exchange, but most hospitals are nonprofit and so are not regulated by the same rules. However, because most hospitals secure financing through debt, or the public bond market, audited financial statements are nearly always required to obtain financing through bond rating agencies. Hospital financial statements can be obtained either directly from the hospital, from the Internal Revenue Service for certain charitable hospitals that file a Form 990, from an organization designated as a nationally recognized municipal securities information repository by the Securities and Exchange Commission, or finally from the Medicare cost report.

The best source of information to use for conducting operational analyses is audited financial statements, which are prepared or reviewed by an independent accounting firm. The independent accountant attests, based on examinations and reviews, that the statements fairly present the financial condition as of a certain period and were compiled in accordance with accounting principles. Audited financial statements give some reassurance that the overall financial statements are presented fairly, which is a potential problem for organizations that do not have to comply with generally accepted accounting principles.

DEBT IN HEALTH CARE

One of the most common ways to finance capital investments for the future is through debt. Debt is recorded on the balance sheet and can be payable in the near term (less than one year) or the long term (amortized over a period of greater than one year). There is a cost to finance the business using debt, as there is with all sources of funds, although some forms of debt are better than others. Simple forms of debt financing entail using organizational purchasing cards from banks with revolving lines of credit and an associated interest charge. Short-term working capital loans are offered by financial institutions to cover short-term imbalances in asset and liability accounts, primarily when AR is slower moving than accounts payable. Hospitals tend to use capital equipment leases for large items when vendors offer very attractive terms, but for very large investments (e.g., new building, new major pieces of equipment), the use of public healthcare bonds is usually the desired debt vehicle.

Bonds are debt instruments issued by a healthcare organization to the public; the organization is obligated to repay the original principal plus interest for the period the debt was outstanding. Bonds can be very complex and often require both external legal and financial assistance in their offers. The amount of interest that organizations must repay is directly related to their credit ratings: organizations that are the most successful, profitable, and the most creditworthy will have the best ratings and, therefore, will have lower interest rates. This is because the public views these organizations as being more stable and less risky; thus, they are willing to take a smaller return. Contrary to this, the more risky firms (i.e., those that have lower credit ratings) will have higher interest.

Credit ratings in healthcare financing are typically done by one of four organizations: Standard and Poor's (S&P), Moody's Investor Services, AM

Best Company, and Fitch IBCA. Each of these organizations has developed separate rating schedules to evaluate the volatility and worth of those seeking credit. For example, S&P uses AAA as the highest overall ratings given to an organization, which represents the least amount of total risk, down to B− for those that are most risky and speculative.

IMPLICATIONS FOR OPERATIONS AND LOGISTICS MANAGEMENT

All departments, functions, and managers play a role in improving the financial condition of hospitals. Understanding the impact of operational activities and how they translate into the financial statements of the hospital (which measure the changes in financial performance over time) are requirements for improving the level of competitiveness and operational effectiveness for a hospital. Operations managers, however, must take the leadership role in this effort.

The relationship between operations and working capital needs to be well defined and managed. When analyzing any project for a department, the working capital consumed needs to be calculated for that area to examine how it contributes, positively or negatively, to the institution. Similarly, operations managers must check that AR and accounts payable align and match to ensure that money is not being paid out faster than it comes in. Exploring changes in inventories for key nursing units and materials management departments is also necessary to ensure that supplies are being used properly and that there is an efficient utilization or turnover in assets.

The linkage between the revenue cycle and the supply chain must also be integrated faster and with less manual effort. There should be real-time integration between supply charges and patient medical records when dispensed so that as new items are added to the item master, they are seamlessly integrated with the CDM, eliminating unnecessary manual steps and reviews.

Also, focusing on increasing the labor productivity for staff in support and clinical areas can mean reducing wait times for patients and lowering labor costs for the hospital. Understanding where these costs are stored in the institution's financial systems and reports is necessary so that operations managers can use the right data in their analyses.

CHAPTER SUMMARY

The role that business operations managers play in improving a hospital's financial condition is a continuous and ever-increasing process. Operations managers must know where financial data reside in their hospitals—in which systems and financial reports—if they are to be able to use them in quantitative analyses focused on operational efficiencies. A hospital's revenue is being constrained by all payers' attempts to reduce utilization of services and use competitive means to reduce reimbursement rates. This translates into lower revenues and profit margins. A hospital therefore has to continually focus on maximizing financial performance to ensure its survival and avoid bankruptcy and other financial distress. The financial condition of a hospital is measured through one of three key statements: the income statement, the balance sheet, and the statement of cash flows. Working capital is an important concept that focuses on operational efficiency. Ratio analyses help analyze whether the hospital is profitable, liquid, burdened with debt, or nearing bankruptcy. Analyzing the impact that operational management has on a hospital's overall performance and financial health is evident only by understanding these statements and by using ratios and metrics that show trends over time.

KEY TERMS

adjusted patient day, asset, balance sheet, bonds, capitation, case mix index (CMI), deductions, diagnosis-related group (DRG), fee-for-services (FFS), income statement, liability, net patient revenues, per diems, profit margins, prospective payment, retrospective, statement of cash flows, statement of financial position, working capital

DISCUSSION QUESTIONS

1. Why should operations managers understand financial statements?

2. What constrains a hospital's revenue?

3. How prominent is bankruptcy in hospitals? What steps can be taken to avoid it?

4. What are the three key financial statements that business managers should be aware of, and how are they related?

5. What is the logic of the order of the assets listed on the balance sheet?

6. What is a financial ratio? What value does it provide?

7. Why do organizations have their statements audited? What assurance does it provide?

8. What is the principal difference between the direct and indirect methods for preparing the cash flow statement?

EXERCISE PROBLEMS

1. A hospital has $25 million in gross revenues and $12 million in net patient revenues. What is the average deduction percentage for that period?

2. The same hospital has $40 million in current assets and $30 million in current liabilities. During a 30-day month, they incurred total operating expenses of $10 million. How many days of working capital did they maintain this period?

3. Using the income statement and balance sheet examples provided in the chapter, calculate the return on capital in 2006.

REFERENCES

Altman, Edward. (1993). *Corporate Financial Distress and Bankruptcy.* 2nd ed. New York: John Wiley & Sons.

American Hospital Association (AHA). (2006). *Chartbook.* Chicago: AHA.

Association for Healthcare Resources and Materials Management (AHRMM). (2005). *Supply Expense Benchmarking Study.* Chicago, IL: Association for Healthcare Resources and Materials Management.

Finkler, Steven, and David Ward. (2006). *Accounting Fundamentals for Healthcare Management.* Sudbury, MA: Jones and Bartlett Publishers.

Healthcare Financial Management Association. (2005). *2005 Supply Chain Benchmarking Survey.* Washington, D.C.: HFMA.

Langabeer, James R. (2006). Predicting Financial Distress in Teaching Hospitals. *Journal of Healthcare Finance,* Winter issue.

Morris, R. (1997). *Early Warning Indicators of Corporate Failure.* Burlington, VT: Ashgate Publishing Ltd.

PART II

Process Engineering and Optimization

Part II of this text describes how hospitals can continue to improve their operations management capabilities through quantitative approaches, projects, and improvement plans that will reduce waste and improve performance.

Chapter 4 concentrates on the role of business processes in operations management. The use of quality improvement practices is explored, and a methodology for continuous process improvement is presented. Operations management professionals should be constantly looking for ways to improve processes, through cycle time reductions, improved flow, and increased productivity.

Chapter 5 focuses on using quantitative tools to improve patient and process flows. Maximizing throughput with given capacity and aligning demand with capacity are discussed in detail. An introduction to forecasting algorithms as a tool for estimating demand is presented, and sophisticated tools for de-bottlenecking wait lines are described.

Chapter 6 defines productivity management. Understanding processes—their resource consumption, costs, cycle times, and outcomes—comprise a large part of a hospital's continually increasing cost structure. One of the most vital roles of operations management is to increase productivity ratios to improve operating efficiency, and the concepts of productivity and their calculations are explored. Staffing models and the use of labor optimization algorithms are explored as ways to minimize total costs. Specific use of analytical tools to manage productivity is also discussed.

Chapter 7 describes the role of project and change management and how to comprehensively develop and manage a portfolio of projects. The role of a department called management engineering is discussed. Methods for improving rollouts of technology or process changes, including Gantt charts and project plans, are also reviewed.

Chapter 8 describes how business plans can improve operational strategy. A plan for analyzing other hospitals, the industry, and the internal environment—and for using this information to improve your own hospital—is described in significant detail.

Chapter 9 describes how to calculate the return on investment from projects of all kinds in hospitals, especially those focused on information technology and automation. To achieve a return on investment, the total benefits derived from technology and other projects must outweigh its cost. Accounting for all benefits and costs in a systematic process is important to quantify financial value, net present value, internal rates of return, and payback. Chapter 9 provides a comprehensive discussion of each of these areas and gives suggestions for maximizing return on investment during all phases of projects.

Process and Quality Improvement

Goals of This Chapter
1. Be able to explain the key goals of process improvement initiatives
2. Understand the terminology and tools of process improvement
3. Use a process improvement methodology to improve business process
4. Understand the key drivers of patient service quality

Central to any hospital's efforts to achieve operational excellence is a focus on continuous improvement. Improvement of processes leads to better outcomes, reduced costs, and shorter cycle times. To *improve* means to make something better, and it takes a process-oriented mindset to maintain day-to-day operations while seeking opportunities for betterment. **Continuous improvement** implies a constant focus on achieving better outcomes. The use of analytical methods and tools can help hospitals achieve better results, while benchmarking allows hospitals to break down their operations into specific processes and compare these results against others to ensure that they are competitive and improving. This chapter discusses the role of process management and improvement as a component of operational management.

STRATEGIC CHOICES FOR OPERATIONS MANAGEMENT TOOLS AND TECHNIQUES

To make improvements in health care, it is important to use the right tool for the appropriate situation. Remember Abraham Maslow's famous quote: "If the only tool you have is a hammer, you tend to see every problem as a nail" (Maslow, 1998). In other words, you can't use a hammer to fix all problems. In the field of operations management, there is a large portfolio of quantitative tools and techniques that can be applied in the appropriate situation to solve problems involving operational efficiencies. For instance, if an emergency room is having trouble with wait lines, a combination of Pareto charts, wait line minimization or queuing models, and process analysis (all of which will be described later) might be applied. **Figure 4–1** matches the types of problems or objectives of operations with possible operational management tools and techniques. All of these are discussed throughout this text.

BUSINESS PROCESS

A business **process** is the set of activities and tasks that are performed in sequence to achieve a specific outcome. A process typically has three high-level phases: inputs, outputs, and transformation. A process includes all activities, tasks, and steps that must be performed to complete something. Inputs are all resources to be used or consumed in a process, such as labor hours, staff, supplies, space or facilities, information systems, and other

FIGURE 4–1 Operations Management—Tools and Techniques

resources. Transformation is the conversion or change process, where the inputs are combined to deliver final results, which are the outputs. Outputs are the result of the transformation or conversion process.

For example, a patient schedules a visit; on the day of his appointment, he arrives at the clinic. Prior to receiving treatment or diagnosis (the output), the clinic uses its staff, systems, space, forms, and records (the inputs) to organize the patient, stage him in the appropriate locations, and allow the physician to provide treatment. **Figure 4–2** shows a sample process flow chart depicting these events.

Using the flowchart symbols shown in **Figure 4–3**, a process map or diagram can be created to show the sequence of tasks and activities from start to finish. This is called a **process flowchart**, and it depicts the flows or activity exchanges among participants and shows the sequencing of activities from start to finish. While this is just a simple example to illustrate the concepts, real process maps can be quite detailed and can run across multiple pages with dozens of interactions among departments.

PROCESS MAPS

There are two major classifications of process maps: current (or as-is) and future (or to-be). An **as-is process** is a version of a process flowchart that depicts the actual, current process in place. The as-is map describes how a process really works in practice—and not just in a standard operating

Cycle Time & Costs

Notes:
• The longer the process, typically the greater the cycle time and the costs
• The more boxes and decision points, typically the more intensive, lengthy, and costly the process
• Rectangular boxes = tasks; Diamonds = decision points; Double-boxes refer to separate processes with their own tasks

FIGURE 4–2 Process Management—Sample Flowchart

In most process flowcharts, there are multiple symbols in use. The most commonly used are the following:

• A **rectangle** normally displays a specific task or activity that is to be performed.

• A **circle** or an oval normally represents the start and the end points of the process.

• A **double-lined rectangle** indicates that the activity is a pre-defined process that has multiple, additional activities below this, which would be depicted in a separate process flowchart.

• A **diamond** or a rhombous indicates a decision point, which usually has at least two lines protruding outward, representing each of the different decision scenarios that could be reached. In many cases, decisions points have at least two lines: one representing a positive or "yes" answer to the decision, and the other a negative or "no" response.

• A **parallelogram**, or rectangle on an angled plane, represents data. This could be stored in a system, record, file, or on a manual log.

There are many more shapes and symbols, but these are the most commonly used in process flowcharts.

FIGURE 4–3 Flowchart Symbols

procedure. It is normally the starting point for process improvement efforts because it shows the roles, participants, functions, and tasks involved in converting inputs into outputs.

The goal of documenting the current process is to find opportunities for reducing steps, interactions, decision points, reports, and the overall length of the process. There are three major opportunities for improving the current process:

1. Increasing the throughput, capacity, or volume that can flow through a process with little or no change in inputs. This requires an identification of the choke point, or bottleneck, that limits the capacity of a process to maximize results. There will be much more detail provided about de-bottlenecking in Chapter 5.

2. Reducing the costs, steps, waste, and resources utilized in the process. This requires scrutiny of individual steps that may be redundant, unnecessary, or do not add value overall.

3. Reducing the variation (or changes from the norm) in performance over time. This requires the use of statistical process control tools such as scatter diagrams and control charts.

Often, as-is maps are carefully designed and documented, yet users do not take the next steps to identify how to increase throughput or reduce resource consumption. In simple terms, the keys to mapping as-is processes is to document the overall cycle time it takes to complete from start to finish; the number of touch points, or interactions, between different participants; and the total dollar amount of all inputs, especially labor. The as-is process should then be redesigned or reengineered to achieve a faster, more efficient, and more effective process flow.

Process engineering refers to the careful scrutiny of a current process to identify value creation opportunities, such as eliminating hand-offs or steps in the process, and it should attempt to find value through the three categories listed earlier (increasing capacity, reducing costs, and reducing variability). Each of the tasks in the current process that does not add value, or that could be replaced by automation or a process change that might reduce other steps, should be eliminated. The **to-be process** represents the future state, after all changes and improvements are designed into the current process.

PROCESS IMPROVEMENT METHODOLOGY

How does a hospital start addressing these process issues? It is important to follow a structured methodology so that issues can be discovered and engineered into the process (Hammer & Champy, 1993). Up to this point we have discussed the issues of efficiency, but health care cannot ignore the impact on quality or service. Sometimes a hospital can reduce steps and increase process speed yet still have low quality or do the wrong things. Doing the right things, or effectiveness, requires organizations to think about the broader aspects of the organization and specifically address issues such as (Harrington et al., 1997):

- Why are we using this process at all?
- What value does it add?
- What quality improvements are necessary to improve outcomes?
- Can multiple processes be combined into a single role?
- If we make this change, will it adversely affect our service quality to patients?

It is important for hospitals to more broadly consider issues of job structure, values, and culture in the organization, as well as business process management. To accomplish this, it is necessary to follow a process improvement methodology. There are many to choose from, including the PDCA model (plan, do, check, act) or Six Sigma (George & George, 2003). Most of the improvement processes today are very similar in many regards. For example, most processes encourage multifunctional participation, encourage planning before action, use testing or piloting of solutions before widescale deployment, and use continuous and rapid measurement as feedback. **Figure 4–4** shows a suggested process improvement methodology.

Plan and Prioritize

The first few steps in process improvement encourage hospitals to think through all areas of the organization and then prioritize and plan the improvement efforts. Typically, prioritization should be based on potential gains in cost, quality, patient satisfaction, or some other performance category. Ranking of the various processes, based on these criteria, can help identify which process to attack first.

Once an improvement area has been targeted, a plan should be created for how to attack the problem. This plan includes project schedule and timelines, team members, and project goals. The team should be cross-functional, or representative of all of the major participants in the actual process. Project goals should be clearly stated, such as "our goal is to take

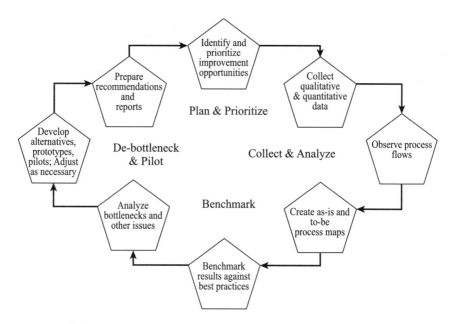

FIGURE 4-4 Process Improvement Methodology

40% of the cycle time out of this process" or "we will reduce at least 15% of the costs in the current process." Establishing quantitative targets helps provide a framework, and eliminates one of the biggest problems in process improvement—identifying only incremental, minimal change.

Collect and Analyze

This second phase involves collecting all key data elements that need to be analyzed. A management engineer or performance improvement specialist, if available, should serve as facilitator of this process, because most data collection requires brainstorming and teamwork that is difficult to get when working with multiple personalities and individuals. Communication barriers often exist and need to be reduced as much as possible, which requires skilled facilitation.

Studying the details of the process work flow and carefully measuring start and stop times for each activity, key deliverables, reports, and interactions between individuals and departments is necessary to fully document the as-is process. Other data, such as work effort or other inputs, help provide a complete picture of the causes and effects for the current process performance. At the same time, once these current processes are diagrammed, the team begins process engineering to develop the future state process. Are there opportunities for eliminating tasks or reducing hand-offs between departments? Can automation help streamline processes? Are there ways to change this to a more exception-based process, which requires effort only if it deviates from some norm? Information on productivity, costs, quality, service levels, staffing, cycle times, number of steps and points of interaction, and key deliverables must all be collected during this phase.

Data collection also requires analyzing process performance over a broad range of time periods and dates to ensure that the sample data collected can be extrapolated and are representative of all times and dates. Consider that work flow peaks at times, and that if you engineer the process for peaks, it is not representative. Plotting the data graphically, on process control charts, helps analyze changes in inputs and outputs over time, normalize the data, and look for process deviations or variations.

The use of **Pareto charts** provides a graphic representation of the most "vital few" issues that exist in a process in a ranked order to show relative priorities. Pareto charts are based on the philosophy that 80% of the effects are caused by just 20% of the problems (also called the 80–20 principle). The first few columns in a Pareto chart represent the categories or problems that are the highest importance or frequency, based on cumulative percentages. These first few issues are causing the majority of the effects, so they should be focused on initially. A sample Pareto chart is shown in **Figure 4–5**.

To create a Pareto chart, there are three simple steps:

1. Use a root cause analysis technique to identify the key issues. **Root cause analysis** is a process for identifying and correcting the major issues causing problems. Brainstorming, observation analysis, cause-and-effect diagrams, surveys, and many other common techniques are used to discover root causes for problems.

2. Through the use of a log or frequency chart, document the frequency of occurrence for each issue or event.

3. Using a graphical software tool like PowerPoint, arrange each of the items on a bar chart, placing those with the highest occurrence in ranked order from most to least.

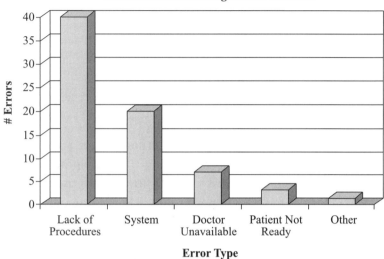

FIGURE 4–5 Pareto Charts Prioritize Problems

Surveys are often used to gather data from both employees and customers of the process. Customers might be patients, or they might be other internal departments of the hospital, since many departments exist only to serve others. Surveys can be administered through the Internet, through sites such as Survey Monkey (www.surveymonkey.com) or Zoomerang (www.zoomerang.com), administered as part of the organization's patient satisfaction surveys, or they can be conducted as personalized interviews with random participants.

Benchmark

Once the business process is completely understood, it should be benchmarked against others. **Benchmarking** is the process of identifying best practices and comparing performance relative to others, with the intent of making improvements to your own organization. Benchmarking takes one of two forms: first-hand observations of other organizations or direct comparisons of secondary published data. Using published data is the most common way to compare against multiple organizations simultaneously, although detailed on-site benchmarking visits of other hospitals often prove invaluable.

Benchmarking involves four primary steps:

1. Select organizations for comparison.

2. Collect or observe data and processes.

3. Identify sources of differential performance.

4. Incorporate these benchmarks into performance scorecards and daily management processes.

The first step is to select the appropriate hospitals or other organizations to benchmark against. This process can either use process and performance data to compare against multiple firms or can use a single site for benchmarking (i.e., contact another hospital, perform a site visit, and directly compare the data).

It is more common to use external data sources for some processes, although this is very difficult in health care because there are not many clearinghouses for performance data, which is more common in private for-profit industries. One of the largest healthcare benchmarking firms is Solucient (www.solucient.com), which offers a number of tools and publications to assist in benchmarking. Other organizations, such as the American Productivity and Quality Center (www.apqc.org) and the Hackett Group (www.thehackettgroup.com), offer benchmarking data across multiple industries. It is not necessary to focus exclusively on hospitals; some business processes are not healthcare specific (e.g., financial processes, such as accounting or reporting). Typically, the hospital with best practices can be discovered through write-ups in hospital news journals or by analyzing the competition's financial or quality performance.

Next, using the data collected, try to determine what makes the benchmark organization's performance different through research and interviews. It may be difficult to get competing hospitals to discuss their processes, but interviews with their patients, payers, and direct observations can all be used to evaluate what makes those hospitals' performance better. Sometimes the use of a specialized competitive intelligence firm can be employed to analyze competition. These new benchmarks should be established as targets in performance scorecards and business plans to help set goals for continual improvements. Finally, hospitals have to apply this knowledge to improve performance. After discovering what makes others successful, hospitals have to adapt these findings to their own unique environments and try to improve overall performance.

De-bottleneck and Deploy Pilot

There are always opportunities to de-bottleneck processes. To *de-bottleneck* is to eliminate constraints, which will be discussed in Chapter 5. Improvement teams need to focus on finding ways to increase process throughput, increase productivity, reduce unnecessary steps, or otherwise improve the process being considered. One way to de-bottleneck is to use statistical process control charts to identify causes of variation. A **control chart** shows data over time, relative to both a mean (average) and control limits. Control limits work on the assumption of standard deviation, which suggest that in normal operations results should be concentrated fairly closely around a mean. **Standard deviation** refers to the spread or dispersion from the mean, defined as the square root of the sums of the distances between the observations and the mean. Deviations greater than a certain amount are considered problematic and characteristic of processes that are out of control. Typically, control limits are represented both above and below the means.

An upper control limit is typically a maximum of +3 standard deviations (represented by the Greek letter sigma, σ) away from the mean for each observation, while the lower control limit maximum is −3σ. Tighter control around variations requires the use of upper and lower control limits that are closer to 1σ, not 3. A sample statistical control chart with −2σ upper and lower control limits is shown in **Figure 4–6**.

Notice in Figure 4–6 that data observations are graphed out in the control chart over time using an x-y axis, where x represents the time periods

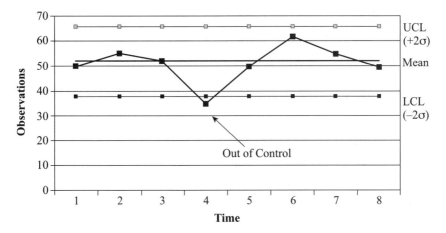

FIGURE 4–6 Statistical Process Control Charts Manage Variability

and y represents the data values or observations. A mean value of these data over time was approximately 52 and calculating 2σ variations or limits on each side kept a tight band from around 38 to 66 (38 is the lower control limit, and 66 is the upper control limit). This implies that when the process behaves normally, there will be a range of values acceptable anywhere in that band. However, in time period 4, a value of 35 occurred. This observation significantly deviates from the norm and therefore is considered to be out of control. Special investigation of this data point needs to occur to learn what changed during this period, so that it can be prevented from reoccurring in the future. If using this statistical control chart to analyze a healthcare process, detailed analysis of all points out of these limits should question what created the variability. Was it:

- Changes in staffing mix or levels?
- Higher demand or patient volumes?
- System or equipment downtime or glitches?
- Modifications in supplies or resources employed?
- Different employees?
- Related to time of day or day of week?

Sources of the variation have to be identified to manage and eliminate the variability.

Developing and deploying the future state in a "pilot" mode is often quite beneficial (Schrage, 2000). **Pilot** is an initial test of the proposed new process, under limited conditions, to help gauge issues and success in achieving the desired goals. The pilot helps identify if the future business process will help achieve the project's stated goals, and it allows for more rapid changes, if necessary, to help streamline and improve. If successful under the pilot, more full-scale deployment should be initiated.

Report and Adjust

Once process changes have been made, a summary report should be prepared that documents the changes, procedures, findings, and performance levels for the process. This should be used as an institution's "memory" to help document why changes were made and what conditions existed prior to the change.

Performance should be monitored and tracked continuously to ensure that the results achieved in the pilot and initial rollout continue, and that if any issues or problems arise they are immediately addressed. This feedback and adjustment process is necessary for at least three to six months following any process improvement initiative.

IMPROVING SERVICE QUALITY

Cost and efficiency are key outcomes of process improvement. However, a focus on efficiency sometimes comes at the expense of "quality," which is unfortunate. **Quality** implies high standards, excellence, and the ability to meet and exceed customers' expectations. As hospitals continue to improve in both areas (cost and quality), they will employ improvement programs and other improvement processes focused on error reductions, process simplification, and patient satisfaction.

Quality in health care revolves around a core set of important service level categories: patient outcomes, patient safety, financial, administrative, and patient logistics flow and facilities.

- *Patient outcomes.* Did the patient receive quality medical care? Did the patient get better during his or her visit or stay? Was length of stay longer than it should have been? What are the facility's overall mortality or morbidity rates?
- *Patient safety.* Were there any medication errors, where pharmaceuticals or supplies were inadvertently administered to the wrong patient? Were there any other medical complications during the patient's stay? Any patient slips and falls to report?
- *Financial.* Was there a billing error or financial complication with the patient's account? Did payer type cause the discharge or reimbursement process to be slower or more painful than normal?
- *Administrative.* Were staff friendly and helpful? Did providers and staff greet the patient with a smile? Were there any issues regarding confidentiality of patient information?
- *Patient logistics flow and facilities.* Was the navigation around the organization easy? Were there excessive wait lines in any area? Did the patient endure wait times because of shortages or stock-outs of drugs or supplies? Did the patient get routed where he or she needed to go in as little time necessary? Were the patient's guests and family members comfortable in waiting rooms?

Customer service and quality cannot suffer as a result of improving healthcare efficiency and productivity, so metrics around each of these core quality outcome categories must be managed simultaneously.

Staffing, technology, improved facility layouts, and education are all critical to improving quality service.

Six Sigma

There are a number of quality management programs that exist. One of the most well known is Six Sigma. **Six Sigma** is a methodology developed at Motorola, and significantly refined and advanced by General Electric, that focuses its effort on improving processes and eliminating defects by focusing on sigma (or standard deviations) that cause volatility and variability of outcomes (George & George, 2003). Achieving a Six Sigma level implies near perfection in an operational process, with around 3.4 defects (e.g., problems, failures, or issues) per million opportunities, or 99.99966% accuracy rate. That is, the numerator is the number of errors or defects in a process, while the denominator is the total number of opportunities for error (number of encounters or output). Each sigma, or standard deviation, represents an exponential level of improvements. Five sigma represents 233 defects per million, 4 sigma represents 6,210 defects, and so on.

In health care, one patient represents literally 50 to 100 opportunities for error during each stay or visit. The moment the patient arrives through the front door is the first opportunity. The parking garage, valet, registration, financial counseling, laboratory, radiology, and clinic all represent opportunities for potential error. When documenting the error or failure rate, it is important to understand both the numerator and the denominator thoroughly if improvements are to be made.

Education on Six Sigma topics covers concepts of process analysis, statistical tools, data collection, and control charts. Students can advance through different "belts" or learning levels, from yellow to green and then on to black. Black belt signifies complete mastery of Six Sigma to improve process and achieve results.

Six Sigma follows a process improvement methodology similar to the one described earlier, but it is typically called DMAIC: define, measure, analyze, improve, and control. This methodology focuses on finding sources of variation inherent in the processes through root cause analyses, and eliminating them to achieve more consistent results. Once the processes are improved, their performance and behavior should be continually tracked, routinely monitoring performance using statistical process control charts and performance scorecards to ensure low levels of variability and deviations. Six Sigma methodologies, like all process improvement processes, are visually represented as a cycle or circle—because the search for perfection is never over.

Quality and Lean Processes

Quality management is defined as the application of quantitative and qualitative methods to ensure that healthcare services and products possess the characteristics necessary to completely satisfy the needs that they are designed to serve.

In recent years, the manufacturing sector has begun to use the term **lean process** to imply a quality process that focuses on improving quality while dramatically changing the operational processes to become faster and more flexible, with less waste, smaller lot sizes, and more highly customized services—all while providing the right goods or services at the specific time required. Central to lean processes are the concepts of speed and reducing cycle times.

Cycle and Transition Times

In healthcare processes, there are several components of time that affect an organization's ability to use speed and flexibility:

- *Process time.* This is the actual time spent performing work; it is true productive time. For example, the time that a nurse spends directly with a patient is productive process time.
- *Idle time.* This is time when patients and staff are not performing work, which could be due to system downtime or breaks.
- *Wait time.* This is time spent waiting because of lines or queues that form in parts of the facility.
- *Transit time.* This is time spent walking from one department or unit to another. For example, the time that a patient spends moving between units is transit time.
- *Transition time.* This is the time interval necessary between productive work where a conversion, cleanup, or changeover prepares a resource to switch from one state to another.

Transition time is one of the largest components of healthcare waste. Reducing transition time supports more rapid response and improved logistical flows. Transition time in health care is one of the largest sources of inefficiencies—and inefficiencies occur everywhere. An example of a transition in health care is when a bed is turned or changed from one patient to another. If a bed is vacated, and 45 minutes later the bed is made ready (sheets are changed, room is sterilized and cleaned), then 45 minutes of productive capacity has been lost. Losing just 45 minutes of capacity in a large hospital can be the difference between 60% and 80% occupancy rates (or utilization). Similarly, when equipment has to be temporarily taken down to make ready for the next patient (e.g., to change out films or cartridges or prepare the computed tomography equipment), this represents transition time. Reducing this transition time is essential to reduce the total cycle time and obtain greater throughput with the same capacity. This is also called "just in time," which will be discussed in more detail in Chapter 10.

Quality Programs

One dominant group that helps evaluate and monitor hospitals' quality efforts while focusing on quality principles is the Joint Commission on Accreditation of Healthcare Organizations (JCAHO). This organization helps hospitals concentrate on process improvement, create performance standards, and manage outcomes. JCAHO provides an evaluation program, complete with thorough criteria and tools for evaluating the overall level of patient care (from clinical delivery of care to support services such as the condition of facilities). Many organizations participate in mock surveys to proactively prepare for real evaluations and continuously improve plans and processes. It is important to familiarize yourself with all of the JCAHO standards governing quality and processes. These are commonly available in a variety of texts and multimedia formats (Bryant, 2004; Taylor & Taylor, 1994).

Another quality program is available through the National Institute of Standards and Technology (NIST), which offers the Malcolm Baldrige National Quality Award. The award covers a variety of organizations, including manufacturing, services, education, and health care. The award application process encourages hospitals to evaluate their level of success in managing quality relative to other similar hospitals. The Baldrige criteria allow hospitals to either self-evaluate or participate in a formal external evaluation program. These evaluations are instrumental in helping hospitals raise awareness of quality and benchmark their programs against other organizations. Additionally, it helps generate ideas and action items for improving quality. Baldrige criteria focus on process management, strategic planning, leadership, and performance, all of which are key components of business planning and process improvement.

Several hospitals and healthcare organizations have won the Baldrige award in recent years, including Premier Inc., Bronson Methodist Hospital, North Mississippi Medical Center, Robert Wood Johnson University Hospital, and St. Luke's Hospital in Kansas City (NIST, 2006). This type of recognition affirms a hospital's plans and provides powerful branding and competitive positioning in the marketplace, both of which help generate positive publicity and hopefully increased financial returns.

KEY QUESTIONS TO PROMOTE DRAMATIC CHANGES

During an improvement process, it is helpful to ensure that all aspects of the problem have been uncovered and identified. Asking the right questions of process improvement teams can help promote dramatic process changes. These questions include:

- How does the change affect our customers?
- How does the change affect organizational job structure, roles, and responsibilities?
- Can we redesign jobs and positions entirely?
- How can we focus more on "exceptions" than transactions?
- Who benefits from the change?
- What other insight or inspiration emerged from the process engineering efforts?
- Do we know the impact on cost and quality of our proposed changes?

These questions need to be discussed openly within the team because the responses will help provide insight to other opportunities and may expose cultural barriers, communication issues, and even organizational politics that historically drive decision making in health care. All of these create processes that are inefficient and oftentimes ineffective.

CHAPTER SUMMARY

Improving operations requires continuous improvement of all business processes. Processes evolve over time, and without continuous scrutiny they can develop into bureaucratic, costly, and ineffective efforts. The process of analyzing processes encourages open dialogue, discovery, and insight about the organization. It helps raise awareness of issues and encourages change. The use of a formal process improvement methodology can help plan and prioritize efforts, analyze and collect data, benchmark, de-bottleneck and deploy, and then report and adjust as necessary. Benchmarking performance against other organizations helps ensure competitive processes and identify areas where improvement is most necessary. Piloting future processes helps ensure rapid feedback and identify issues on a smaller scale so that they can be addressed quickly.

KEY TERMS

as-is process, benchmarking, continuous improvement, control chart, lean process, Pareto charts, pilot, process, process engineering, process flowchart, quality, quality management, root cause analysis, Six Sigma, standard deviation, to-be process

DISCUSSION QUESTIONS

1. In which three categories can process reengineering improve performance?

2. Define and describe the key shapes used in process flow charting.

3. What is the difference between a Pareto chart and a control chart? When should each be used?

4. What are the major phases in the process improvement methodology?

5. What are the major types of customer or patient service level issues that exist in health care?

6. When should hospitals benchmark against non-healthcare organizations? Under what circumstances?

REFERENCES

Bryant, Steven W. (2004). *JCAHO Coordinators Standards*. Marblehead, MA: HCPro Inc.

George, Michael L., and Mike George. (2003). *Lean Six Sigma for Service*. New York: McGraw-Hill.

Hammer, Michael, and James Champy. (1993). *Reengineering the Corporation: A Manifesto for Business Revolution*. New York: Harper Collins.

Harrington, H. James, Erik K. Esseling, and Harm V. Nimwegen. (1997). *Business Process Improvement Handbook: Documentation, Analysis, Design and Management of Business Process Improvement*. New York: McGraw-Hill.

Maslow, Abraham H. (1998). *Maslow on Management*. New York: Wiley.

National Institute of Standards and Technology. (2006). www.nist.gov. Accessed July 2006.

Schrage, Michael. (2000). *Serious Play: How the World's Best Companies Simulate to Innovate*. Boston: Harvard Business School Press.

Taylor, Robert J., and Susan B. Taylor. (1994). *The AUPHA Manual of Health Service Management*. Frederick, MD: Aspen Publishers.

Optimizing Patient and Process Flows

Goals of This Chapter
1. Understand how to identify and eliminate bottlenecks
2. Use forecasting methods to estimate patient volumes and demand
3. Understand the concept of capacity and its relationship to demand
4. Explain why tracking systems can improve process flows
5. Describe bar codes and RFID and their role in operations management

Healthcare facilities are busy places with hundreds of people constantly buzzing around. To maintain efficient operations, organizations need to optimize patient and other process flows. This entails:

- Understand patient demand.
- Align capacity and resources with demand.
- Use de-bottlenecking approaches to improve throughput.
- Manage patient and asset flows through tracking systems.

The use of quantitative tools, such as wait time minimization models and forecasting algorithms, helps support improvements in flows. To make informed decisions about changing processes, decisions must rely on data, not just subjective gut feel. This chapter discusses these concepts in detail.

DE-BOTTLENECKING

Assume that a hospital admissions department has two full-time employees who admit patients in the hospital during the 8-hour day shift. Each employee has a computer and monitor with access to the admission system, which takes approximately 30 minutes to complete for an average new patient admission. Therefore, the maximum capacity of this process is 32 new patient admissions daily (2 employees × 8 hours × 2 patients per hour). This 400-bed hospital has a 72% occupancy rate and frees up approximately 40 rooms daily. The challenge of this hospital has always been to get more patients into the process earlier.

As described in this example, only 32 patients can be admitted based on current capacity at the entry point of the process, even though 40 is the actual demand or theoretical capacity further downstream in the process. Therefore, if more than 32 patients arrive, a bottleneck would exist (Demand < Capacity). A **bottleneck** is a choke point, or a point in a process where demand exceeds available capacity. In other words, a bottleneck can occur at any point where capacity is insufficient to meet demand due to physical or logical constraints. A bottleneck can also be a person, a role, or any other barrier or obstacle to cooperation and work performance among departments.

One of the keys to increase throughput or capacity is to remove these obstacles or bottlenecks, which is called **de-bottlenecking**. In the preceding example, potential solutions for reducing the bottleneck might be to add labor (recruit additional employees), reduce the process time below 30 minutes (invest in systems and procedures that allow for faster processing), or remove forms or tasks that are redundant. All of these should be considered. **Figure 5–1** provides an example of a bottleneck, shown visually as a funnel. In a funnel, the neck of the funnel limits volume throughput. In other words, the narrowest part of the funnel determines how quickly volume can be moved through the process, thus creating a bottleneck.

The key to being able to de-bottleneck is to thoroughly analyze both demand and capacity to determine where the bottleneck exists. To be successful in improving processes, it is important to determine if the bottleneck is the result of an inability to handle demand at all times, or just at a specific point in time, as well as to discover if other barriers to throughput exist.

Bottlenecks can occur at any point in the process: where a patient enters the hospital, at registration, during transition time of equipment, and at time of discharge. The earlier the bottleneck exists in the process, the fewer the number of patients (or throughput) that can be pushed through

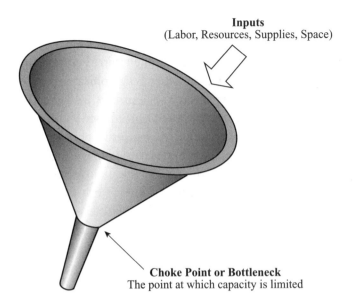

Inputs
(Labor, Resources, Supplies, Space)

Choke Point or Bottleneck
The point at which capacity is limited

FIGURE 5–1 Process De-Bottlenecking

the system. Alternatively, a bottleneck at the end of the process typically results in wait times and inefficiency that can eventually affect the entire system. Eliminating a bottleneck at the beginning, only to discover that more exist in the middle or end of the system, will not help increase throughput. That is why it is important to study all processes systematically and to identify those obstacles that really limit capacity.

FORECASTING PATIENT DEMAND AND VOLUMES

Forecasting patient demand is the first step in being able to thoroughly understand changes in activity levels over time. Comprehensively defining patient logistic flow involves tracking volumes intraday, as well as throughout the week, using time-series data. If a hospital does not exhaustively know patient volumes and traffic levels, it cannot project volumes for individual departments and services throughout the day. Without understanding demand, it is nearly impossible to align resources and capacity with demand.

Forecasting is a collaborative process that estimates the volume of patients that will be served over a specific time period. More precisely, it is a projection of demand that will occur along three dimensions: service type, location, and time dimensions. Service type includes the specific procedures performed or the staff involved in the effort. Location includes the specific department, unit, floor, or other geographical location that performs the service types. Time refers to the hour, day, week, and month that the demand was met. Forecasts are based on time-series data. **Time series** refers to a set of values or observations at successive points in time.

Forecasting by definition is the practice of making a prediction or estimation about the future (Makridakis, 1996). It involves modeling the past to define the future. Demand forecasting then is the practice of predicting future demand to accomplish specific business goals, such as more accurately planning how many beds or clinics are needed or how much staff to hire. Performing forecasting really well allows managers to minimize unproductive wait time, maximize customer service, and in general improve operational efficiencies—the goal of operations management.

There are two major types of forecasts: qualitative and quantitative (Armstrong, 2001). Qualitative methods include mainly market research, executive opinion, or Delphi methods to make subjective or judgmental decisions about the future without relating demand to historical performance quantitatively. Qualitative methods for demand forecasting might be useful for gauging potential demand of entirely new products that have no relationship with other products and cannot be reasonably estimated statistically. Qualitative forecasts of new products that a surgeon or specialty area requires might be the best use of these types of forecasts.

In health care, forecasting should primarily be based on quantitative methods. Quantitative forecasts can be broken down into two major types: univariate and multivariate methods. **Univariate** can be defined as dependence on a single variable; univariate methods attempt to forecast demand by exploring historical data relative to a single variable, such as number of patients, procedures, or items. In standard hospital environments, all of the transactional details for patient volume are captured in the clinical scheduling or information system, such as the number of admissions or the number of surgeries. In addition to this, clinical systems also capture the date patients are admitted and discharged, which procedures were given, the drugs and supplies administered, and prices charged. Reliance on any one of these transactional data elements is a univariate method, which reflects the single variable that will be analyzed to assess historical usage levels and then, based on this analysis, used to make a projection about future values.

With univariate forecasting, there are a number of different statistical models that are often called upon to assess patterns in the data. These include such methods as Box-Jenkins, linear trend analysis, exponential smoothing, moving averages, least squares, and many others. These models all have specific advantages and disadvantage that make them useful for single variable forecasts. We discuss some of these methods in the rest of this section.

Moving Average Forecast

A moving average calculates an average historical figure for a specific time period, such as the last 3 rolling months, and then extrapolates this average forward. This is a very imprecise type of forecast because it actually lags the relevant time period. In a constantly growing environment, moving average can be too conservative, and it is underbiased in its predictions. The mathematical calculation of a moving average forecast is:

$$F = \frac{\Sigma(n \text{ data values})}{n}$$

The term "moving" indicates that as a new data point becomes available, the oldest data value drops off and is replaced. In other words, if you were calculating a 3-month moving average, the calculation would sum the last 3 months' actual historical data values and divide the total by 3. For example, if historical data values were 10, 20, and 30, the moving average forecast would be 20, calculated as following:

$$F = \frac{(10 + 20 + 30)}{3} = \frac{60}{3} = 20$$

Trend Forecasting

Another type of forecasting algorithm is based on simple trend analysis. Trend analysis looks for linear upward or downward movements in data and then extrapolates them going forward. Trend models are effective when demand for a product exhibits fairly consistent demand over time. The basic formula for calculating trend forecasts uses the initial starting point or intercept and adjusts for slope (or angle of the trend) over time. This is often called "rise over run," and it is mathematically calculated as follows, where Y is the forecasted value, a is the y-axis intercept, b is the slope of the regression line, and x is the independent variable.

$$Y = a + bx$$

Other Methods

Smoothing methods in demand forecasting are useful because they use a factor to weight the most recent demand observations more than in previous periods and they help account for errors in previous periods. Smoothing, whether it is exponential (i.e., discounts previous periods with a higher magnitude as the observations age), double exponential, or third-order, focuses on improving forecast accuracy by giving more weight to the most relevant historical periods.

Box-Jenkins is a slightly more complex model that uses regression or curve-fitting techniques at predefined time intervals for the single variable being analyzed. It combines single-variable linear regression with a moving average technique to achieve good results from univariate methods.

A much more comprehensive set of forecasting methods falls within the category called "multivariate." **Multivariate** methods attempt to use more than one variable to help better explain or model the past to make more accurate forward projections about the future. Although factors such as seasonality and cyclicality (i.e., business cycles that repeat similar patterns over time) can be detected and modeled using advanced univariate methods, they are much more common in multivariate methods. Using multiple variables to help make predictions about the item being forecasted allows seasons and cycles to be combined with other causal factors (e.g., pricing, promotions, events) to model relationships with other variables and improve forecast accuracy.

The most common form of multivariate demand forecasting in large-scale causal forecasting is multiple regression. Multiple regressions use other contributing factors to help better explain the past and predict the future. For example, when forecasting demand for a downstream department (e.g., radiology), we might find a causal relationship with number of admissions, number of square feet in the hospital, patient acuity levels, case mix index, or other variables.

Excel and other spreadsheet packages can be used to create both univariate and multivariate forecasts. The Excel functions—trend, forecast, growth—and many others allow users to create forecasts with time-series data for linear trends, exponential curves, and moving averages. They are fairly simple and straightforward. The transactional data can be organized to show the time dimension, or periods, and the corresponding item usage. Then use of Excel's "=forecast" or similar function can be used to point to the known dependent and independent variables, which will then plot the forecasted value. This can be shown in spreadsheet or graphical views, as **Figure 5–2** illustrates.

Similarly, analysts can use Excel to simulate multiple regressions, using the data analysis add-in package. These regressions are a bit more sophisticated than simply using linear trends because regressions attempt to fit or model the historical transaction data to predict more probable future estimates.

The Forecasting Process

The process of forecasting demand involves four key steps, which are shown below:

Identify >> Model >> Analyze >> Adapt

These steps are typically performed in a wide range of time intervals, from short range (next day or week), intermediate (next month), or long term

A	B	C
Month	Usage	Forecast
1	150	
2	135	
3	162	
4	175	
5	161	
6	191	
7	182	
8	199	
9	200	
10	185	
11	205	
12	225	
13		223
14		231
15		231
16		237
17		247
18		241

Step 1: Capture historical data for item to be forecasted, such as patient volumes or item usage (in this case, 12 months usage)

Step 2: Use built-in Excel functions (e.g., TREND or FORECAST) =FORECAST(13,B1:B12,A1:A12) Populate cells C13–C18 using same function

Step 3: Graph Results using line charts

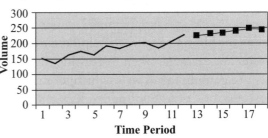

FIGURE 5–2 Forecasting Volumes in Excel

(next year or two). For demand forecasting as it relates to patient volumes in health care, forecasting is typically done in short and intermediate time intervals. Longer-term forecasting is typically done for strategic planning purposes, such as for adding bed capacity or capital investment in new space or equipment.

The process starts with an analyst, operations manager, or planner identifying or isolating what is to be forecast; patient admissions, appointments, visits, clinic registrations, research protocols, supply usage, and pharmaceutical sales are common forecasting applications. Typically, forecasting is used to make specific business decisions, such as how many of each type of pharmaceutical to order next week or how many outpatients to expect next month. Most healthcare forecasts tend to focus on univariate methods, where time-series data are forecasted.

Once identified, the planner needs to gather all historical data for this variable. Data collection might come from a variety of systems, depending on the time-series data selected. For example:

- Appointment data reside in the organization's scheduling system.
- Admissions data come from the admission discharge transfer system.
- Pharmaceutical or supply information is stored in an enterprise resource planning or other purchasing system.

Once the system has been selected, either an interface or a download of historical data will have to be requested from the information systems group, unless the data are available for export directly. A choice of any attribute or other characteristic that describes the data values might also be collected. Time-series data, which represent values over time, are necessary for most mathematical forecasts to predict for the future.

Once these data are in place, they should be incorporated either into a spreadsheet solution (for simple forecasts) or a sophisticated forecasting package. There are a number of excellent software solutions that can inexpensively and simply model and analyze the historical demand patterns to help understand the past and make accurate projections for the future.

The planner then needs to analyze the data to make sense of the forecast and to ensure that the results seem appropriate. Closely examining the forecast and history will ensure that there were no issues with the data and that the forecast is reasonable. Finally, the analyst must continually monitor and adapt the forecast to ensure that forecast accuracy increases over time (or, alternatively, that the error rate decreases). This can be accomplished using tracking signals or by monitoring forecast errors such as mean absolute percent error. Error rates should be used in the monitoring process to adapt or refine the model to obtain better projections the next time.

It is important to focus on the data variation, whether it is random or predictable. One of the goals of demand forecasting is to reduce the uncertainty or variability that inherently exists. Ways to do this include looking at the source of the data, examining the frequency of the process, looking for patterns in volumes or demand behaviors (e.g., spikes due to purchasing increases to draw down operating budgets at year-end by departments), and looking for the best level at which to forecast.

BASIC PRINCIPLES OF FORECASTING

There are some principles of forecasting that should be kept in mind to improve results. First, forecasts are always inaccurate. There is no process that will repeatedly match forecast to actual. That is why it is important to quantify the error and use it to adapt the forecasts for the future. Forecasts made at high levels (e.g., total number of inpatients weekly) are always more accurate than at the lowest levels (e.g., outpatient appointments in a specific location at a certain time). The more granular the forecast, the less precise it will be, but that is typically where the value of forecasting really can be found. Creating forecasts at the lowest levels and then grouping them accordingly for planning purposes is vital to a healthy process. Finally, it must be remembered that forecasts are only the starting point for the planning process—forecasts help provide a basis for further refinements and the selection of a most likely scenario for the future. Here are some additional guidelines and principles.

Level of Hierarchy

Decide on the level at which you wish to forecast. Forecasting at the lowest levels (typically, a patient procedure at an individual location in the hospital) provides significant levels of details, but if this detail is not necessary it should not be used. Aggregation of the data allows for more strategic viewing, but some of the richness of the underlying data is lost. Thus, a trade-off exists between the details gained and the additional level of effort required. Forecasting attributes allows a different perspective, which might be useful during negotiations with suppliers. As much as practical, use downstream transactional data. The best source of demand is actual customer requisitions or items that have been directly issued or charged to patients, not warehouse orders or inventory movements.

Decompose the Forecast

Understand the real demand-forecasting problem first; then break it down into smaller, less complex parts. This is the principle of decomposition, which uses a general approach to drill down into more specific, narrower areas.

Time Horizon

Decide on a realistic forecasting horizon. Although the business process should dictate the forecasting horizon, shorter time horizons provide more reliable results. For most demand forecasts, forecasting out more than 3 to 6 months is not optimal.

Apply Quantitative Techniques

Utilize a mathematical or statistical forecasting application if at all possible, preferably one that is integrated with the hospital's existing information systems. More advanced tools can help to automatically isolate the impacts from seasonality, pricing, operating cycles, or other causal factors and apply appropriate algorithms without significant manual intervention. Also, use combination approaches if possible. Weighting of specific statistical models based on their historical standard errors, such as the Bayesian approach, tends to generate significantly better forecasts than single forecast methods. Some excellent solutions that are widely used in various industries include Forecast Pro (www.forecastpro.com), SAS (www.sas.com), and Logility (www.logility.com).

Simplicity First

Try forecasting in the simplest fashion possible, and add complexity only if necessary. If multiple demand patterns, generate poor forecasts due to complexity or scale, look for causal relationships and better statistical models to build a more robust solution. Be careful to not "overfit" the forecasting models. In many cases, too many variables are used in multivariant forecasting. Adding this complexity does not always result in improved forecasting accuracy, so be careful to challenge the concept that "more is always better" by validating each variable used in the model.

Reliable Data Sources

Utilize reliable data sources. Data coming from hospital resource planning or other clinical systems tend to be the most accurate. It is important not to use any systems or data points that are incomplete or have errors or missing data. Look for alternative sources of data that can reliably feed the demand forecasting system to generate the most valid, reliable results.

Cleanse the Data

Cleanse or scrub the data using business rules. Data coming from most hospital systems or business warehouses today tend to be inaccurate in some manner. Cleansing or scrubbing the data by applying logic and business rules (such as, "do not import any history that has negative values") results in higher-quality forecasts.

Causal Relationships

Avoid making predictions on predictions. Causal relationships that are highly judgmental about the future (e.g., expected changes in interest rates or weather) tend to serve as poor causal factors because their forecast is usually inaccurate and unpredictable. Basing your product's demand forecast on these forecasts often yields unreliable results.

Exception Reporting

Make use of exception reporting to flag problem areas. Specific forecast combinations that might be problematic should be flagged based on specific business rules (e.g., where forecast error is greater than 15%).

Graphical Analysis of Trends

View forecasts graphically, since visual representation of data allows users to better interpret results and identify inconsistencies. Graphical analyses allow patterns to emerge more readily than in straight tabular forms.

Apply Insight and Intuition

Never use statistical results without applying business intelligence. We know that forecasts are always wrong, so it is important to apply human business intelligence to ensure validity within the current context. For example, a statistical forecast might generate specific values, but if the models applied did not know that a clinic is closed on Mondays, the demand will be overstated.

Use Unconstrained Data

Do not forecast based on constraints. For example, if historical patient visits were down last month because of a major snowstorm that limited patient volumes, this constrained or reduced demand is artificial and biases the forecasts. Forecasting based on these artificially low figures should be explained through a causal event, by adding "pseudo" sales to account for an unrealistic month or by eliminating that period as an outlier.

Measure Errors and Accuracy Levels

Measure forecast accuracy in multiple ways. Use multiple measures of forecast accuracy or error to help remove the distortion that occurs when firms become fixated on a single measure. Use the forecasting error to improve the next forecast so that the errors generated in the last forecast are fed back into the next one to improve the quality of the forecast. Typical forecasting software or spreadsheet solutions will provide at least the mean square error rates, which is a simple statistical calculation that squares the difference between the forecast and the actual values. Another similar calculation is the **mean absolute deviation (MAD)**, which is the sum of the absolute difference between the average of the actual values and the forecast, divided by the number of observations. Mathematically, this is calculated as follows:

$$MAD = \sum_{i}^{n} | Fn - \overline{\chi}_n |$$

For example, if the time-series forecasted values were 10 in August and 8 in September, and actual values observed for those months, respectively, were 9 and 7, the *MAD* would be 1. The first step is to calculate the mean value of the actual data, which would be 8 in this case ([9 + 7] ÷ 2). Second, subtract the mean from the forecast value for each observation. Third, take the absolute value (the value regardless of the positive or negative sign) of the difference. In this case, that is 2. Fourth, divide this by the number of observations (2). Therefore, the *MAD* is 1.0, calculated as follow:

$$MAD = \left(\frac{(10 - 8) + (8 - 8)}{2} \right) = \frac{2}{2} = 1$$

Tracking the mean absolute deviation or the mean square error allows forecasters to compare how accurate their forecasts are over time to continue to refine and improve the calculations and methodologies.

CAPACITY ANALYSIS

Once demand is known, it is extremely important to understand how much capacity exists. **Capacity** refers to the amount of resources or assets that exist to serve the demand. In health care, capacity can be measured in terms of multiple resources, including:

- The number of available beds, treatment or examination rooms, and clinics.
- Labor availability of physicians, nurses, and other providers.
- Availability of key medical technologies and equipment (e.g., diagnostic imaging, X-ray).
- Supplies and other resources.
- Elevators, hallways, and other facility space.
- Cafeteria, parking, and other support services.

Capacity analysis requires detailed understanding of the organization's resources, including labor, technology, and facilities. Documentation of this capacity should be done using time-series data, similar to how demand-series data were treated, to track capacity changes over time.

For example, if a hospital has a magnetic resonance imaging (MRI) machine, the assumption might be that it could operate 24 hours per day, 7 days per week. This is called the **design capacity**, which is the maximum stated or theoretical output for a resource. However, when closely analyzing the equipment over a period of time, it would be discovered that there is necessary downtime for maintenance or repairs or other reductions to stated capacity. Therefore, the more important capacity term is called effective capacity. **Effective capacity** adjusts the design capacity with average expected utilization rates. For example, if average operating efficiency or utilization is 75% on the MRI machine, then the effective capacity is 18 hours, calculated using the following equation, where C_e is effective capacity, C_d is design capacity, and U represents utilization rates:

$$C_e = C_d \times U$$

Consider this example. A hospital clinic has two treatment rooms and offers services that typically require 30-minute appointments. Therefore, approximately two patients can be seen each hour in each room. The daily design capacity of this system, based on an 8-hour day, is therefore 32 ($2 \times 8 \times 2$). This is the design capacity given "average" procedure types for the clinic and standard cycle times (the process for calculating normal times will be discussed later in this chapter as part of time and motion studies). However, these averages do not take into account any deviations, such as scheduling problems, patient delays, or transition times in between patients. Historically, the average clinic room utilization is 72%. Therefore, the effective capacity is really only 23 patients per day.

CAPACITY PLANNING: ALIGNING CAPACITY WITH DEMAND

Capacity planning refers to the planning process for aligning capacity with demand, analyzing if resource constraints (shortages) or surplus (excess) exist at all points in time. If 100 hours per week of physician labor is available to a specific clinic, yet demand forecasts suggest 1,400 procedures and 120 hours of potential patient demand, there is a mismatch or lack of alignment between capacity and demand. This is very common in health care, where either demand or capacity is limited (or both). Creating a strategy for effectively dealing with this takes five key steps:

1. Forecast patient demand at detailed levels (by hour, location, etc.).

2. Using productivity estimates, translate this demand into capacity requirements (where patient flow exists; which resources will be used).

3. Analyze current level of capacity in terms of hours of labor or equipment available or numbers of other resources. Translating capacity into a per-hour basis is the most common measurement (e.g., 11 hours of available equipment time available on an MRI daily, or 362 hours of nursing labor).

4. Estimate the delta (or change) between capacity and demand on a per-hour or other basis.

5. Develop a strategy for aligning capacity with demand.

Typically, this involves mapping supply and demand over time, graphically analyzing the data, and then developing plans for adding or removing capacity. The most common strategies for dealing with capacity constraints are as follows:

1. *Increase capacity,* where capital or operational dollars allow. Adding capacity suggests purchasing new capital equipment that could allow the facility to perform more procedures or operate longer hours. Organizations also add capacity by hiring more labor, adding swing beds, or increasing total square footage for new clinics or rooms. Other options include contracting with other facilities to provide additional capacity or subcontracting certain service lines. The use of return on investment models, which will be covered in Chapter 9, should be utilized to ensure that the benefits of adding capacity are greater than the marginal costs to invest in the capacity expansions.

2. *De-bottleneck,* which might free capacity. The use of process engineering tools described earlier can identify bottlenecks, and targeted improvement methods can eliminate them.

3. *Reduce demand,* where possible and profitable. This might include reducing the services or procedures provided or re-directing patients to other competitor or partner's facilities.

4. *Transfer capacity from other areas* (i.e., sometimes capacity exists in certain areas or departments that is often not needed, which can be used to fund capacity expansions in other areas). For example, if

facilities or space is the issue, square footage can be reduced in one department and provided to another.

MINIMIZING WAIT TIMES

Typically one of the biggest bottlenecks in health care involves the issue of wait times. **Wait time** is defined as the time interval during which there is a temporary cessation of service. Alternatively, it is the amount of time that has elapsed or has been delayed from the start point until some action occurs or until service is provided. Most of us experience wait times everywhere in our daily life, even if they are brief—at the gas station, restaurant, convenience store, or coffee shop.

In health care, wait times are frequently a source of poor patient satisfaction and process inefficiency. In emergency rooms, for example, wait times of up to several hours are quite common. Some waits are more acceptable than others. Another common example of wait time is when patients arrive at a clinic but spend time waiting to get registered or checked in.

Wait lines occur in all areas of the hospital—such as patient admissions, financial services, physicians' lobbies—and are generally considered to be routine and just a part of everyday business in health care. This is inaccurate. Understanding wait times is a required step to model process and staffing changes to improve service. Wait times are generally one of the most controllable and significant variables driving waste and inefficiency.

Wait lines form because people are seeking service faster than they can be served. There are several situations where queues typically form in health care:

1. Point of admission (entry).
2. Financial services.
3. Point of discharge (exit).
4. In the front lobby.
5. Treatment or exam rooms.
6. High-volume departments, such as emergency departments (EDs) or operating rooms.
7. Point-of-use for key clinical technologies (e.g., MRI, computed tomography, position emission tomography).

8. In common clinical ancillary services (laboratory, pharmacy, blood bank).

9. Elevators, hallways, or other common spaces.

10. In the individual physician's office.

11. At supporting services (cafeteria, gift shops, social work).

Wait lines can be minimized using advanced quantitative tools. They can be modeled to improve service, align staffing with projected volumes, and control the service levels (or minutes spent in a queue). Wait line simulation models can be built around all aspects of an organization to improve service and process efficiency.

There are three key components of wait line simulation models: arrival rate, service rate, and queue structure. The speed at which patients arrive is called the arrival rate. Arrival rate is represented by the Greek letter lambda (λ) and is always defined as X per unit of measure (e.g., 12 patients per hour). The speed at which employees can serve them is called the service rate. Service rate is represented in most equations by the Greek letter mu (μ). The queue structure is defined by a few subvariables, including number of simultaneous servers or channels, which represents the employees who offer assistance to guest or patient represented by the symbol (c), and the number of phases in the process (p). Most healthcare wait lines are considered to be a finite problem. Therefore, finite wait time minimization models can be defined generically as:

$$\text{Wait time} = f(\lambda, \mu, c, p)$$

There is a lot of complexity that can be built around queuing models, but for purposes of this text we discuss one primary model—that of multiple channels (or multiple servers) providing service through a single-phase process. For instance, at a clinic waiting room, there are two employees at the front desk who check in patients, register them, ensure that updated medical insurance is on file, and ensure that all other forms for registration are completed. This is represented in **Figure 5–3**.

In the example in Figure 5-3, there are currently three servers or channels that can provide service to the customers. All three of them are on the phone, and only one person is currently providing service to one of the waiting guests. There is a buildup of four customers in the waiting line. There is only one phase, in that the next step after receiving service

Single Phase□
(After check-in they enter treatment room)

Wait Line□
(4 patients in the queue seeking service)

FIGURE 5–3 Wait Time Simulation Models

is to visit the physician. In many processes, however, there are of course multiple waiting rooms, or phases.

A key indicator for managing customer service is the number of minutes that a patient has to wait in the queue. This can be modeled using the following equation, where W = wait time, L = the number of customers in the system or queue, and λ represents the arrival rate, or the speed at which new patients arrive in the clinics:

$$W = \frac{L}{\lambda}$$

For example, assume that there are currently five people in the system, and they arrive every 2 minutes (or 30 per hour). The average wait time would be 10 minutes, solved as follows:

$$W = \frac{L}{\lambda} = \frac{5}{30} \, (60) = 0.166667 \times 60 = 10 \text{ minutes}$$

However, in practice, the number of people in the system is a complex calculation and solving for L requires a number of calculations that are best done in a spreadsheet solution. The formula that follows shows how to solve for L when it is not given as an assumption. In this calculation, L = total number of customers in the system, P_0 = the probability that no customers are in the system, and all other variables are as defined earlier (Anderson, Sweeney, & Williams, 1997).

$$L = \frac{\lambda\mu\left(\frac{\lambda}{\mu}\right)^s}{(s-1)!(s\mu-\lambda)^2} P_0 + \frac{\lambda}{\mu}$$

To calculate P_0, the mathematical calculation is also quite complicated:

$$P_0 = \left[\sum_{n=0}^{n=S-1} \frac{1}{n!}\left(\frac{\lambda}{\mu}\right)n\right] + \frac{1}{s}\left(\frac{\lambda}{\mu}\right)\left(\frac{s\mu}{s\mu-\lambda}\right)$$

Average number of customers waiting inline is calculated as:

$$L_q = L\left(\frac{\lambda}{\mu}\right)$$

Finally, another important calculation is to define how long it takes for a patient to wait in the line versus the total time spent in the system (W_q; both receiving service and waiting in the queue). This can be calculated as follows, which basically subtracts the inverse of the service rate from the total waiting time:

$$W_q = W - \left(\frac{1}{\mu}\right).$$

Wait Time Example

A patient arrives at the Solder County Hospital emergency department (ED) and finds a waiting line that is currently 60 patients long. A number of negative comments are passed on to the front desk employees, which are then communicated to the director of emergency department (ED). When she looks out in the waiting area, she too becomes annoyed with this situation, and she makes up her mind at that point that something must be done to help improve the situation. She decides to engage the hospital's management engineering department to study the situation and recommend possible solutions. The director wants to comprehensively understand current waiting times and determine if staffing levels are appropriate to meet these stated service levels or analyze what changes might be made.

The process has only one phase—patients are registered and then transferred back to a primary treatment or exam room (this is a simplification of course, for illustrative purposes only). The potential population or number of patients is finite, and most importantly there are three employees at the front desk to handle all admissions and registration, so it is considered multichannel. The ED director has defined a service level policy of 45 minutes, suggesting that each patient should have to wait no more than this time prior to being moved to an exam room before being seen by a triage nurse or other provider, although admittedly they have never comprehensively monitored total cycle time or wait time.

After careful analysis over a 1-week period, the management engineer assigned to the project conducted several detailed cycle time studies. He discovered that on average during the morning shift there are approximately 50 patients arriving every hour and that the front desk personnel can register a patient in approximately 3.5 minutes, or 17 patients per hour.

Using the formulas provided earlier, the probability that there are patients in the system is very high, and the P_0 (or probability of the waiting queues being completly cleared) is less than one-tenth of 1% (0.004). Therefore L (average number of customers in the system) is around 51, which is similar to the 60 that the ED director found on the day this project was kicked off. The total wait in the system is found to be a little over 1 hour (61 minutes). Because registration time is only 3.5 minutes, the total time spent waiting in the line is nearly 58 minutes (i.e., $61 - 3.5$). This is significantly higher than the 45-minute service level that the director expected.

How can this situation be improved? There are a few key options:

1. Streamline, or reduce, the number of checks or steps that the front-desk personnel are required to perform, to increase throughput and shorten the registration time to less than 3.5 minutes. For example, if the process can be shortened by just 5% (to have a service rate of 18 patients per hour, or 3.33 minutes per check-in), the total waiting time would fall to just 13 minutes in line!

2. Add another employee (additional capacity). Recruiting one more employee (or channel) would cause the total waiting time in the line to fall to just 2 minutes. Of course, the costs of that additional

employee need to be evaluated relative to the benefits of reducing the queue.

Wait Time Decision Making

Depending on the system, it might be necessary to use different optimization algorithms. The algorithms are different for each of the four types of systems:

- Single channel, single phase.
- Single channel, multiple phase.
- Multiple channels, single phase.
- Multiple channels, multiple phases.

In this text we covered only the third type of system. For a more comprehensive discussion of the optimization models for all four systems, consult *Introduction to Queuing Theory* (Cooper, 1981).

Wait times create poor service levels and are bottlenecks for system throughput. As much as possible, and as long as total benefits exceed costs, they should be minimized. In reality, however, there is no such thing as an optimal solution with wait lines. They can be minimized, but the total cost of adding new channels needs to be carefully weighed against those gains. Similarly, if we eliminate a bottleneck in registration, it might just move that bottleneck to the physician's or nurse's treatment rooms. Moving a choke point back one step in the process does not create any system benefits, so it is important that the total system wait times and process be analyzed carefully.

TIME AND MOTION STUDIES

One of the best ways to minimize wait time, is to increase speed of processes through time and motion studies. All process engineering analyses require detailed understanding of the business process. Key characteristics include an estimation of the following:

- Total cycle time (Δ or difference between the start and the stop times).
- Number of activities, tasks, or motions performed during this period.
- Details about the specific transaction or activity performed (e.g., document identifier, person performing task, time of day, day of week, number of observations).
- Analysis of inputs received and outputs delivered to the next phase.

Careful analysis of the details of each process to identify and reduce the total amount of time it takes to perform a specific procedure or achieve a deliverable, while reducing the number of motions or tasks performed, is called a **time and motion study** (alternatively called simply *time study*).

Proper time and motion studies need two things: a stopwatch or timer and a log sheet. All of the characteristics defined earlier need to be recorded in a simple log. Obviously, the most critical information is to identify the specific start and stop times for an activity, but there are many other factors to consider and document.

For example, assume a nurse arrives in a patient room at 11:32:00 A.M. At 11:34:25, the vitals have been taken and recorded. At 11:38:40 A.M., an infusion pump is connected and recorded in the medical record. At 11:40:10 A.M., the nurse leaves the patient's room. What is the total cycle time for this process? Using a stopwatch and observations, this specific process has a total cycle time of 8 minutes and 10 seconds (or 8.17 minutes). Similarly, each of the elements or subcomponents of the process can be monitored as well.

A good time and motion study follows these steps:

1. Select a random sample of participants who will perform the procedure, temporally distributed so that they are representative.

2. Observe the transactions or procedures being performed. Using the stopwatch and the log, observe all specific details of work being performed and total time for each step. Document any noticeable or unusual aspect of the environment, the employee, or the process that might skew results.

3. Document the procedures performed and all other details in a log.

4. Document the process activities in a flowchart, using the flowchart symbols described in Chapter 4.

5. Plot out all observations over time on an x-y graph.

6. Calculate the mean for the observed cycle time and standard deviations for both upper and lower controls. Try to identify root causes or sources of any extreme values (i.e., those outside of the upper or lower controls) and determine if any outliers need to be omitted from the average calculations. Average observed cycle time can be calculated as the sum of the total times recorded for all observations, divided by the total number of cycles observed:

Avg. observed Cycle time $\bar{x} = \dfrac{\sum T}{n}$

7. Adjust the mean, if necessary, for nonproductive times, such as breaks or work delays. Nonproductive time might require up to a 10% or 15% allowance factor to obtain a "standard time," based on all cycles and employees observed. This can be calculated as:

ST = std. time
A = allowance factor $ST = \dfrac{\bar{x}}{1 - A}$

For example, assume that the total observed cycle time for a procedure was 25 minutes, but the employee had an average of 85% productivity or, alternatively, a 15% allowance factor was given. This means that the standard time would be 29.4 minutes (25 ÷ 0.85).

8. If necessary, you can also make adjustments for individual performance level variances, because some employees perform differently and time studies might wish to adjust for these ratings.

Common Problems in Time Studies

There are a few common pitfalls made by operations managers in time and motions studies. First, they do not observe a sufficient quantity of transactions or procedures. Simply observing the nurse performing one task, as described earlier, may not be representative of other nurses or the same nurse with other patients. Effective time studies represent the entire population, not selected individual samples. Second, time studies are highly dependent upon the specific individual performing the task. Observing the same procedures for multiple providers or employees ensures statistical representation. Third, because both patient demand and provider capacity changes from hour to hour, and from day to day, it is necessary to observe processes over an extended time period, or on a **longitudinal basis**. Finally, all procedures or transactions performed must be verifiable—that is, they need to be recorded with an audit trail that can be referred to later.

Time and motion studies can be highly biased by a number of factors if they are not statistically representative, conducted over a sufficient period of time, and temporally distributed. One common bias is the

Hawthorne effect, which is a phenomenon in which individuals perform differently when they know they are given attention or being observed than in other situations (Landy, 1989). Observing individuals repeatedly over extended time periods helps reduce this bias.

IMPROVING FLOWS WITH TRACKING SYSTEMS

Operations management relies heavily on advanced methods and technologies to improve operational excellence, reduce costs and waste, and improve cycle times. Doing this requires management of a variety of resources and assets, including patients, equipment, materials, and employees. Technology that can help automate, simplify, and streamline business processes in these areas will help improve labor productivity and operations effectiveness.

For any resource to be closely managed, it must be observable and visible. Yet this is difficult in large hospitals, which might have 5 to 10 floors and more than 150,000 square feet. There are many places for patients and assets to hide.

For example, infusion pumps are very common in hospitals (an infusion pump infuses, or administers, medications intravenously through fluids to patients). An average hospital might have 200 or more pumps, many of which are never in use. If measured in terms of utilization rates, the average utilization hovers around 35%. This is an issue of effective capacity, in that at any given point in time, there are three times more pumps on hand than necessary. At several hundred dollars each, this represents significant costs and waste. If these pumps could be tracked better, they would allow for fewer inventories on hand and higher overall utilization rates. If a pump on one unit on a floor was not being used, it could be moved to another unit where it would be used appropriately.

The same holds true for all resources: emergency crash carts, IV poles, beds, and computers. To effectively use these resources, it is necessary to have tracking systems in place. **Tracking systems** are tools that monitor the position, flow, and movement of resources. Asset tracking typically involves a system that consistently allows hospitals to locate key assets. Tracking systems require two key components: software to support tracking and automatic identification of the resource by that software. To achieve these second components, it is usually necessary for items to be tagged, with a unique fingerprint.

BAR CODES

A bar code is one such fingerprint, often called a "license plate," and it allows a resource to be tagged with key information and then monitored. Bar codes have been around for many years. The Automotive Industry Action Group used them early on for parts identification, and the retail industry uses them to track items through universal product codes.

Bar codes vary by the industry they serve. Standards exist for most industries about the descriptive information that bar codes should contain, what data format should be used, and any other standards. In health care, however, because the industry is quite fragmented, standards have been slow to be adopted. In healthcare pharmaceuticals, the national health-related items code has been somewhat adopted by most manufacturers, although not all comply. In medical supplies, the use of a health identification number has been discussed, as well as a global location number for health care through the Uniform Code Council. The most traction for standardization is coming from the Coalition for Healthcare eStandards, which promotes the universal product number (UPN) for all medical surgical suppliers. In practice, however, many vendors set their own practices and do not follow any standards.

This makes the use of bar codes very difficult, because they rely on standardized data that are understood and used by both the sender's and the receiver's systems (e.g., vendor and hospital). A **bar code** is a single- or two-dimension machine-readable code that contains a number of key pieces of information. Previously, a bar code appeared as just a linear, unique serial number that was coded in an array of parallel, black and white bars containing keys with detailed information. A **bar code reader**, or scanning device, could then be used to scan, decode, and interpret the contents.

In Chapter 15, we discuss the use of national drug codes (NDCs) for all pharmaceuticals. A sample drug, Merck and Company's Vytorin product, sold in 10-mg-strength bottles, could be bar coded so that, when received on hospital premises, it could be scanned and instantly logged into the hospital receiving and order fulfillment systems. Then, when the drug is dispensed to the nursing unit, it could be tracked, and finally, when administered to the patient, it could be scanned to complete the cycle. Scanning in this case ensures that the patient receives the right product and that electronic documentation of the drug administration occurs. A sample representation of that barcode is shown in **Figure 5–4**.

In addition to different standards for coding items, there are also a number of different bar code symbols or technologies. Different codes, such as 39, EAN, UPC, Code 128, Code 93, and many more exist, all of which are represented differently. The different standards for coding and different symbology practices cause the use of bar coding to be highly difficult. If the industry is to achieve better integration, more efficient response, shorter lead times, and improved operational efficiencies, one standard for coding and technology will have to exist. This could likely take a decade—or longer—to come to fruition.

Figure 5–4 is a traditional single-dimension, or linear, bar code (barcodemill.com, 2006). A major limitation to this is that it cannot hold enough information to make it relevant enough for widespread penetration. For example, the bar code might have an NDC or UPN number on it, but it fails to show obsolescence date, price, origin, precise unit of measure, and many other pieces of information that would be quite useful to an organization. To hold more information, linear bar codes can expand only their widths, because the height of a bar code has no significance. As bar code widths expand, however, they cannot be easily scanned, and they often result in taking more time to be recognized than manual processes. Redundancy is built into single-dimension codes that, if they are short enough, allow for fast scanning. But as they grow longer, the result is a much lower first-pass scan rate and more frustration on the part of users of bar code readers.

To improve on this weakness, modern bar code symbologies are moving toward two dimensions, where the codes no longer look like single rows of bars but more like black dots dispersed throughout a white space. These two-dimension codes can manage significantly more information and have greater overall capacity. Instead of holding 10 characters, as

FIGURE 5–4 Bar Code Symbology

most linear bar codes do, the best technology can hold many times that number.

As the healthcare industry standardizes item nomenclature and the technologies used for stamping items, the use of bar-coding technology is one of the most efficient ways to ensure that assets are quickly scanned and monitored throughout the hospital.

RADIO FREQUENCY IDENTIFICATION

Another limitation of bar codes is that they require each item or asset to be "touched," or to have a direct line of sight, in order to be scanned. Typically, this means the reader must be within at least 1 foot of the item. If an item is going to be monitored, it has to be scanned into the system, requiring a user to scan the item and then move to another asset.

A newer technology, which does not rely on line of sight, is radio frequency identification. **Radio frequency identification (RFID)** is a technology that uses small radio transponders to read and transmit data over existing wireless standards and frequencies. Instead of relying on a direct scan through a visual pattern on a label, RFID uses electronic tags that can store data and then be used for sending and receiving.

RFID comes in two forms: active and passive. Active tags have a battery, continuously transmit data, and can store more information. They can be read and transmitted throughout the hospital, assuming ample supply of antennas and readers, and thus have the advantage of less human interaction. Passive tags do not contain a battery and can only be read when a reader calls for a signal or is nearby. Active tags are much more useful from an operations management perspective, but they come with a higher price—typically several times the cost. The costs of RFID systems are primarily in the infrastructure, with the cost of deploying wireless antennas and ensuring frequency capacity throughout the facility. The cost per chip has been decreasing significantly over the last few years (about $0.30 per chip or less at present), but prices are expected to fall to less than $0.05 per chip in the near future (Markelevich & Bell, 2006).

Uses of RFID

RFID has a number of very practical uses. It can be embedded in or on the packaging of certain pharmaceuticals, especially those that have a high dollar value or a high risk of abuse or theft. It can be used on expensive, durable medical equipment, such as infusion pumps or crash carts. RFID units can be placed on transportation equipment, such as beds or wheelchairs, or they can be used to help track patients themselves, embedding chips on the traditional patient wristbands. A sample RFID tag is shown in **Figure 5–5**—magnified significantly because the size of the smallest tags is measured in millimeters (or fractions of an inch).

Each of these applications of RFID helps improve utilization of resources and supports real-time tracking. Of course, these benefits will not be realized unless a hospital organizes its personnel and business processes to take advantage of the information. One way to do this is to create dashboards that can be monitored by operational personnel and used to analyze flow and movement patterns for key resources. Many hospitals fall short by implementing a simple RFID tag and then doing nothing with it. To be successful in improving asset utilization (which effectively drives up capacity), organizations need to implement RFID on patients or equipment, monitor the logistics patterns and flow, and then make layout and process changes accordingly. This will allow increased utilization and throughput. Additionally, clear performance metrics and goals should be established to determine pre- and post-implementation expectations of

FIGURE 5–5 Radio Frequency Identification Tags *Source:* Courtesy of Philips

benefits. Defining the expected post-implementation level of performance, and then managing toward those ends, is something most hospitals do not typically do well.

RFID Infrastructure

RFID works primarily on the existing Wi-Fi, or wireless network, standards of the Institute for Electrical and Electronics Engineers, specifically, IEEE 802.11. Within this set of protocols, there are a number of different frequencies, data transmission rates, and ranges that are operable—including the popular 802.11a and 802.11g. The newest uses 802.11n, which can operate at frequencies of 5 GHz. When implementing RFID, it is important to conduct a radio frequency spectrum analysis. The **spectrum analysis** uses the electromagnetic spectrum to assess waves, ensure that there will be no interference from other equipment or devices, and ensure that the channels and frequencies are clear and will produce optimal results.

Wal-Mart and RFID

Most business and logistics technologies that are in use in retail or consumer-driven industries today will eventually find their way to health care. RFID is one such technology. Today, the primary reason so much buzz and attention centers on RFID is due to the innovation and commitment to its use and value by major retailers such as Wal-Mart. Wal-Mart has proven itself to be the dominant player in using RFID tags to embed product data so that the data can be used for a broad range of purposes, such as removing excess inventory, improving replenishment, and understanding promotional and consumption patterns (Wailgum, 2006).

Wal-Mart's pilot usage of RFID in many of their stores suggests that they have been able to find a way to integrate RFID tags and infrastructure to generate real business value. As a result of their efforts, the price of tags has dropped exponentially over the past decade. The healthcare industry will benefit enormously from these efforts. Similarly, RFID infrastructure is now using standard wireless networks, which reduces costs considerably. Still, most other organizations are still struggling with how to use the data, how to deploy the technology in appropriate areas, and how to change roles and responsibilities to make the most of the technology.

Value from RFID

Hospitals will continue to benefit from the investment that major retailers are making in RFID technology and applications. Retail industry adoption will create cost efficiencies for the tags and help work out the issues with the technology that would otherwise be borne by the healthcare industry. Savings from radio frequency identification come in terms of higher capacity, higher utilization, reduced inventories, lower operating expenses, and labor savings. Considerable time reductions can be seen when employees do not have to seek out items to be scanned or replenished but can allow the systems to continuously monitor themselves. Inventories can be perpetually monitored and will not require employees to perform manual cycle counts to check inventory levels or create requisitions for new items. In summary, if used appropriately and on the right projects, RFID can save hospitals significant amounts of time and money.

Other improvements from RFID might include improved clinical safety and efficacy. The Georgetown University Hospital is using RFID to automate the blood transfusion process and using RFID-encoded in wristbands to ensure the right treatments are given to the right patients, thereby reducing clinical errors (Schuerenberg, 2006). Imagine if every patient had RFID-embedded wristbands—their physical movements, details about cycle time, and details about usage of resources could be monitored comprehensively. Once these data exist, it would be possible to model this and improve the alignment of capacity with demand.

In many ways, passive RFID is very similar to bar codes. While the most functional system might be passive, the benefits may not outweigh the costs at this point in time, but at some point in the near future the economics will shift in their favor. Currently, the primary discussion in tracking assets centers around the use of passive versus active RFID tags, as well as the use of two-dimension versus three-dimension bar codes. Regardless of the route taken, one of these methods needs to be deployed if hospitals are going to continue to improve their operations management capabilities.

CHAPTER SUMMARY

There are four steps to improve patient and process flows: understand patient demand, align capacity and resources with demand, use de-bottlenecking approaches to improve throughput, and then manage patient and asset flows through tracking systems. Each of these require the application of quantitative techniques that use data to drive decision making. Bottlenecks cause patients to wait, resources to pile up, and operations to slow down. De-bottlenecking processes—and identifying strategies for changing demand, expanding capacity, or removing barriers—is critical to improving flows and throughput. Time and motion studies help operations managers understand the bottlenecks by breaking down processes so that cycle times can be thoroughly defined. Forecasts are essential to understand demand over time and to predict changes in volumes. Demand forms the basis for aligning capacity (staffing, supplies, space, equipment) and ensures operational efficiencies. The use of wait time optimization models can help make critical decisions about how to remove one of the most common complaints in health care. Finally, asset-tracking systems help improve asset utilization, which effectively increases effective capacity of key resources.

KEY TERMS

bar code, bar code reader, bottleneck, capacity, capacity planning, de-bottleneck, design capacity, effective capacity, forecasting, Hawthorne effect, longitudinal basis, mean absolute deviation (MAD), multivariate, radio frequency identification (RFID), spectrum analysis, time and motion study, time series, tracking systems, univariate, wait time

DISCUSSION QUESTIONS

1. Define de-bottlenecking. Does it have a role in health care, or should it be used only in industrial manufacturing settings?

2. What are four scenarios in health care where lines or queues exist?

3. How important are bar codes or RFID in tracking assets and resources?

4. What are some of the decisions that must be made prior to investing in RFID?

5. What are the key characteristics analyzed in a time and motion study? Why is it important to have a stopwatch and a written log?

EXERCISE PROBLEMS

1. Patient volumes for a radiology clinic are observed to have the following time-series data: Monday = 25, Tuesday = 28, Wednesday = 32, Thursday = 26, and Friday = 30. Using a 5-day moving average, and ignoring weekend volumes, what is the projection for the following Monday? If you used a 3-day moving average, using Wednesday through Friday values, how would the forecast change?

2. Assume that a hospital has a single-phase, multiple-channel waiting line. There are two employees, and new patients arrive at the rate of approximately 40 patients per hour. Calculate the average wait time.

3. Ten observations of cycle time were made, and the average observed cycle time was 17 minutes. Using an allowance factor of 20%, calculate the standard time for this process.

REFERENCES

Anderson, David R., Dennis J. Sweeney, and Thomas A. Williams. (1997). *An Introduction to Management Science: Quantitative Approaches to Decision Making*. Minneapolis: West Publishing Company.

Armstrong, J. S. (2001). *Principles of Forecasting*. Norwell, MA: Kluwer Academic Publishers.

Barcodemill.com. (2006). Website accessed November 2006.

Cooper, R. B. (1981). *Introduction to Queuing Theory*. 2nd ed. New York: North-Holland.

Landy, Frank J. (1989). *Psychology of Work Behavior*. 4th ed. Pacific Grove, CA: Wadsworth, Inc.

Makridakis, S. (1996). Forecasting: Its Role and Value for Planning and Strategy. *International Journal of Forecasting*, 12:513–537.

Markelevich, Ariel, and Ronald Bell. (2006). RFID: The Changes It Will Bring. *Strategic Finance*, Institute of Management Accountants, August 2006:46–49.

Schuerenberg, Beckie K. (2006). *Bar Codes versus RFID: A Battle Just Beginning*. Health Data Management.

Wailgum, Thomas. (2006). RFID Decision Time. *CIO Magazine*, September 15, 2006, pp. 37–38.

Productivity and Performance Management

> **Goals of This Chapter**
> 1. Define productivity
> 2. Describe the value of tracking productivity over time
> 3. Understand how to calculate capital versus labor substitutions
> 4. Understand analytical models for staffing
> 5. Create a productivity and performance scorecard

Operations management requires efficient conversion of inputs into outputs. **Efficiency** is defined as performing tasks with minimal waste and resource consumption. Delivering healthcare services efficiently requires achieving the same or higher levels of output from employees, at the same quality standards, with fewer inputs over time. If a hospital requires three full-time employees to schedule 21,000 patient appointments this year and had two employees handling 18,000 appointments last year, usage of resources was 22% less efficient from one year to the next. The relationship between capacity and output is called *productivity management*. This chapter lays the framework for using healthcare operations management to help reduce costs and improve overall efficiencies in the utilization of labor, capital, and other resources.

THE QUEST FOR PRODUCTIVITY

Productivity is defined as the ratio of outputs to inputs or:

$$P = \frac{O}{I}$$

There are two key components of this equation: **Outputs** are the level of production or yield (of goods and services) that results from the operations management or conversion process. Outputs are the result of the work conducted through processes and automation. **Inputs** are all the time, costs, labor, materials, capital, and other resources utilized in the delivery of these services. For example, if a nurse can visit three patients in a 30-minute time frame, then three visits (or however many clinical procedures performed) would be the output and the input would be 30 minutes of labor with the associated cost equal to that time multiplied by his average hourly wage. If any supplies or other materials were given to the patients during this time frame, those would also be added to the inputs. In other words:

$$\frac{O}{I} = \frac{\Sigma(\text{Procedures, Visits, Units, Activity})}{\Sigma(\text{Time, Cost, Labor, Materials, Capital})}$$

In many industries, there is a standard measure of productivity that industry analysts, investors, and other stakeholders use to monitor the changes over time. For example, in the oil and gas industry, millions of barrels of oil output are divided by total labor hours to arrive at estimated labor productivity. This figure is well known in the industry and is benchmarked by other firms to gauge the extent of technology automation and the total productivity added by each incremental employee.

Unfortunately, in hospitals this is less common. Comparisons of labor productivity among healthcare organizations are not widely done for two primary reasons: (1) lack of publications and research on the subject and (2) the perception that health care is "different" and does not lend itself to productivity monitoring. Both of these reasons will be discussed in more detail.

First, there are very few published industry reports for utilization and productivity. More than 85% of all hospitals are not publicly traded on stock markets; thus there is no central governing body that requires financial statements to facilitate sharing within the industry. Although some organizations conduct annual surveys (such as the American Hospital Association [AHA]), as with most voluntary surveys, the results are somewhat limited. They also require significant interpretation and cleansing before the data can be used reliably. For financial data, any hospital that receives Medicare reimbursement must file the Medicare Institutional Cost Report to itemize all costs, labor, and income statement accounts by major service line, as well as provide balance sheet information. Unfortunately, however, although these data are the most complete for the industry, most filings are often incomplete and inaccurate which, make bench-marking productivity difficult.

Second, there is a perception among many hospitals that the differences that exist, because of region or specialty, do not allow for comparisons to be made. This is an uninformed position. If not required by external or regulating bodies, then hospitals must have their own internal desire to measure productivity and see improvements over time. Operational scorecards that track productivity and performance for key business processes are needed to track performance internally over time.

MEASUREMENT ISSUES

It is possible for everything important to be quantified and measured, even if the people performing the tasks may feel that the nature of their work does not lend itself to measurement. There is a common expression that "What gets measured gets done." In other words, if productivity is measured and made important, there can be improvements over time.

In health care, physicians and researchers (in the case of academic or teaching hospitals) often feel that a measurement problem exists— delivering quality medical care and research does not fit the normal definition of production of goods and services. Physicians are not typically trained in business or administrative matters, so they do not often see the usefulness in managing productivity of their time. In many cases, however, hospitals should try to look for ways to manage productivity across all areas and job categories.

Can clinician or researcher productivity be measured? Is it possible to compare one study that a cardiac surgeon is conducting to a study by an oncologist? Can hospital administrators examine a metric, such as number of procedures per day or research studies per full-time employee, to manage areas that require significant intangibles and high levels of thinking? In other words, is it only manual transactional processes that can be captured and measured? The answer is clearly no. All types of work can be broken down into outputs and inputs, and these can be tracked to see changes in performance over time; however, it is definitely easier and probably makes the most sense to start with the operational and transactional productivity measurements and focus on the more complex measurement areas last.

Another common issue in productivity measurement is a lack of data availability. In hospitals, internal systems that measure outputs and inputs over time may not be available. Measuring productivity should be conducted frequently, which requires tracking both sides of the formula. If measuring the number of patients moved via wheelchair through the hospital, there is probably no information system in place to record these transactions. Establishing shadow or supplemental systems that can be updated daily with activity information, or summarized weekly or monthly, is a way to begin measuring such activities.

Quality is often another concern with measurement. While outputs might not have changed, the level of quality of the output might have increased. For example, if a physician performs five valve reconstructions over a week, the productivity ratio is easy to calculate. However, how does the quality of the work factor into the equation? The ultimate health outcome can be measured in terms of mortality and morbidity, but that is not a factor in most productivity ratios. The same goes for all areas, whether they are clinical or operational. When managing supply inventories, it is easy to see how many requisitions were managed per employee, but if the hospital is now better equipped to offer the right products at the right location at the right time—this change in quality is not necessarily reflected in the productivity ratio without adjustments. The important part is not to ignore productivity measurement but to make sure such a measurement is balanced and represents the entire picture (e.g., quality of service, in addition to quantity).

SINGLE VERSUS MULTIPLE FACTORS

Productivity can be measured in a very basic way—using only one variable for output relative to the inputs. Alternatively, it can be measured in a more complex manner—using multiple factors, where the ratio of total outputs is applied relative to resource inputs. For example, if a hospital analyzes the movement of patients through wheelchairs, it could look at single-factor productivity using the ratio of number of patients transported as the output measure, and the number of labor hours required as the inputs. If 50 patients were transported in a single day using four full-time employees (average of 8 hours per day), then the ratio would be:

$$P = \frac{50}{(4 \times 8)} = 1.56$$

In other words, 1.56 patients were transported per hour in operation. How does the hospital know if this is efficient? There are only two ways to judge this: Is the figure improving over time, using trend analysis? How does this figure compare with other hospitals? The answer to the second question is often difficult and requires external analyses or benchmarking. **Benchmarking** is the comparison of a key performance measurement relative to the competition or the process of seeking best practices with intentions of applying those within an organization. Only by continuous measurements over time, internally and externally, can a hospital determine if a 1.56 productivity ratio is "good" or "bad."

Now assume that the total of 50 patients are still the output, but the input included four full-time employees at an hourly rate of $8. In addition, there are two additional inputs of $25 of materials for an oxygen tank and a daily system charge of $100 (that represents amortized costs for the new transportation information system that was recently deployed). In this multiple-factor example, the total productivity would be equal to:

$$P = \frac{O}{\Sigma I}$$

That is, productivity is calculated as total outputs divided by the sum of all inputs, where inputs include Labor + Supplies + Capital + Miscellaneous resources. Therefore, productivity can be calculated as:

$$P = \frac{50}{(256 + 25 + 100)} = 0.131$$

In other words, multifactor productivity was equal to 0.131 patient per dollar. Notice that 0.131 is also neither good nor bad at first glance—it is impossible to tell without benchmarking or using trend analysis to compare internally over time. Also keep in mind that in this example of multiple factors, all of the inputs used the same scale or unit of measure (i.e., dollars). All of the units of measure have to be consistent to sum them, which is why the 8 labor hours were converted into salary costs of $256 to keep the same units.

In most cases, multiple factor productivity analysis is probably the most realistic and comprehensive, but it is also more complex and requires more variables and better tracking of information. To make productivity management work, the cost of productivity measurement cannot exceed the benefits derived from tracking the calculations.

COMMON HOSPITALWIDE PRODUCTIVITY METRICS

As stated earlier, there are very few data sources for external benchmark comparison of productivity ratios. Although productivity metrics are most useful and most actionable if they are applied to a specific business process, unit, or service line, the most common high-level metrics for analyzing hospital productivity examine one of the following:

- Number of nurses or physicians per bed.
- Hospital man-hours per discharge or visit.
- Capital cost per discharge.
- Total general service cost per discharge.

Most of these metrics, however, are purely activity indicators, which are different than productivity indicators. Activity indicators merely describe the volume of work, but do not accurately capture all inputs.

It is important that all figures such as these are adjusted for both the severity of the cases served and the prevailing wage rate in the area to avoid any data biases. Case mix adjustments are necessary because patient acuity and severity of the illness dictate the intensity of the service and the amount of resources necessary to treat the patient. Similarly, wage rate fluctuations arbitrarily make certain geographic areas appear more costly, and thus less efficient, when in fact these figures are partially dependent on the prevailing local salary rates, which are outside of the hospital's control.

Regardless of whether these metrics are high level and not immediately actionable, it is an initial attempt to evaluate one hospital's productivity relative to others. If a hospital evaluates its facilitywide productivity and finds that it is less productive than its peers, then the hospital will be more inclined to drill down further into each department and business process to find which area is contributing more to the productivity shortfalls and develop action plans for targeting improvements in the right departments.

Suggested data sources for benchmarking hospitalwide figures include the AHA (www.aha.org), Ingenix's (www.Hospitalbenchmarking.com), and Solucient (www.Solucient.com). Each of these has fee-based publications and online databases that use Medicare cost reports, surveys, and published institutional financials to allow hospitals to benchmark their productivity against others in the industry. Consulting firms also provide benchmarking services, where they use their experience with multiple organizations to benchmark performance relative to others.

IMPROVING PRODUCTIVITY

Productivity management assumes that hospitals want to continue improving the ratios of outputs to inputs; that is, they want to become more efficient and cost effective. Achieving this requires a plan for enhancing productivity. Productivity can improve one of four ways:

1. Output expands with no change in inputs.
2. Output increases with a decrease in inputs.
3. Inputs are reduced, downsized, or streamlined with no change in outputs.
4. Technology or process breakthrough eliminates inputs with no change in outputs.

The quest for productivity is to continuously find ways to improve the ratio of outputs to inputs, while improving service levels, outcomes, and other performance metrics. Productivity management assumes that hospitals are always looking for improvements in process and performance and that maintenance of the status quo is not sufficient.

Technology plays a major role in improving productivity. New software and systems help automate processes and remove entire tasks and activities. In electronic commerce, which will be described in greater detail in Chapter 11, systems can automate the entire purchasing and receiving process. Electronic commerce systems allow a requisition to skip the purchasing department, assuming that appropriate internal controls are developed into the system, which can eliminate a number of tasks and employees and might even increase the volume of outputs. The result is a change of the total productivity ratio through automation, which changes the input cost structure relative to the outputs.

The three major variables of productivity are labor, capital, and management. **Labor** is the basic element, defined as the productive work being performed by employees. Labor has a number of dependencies, such as the education and skill level of the employees performing the work, as well as motivation, work environment, and leadership. Typically, a change in education will have an impact on the amount of labor necessary.

Capital is the second factor of production; it represents investments in assets to offset labor or assets used to produce even more assets. Capital investment in health care is typically focused on investments in hardware, software, computer services, automation, and new equipment and devices, among others. In most well-run hospitals, investment in capital is done by performing return on investment (ROI) analyses to ensure that the capital to be deployed will ultimately change the productivity ratio, either by increasing output or decreasing the level of inputs required.

Management is the final variable. Management makes the basic decisions about staffing levels and mix, compensation and motivation of employees, locations to serve, technology to put in place, and where to focus efforts. Management decides on the trade-off between capital and labor and which to invest more heavily. Utilization of capital and labor, rather than just investing in additional units of both, is one of management's key tasks. Management is both a science and an art, but it requires somebody to make decisions that will help drive productivity increases.

Example

Trinity General Hospital has six cashiers in its food service operations, plus three cooks, four prep technicians, and two supervisors. Average hourly wage is $7, and each employee averages 8 hours per day, which is the total number of hours the cafeteria remains open daily. Total food supply expense is $500 per day, Monday through Friday, and averages 50% of this on both days of the weekend. Computerized food purchasing and inventory information systems were purchased last year at a cost of $100,000, and the amortized cost of this is about $500 daily. The cost of the real estate, including utilities, taxes, and lease, is about $400 daily. More than 1,400 patient and guest meals were served today. Calculate both the single- and multifactor productivity ratio for a workday. **Table 6–1** presents the results.

Thus, using all of the productivity factors (e.g., labor, capital, materials, and other miscellaneous resources), the total multifactor productivity ratio is 0.625. This figure is meaningless, however, without internal trend comparisons over time and external benchmarks against other leading organizations. Using a single factor, such as in this example (number of hours worked), the productivity ratio is 11.7 meals or guests served per hour. Both of these are useful productivity metrics to ensure that productivity increases over time.

Again, the only way to ensure that productivity is improving over time is to monitor productivity metrics relative to themselves (using trend analysis) and to external benchmarks or targets that are considered to be

Table 6-1 Multi- and Single-Factor Productivity Example

Multiple Factor Productivity

Input/Resource	Number of Hours	Average Hourly Rate	Labor Cost
6 cashiers	48	$7	$336.00
3 cooks	24	$7	$168.00
4 prep	32	$7	$224.00
2 supervisors	16	$7	$112.00
Total Labor	120		$ 840.00
Total Materials			$500.00
Total Capital			$500.00
Other Costs (energy, space)			$400.00
Total Other Costs			$1,400.00
Total Inputs			$2,240.00
Total Outputs (# of Meals Served)			1,400
Multifactor Productivity Ratio (Meals Served per Dollar)			0.625

Single Factor Productivity

Output	1,400
Input (Number of Hours Worked)	120
Single Factor Productivity Ratio (Meals served per hour)	**11.7**

the best practice. **Figure 6–1** is a graphic representation of how this analysis shows that a hospital is more productive today than several months earlier, but still not as productive as the best-in-class hospitals.

PRINCIPLES OF PRODUCTIVITY MANAGEMENT

There are five basic principles for measuring and managing productivity that need to be applied. Measurement systems must be consistent, reliable, measurable, quantitative, and comprehensive.

Consistent

Consistency is a requirement in productivity management. **Consistent** means to do the same things the same way repeatedly over time. Hospitals need to measure activity (output) and resources (inputs) consistently to make trend comparisons. If a hospital measured both outputs and inputs in September, but forgot for 3 months and then picked it back up in December, the results are inconsistent and therefore problematic. Similarly, if a hospital changes the formula or basis for calculating costs, then

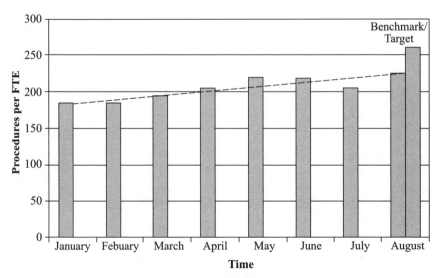

FIGURE 6–1 Trends and Benchmarks in Productivity Management

the results are not reliable. What if December, a holiday month, skewed the output so that it could not safely be compared against September? Managing productivity means measuring consistently over time, building the tracking process into overall management work flow, and then just sticking with it over time.

Consistency also means adhering to the same units of measure. Consistent use of the same definitions month after month allows comparability between numbers. If one month a department uses all factors as inputs and then the next month uses only labor costs, the numbers are not consistent and comparable and therefore cannot be relied on for meaningful results.

Reliable

Reliability is related to consistency. **Reliable** means that the productivity figures yield stable and uniform results over time. For this principle to be upheld, hospitals must ensure that systems used to generate volumes and costs do not change, that they are measured over the same time period (i.e., end of each week or at the month-end close), and that they consider all resources. For example, one hospital department measuring labor productivity chose not to count a specific supervisor's time in its calculation for inputs because, it decided, she played a large role in marketing and not as much in operations. Making the data subjective and open for interpretation creates data consistency and reliability problems, and therefore the results can easily be questioned.

Measurable

Measurable refers to how inputs and outputs are readily observed and calculated. A payroll clerk who processes paychecks clearly has measurable outputs (number of paychecks processed). A manager who oversees multiple functions, such as advertising or market research, may have less measurable work attributes. The use of tracking systems to manage all inputs and outputs is necessary. Often, payroll systems are used to track hours, general ledgers are used to track expenses, and other departmental systems are used to track outputs. Ensuring that these systems are in place, can routinely print reports with data that occurred during specific time periods, and that the data are complete and accurate is vital to having measurable, reliable, and consistent results. Productivity management must ensure that the business work flow is readily measurable and can consistently be calculated.

Quantitative

Quantitative means that data and numbers are used for measurement purposes. Subjective or qualitative assessment does not translate well into productivity metrics, which require numerical expression of value to calculate ratios. There must be secondary ways to measure the quality of a service, and this is equally as important as the productivity. To remain focused on cost and efficiency, though, productivity management must adhere to quantitative calculations.

Comprehensive

Finally, productivity should be simple but **comprehensive**. If multiple factors more accurately describe the cost behavior and resource consumption of a process or function, then all such data should be included in the ratios. Knowingly simplifying the calculation, at the expense of meaningful and reliable data, violates this comprehensive principle of productivity. In addition, use of scorecards that reflect quality and subjective views of performance (such as customer satisfaction, errors, or rework) must be taken into consideration to ensure a comprehensive view of performance.

ROI: CAPITAL VERSUS LABOR SUBSTITUTIONS

ROI models are very common in most industries today. The benefit of capital (which, in many cases, is new information systems, facilities, automation, or equipment) is it can substitute for labor (i.e., technology can often displace human effort). For example, in the household trash collection business, it used to take three employees to go on each route—one driver and two helpers to pick up the trash bags and cans and load them into the truck. At some point many years ago, equipment and automotive manufacturers determined that an automated loading device could replace both of the helpers. Now on many routes, only a driver remains.

The same concept applies in health care. Team-based nursing allows for less specialization of labor and fewer employees. Picture archiving and communication systems have replaced a number of health information management professionals. Electronic commerce has streamlined the payer/provider reimbursement process, thereby increasing productivity.

The decision to undertake **capital substitution** requires careful examination to ensure that the benefits are fully realized. Most ROI models, or cost-benefit analyses, are based on a simple calculation: Expected returns or benefits from capital less expected costs to acquire it; that is, benefits must be greater than the costs:

$$ROI = B > C$$

ROI models should detail all cost savings and avoidances, including current labor costs, and then compare these with the full benefits expected with the new capital deployed. Significantly more detailed explanations are given in Chapter 9.

Example

Consider the following example. A clinic maintains three supply technicians at a total labor cost of $150,000 per year to perform basic inventory functions, such as creating requisitions for supplies as they are used, counting inventory prior to requisition, and stocking shelves. Historically, there were no supply systems in place, and all processes were manual. A vendor has submitted a proposal for an automated, inventory point-of-use dispensing system. It is estimated that this will replace 1.5 full-time equivalent positions; there will be no further need for counting products or creating 10,000 annual requisitions because these functions will be automated. The total lease payment for this system is $40,000 annually. Is this a wise decision for a capital substitution over labor? The quick calculation clearly suggests that it is, ignoring cash flow and time value of money, which will be covered in more detail in Chapter 9. The calculation compares current versus future inputs, assuming outputs do not change:

$$\text{Current labor costs} = \$150,000$$
$$\text{Proposed capital and labor costs} = \$40,000 + \$75,000$$
$$(0.5 \times \$150,000)$$
$$= \$115,000$$
$$\text{Capital costs} < \text{Current labor costs}$$

Because the capital (or technology automation) would replace $75,000 of labor, and because total costs in the future would be $35,000 lower using a combination of factors (labor and capital), then the decision to invest in capital would wise. Converting this into a productivity ratio, the current ratio would be 10,000 ÷ 150,000, or 0.067 requisition per dollar. After capital investment, the productivity ratio would be 10,000 ÷ 115,000 or 0.087 requisition per dollar spent. The delta or change between the before and after is 0.02, which represents about a 30% operational improvement after capital substitution for labor (i.e., 0.02 ÷ 0.067 = 29.85%).

STAFFING AND LABOR SCHEDULING MODELS

As a service organization, labor contributes between 50% and 60% of all operating expenses for an average clinical department in a large hospital. To improve productivity ratios, it is important to develop quantitative staffing models to optimize the mix of employees needed and total labor hours for each period. Most hospital departments develop schedules (sometimes called rosters), however, based on history and gut feel (e.g., "on Tuesdays we need more people because it is usually busier" or "We have always had 10 people in that area").

Trial and error is common in developing labor schedules, but rarely does it produce efficient or optimal labor costs. To illustrate, what happens if the patient volume is 20 on one day and 10 the next? Or, what if the hospital occupancy rate goes from an average of 65% to 90%? Does a hospital or department need to employ the same level of employees regardless of output or workload? Obviously not, but that is exactly what most hospitals do—they build labor schedules based on handling either peak or average workload, and these labor budgets become fixed permanently. Any variability from the norm is difficult to manage, because capacity and demand are not forecasted sufficiently, and therefore, no flexibility exists in labor schedules. Labor is one of the most controllable costs; as operations managers continue to drive toward productivity gains, there are better ways to approach this issue. Several sophisticated mathematical approaches can be used to quantify the labor requirements and to turn them into weekly operation schedules.

Other service industries (e.g., retail and restaurants) have widely adopted the use of mathematical labor scheduling software tools. Given the right information, commercially available software can integrate with both "time and attendance" and payroll processing software to use historical information to drive optimal results. In fast-food restaurant chains, where average profit margins are less than 3%, the more sophisticated restaurant managers have statistically predicted when their busiest demand periods are, and they use this forecast to drive labor mix (i.e., cashiers, prep, cooks) and labor schedules (i.e., which specific day and time each employee is due at work). If demand is low, staffing is low, and as demand increases, labor is increased—creating an alignment between capacity and demand.

As far back as 1990, Taco Bell has employed optimization models in establishing labor requirements for each store (Godwart & Swart, 1994). Similarly, Burger King used optimization techniques in labor scheduling as far back as the 1980s (Swart & Donno, 1981). Restaurant managers know that for every hour they do not have to employ an individual, the operating margin increases exponentially. An optimized labor schedule in industries such as fast food, where efficiency is required and margins are minimal, does not happen accidentally. It is well planned and mathematically generated.

There are two major types of mathematical approaches used in the labor optimization software systems available today: simulation and linear programming. Both have been used successfully. Linear programming models are probably the most common. **Linear programming** refers to an optimization technique that seeks to either maximize or minimize an objective function, given a set of variables and constraints. In staffing models, there are typically five sets of variables that drive the quantitative models:

- Forecasted demand and patient volumes/flows (D) (e.g., 18 patients per day).
- Per-unit labor cost (C) (e.g., \$9 per hour).
- Resource or job type and mix (R) (e.g., accountant, nurse).
- Average transaction cycle time (T) (e.g., 17 minutes per function performed).
- Other constraints (e.g., actual capacity constraints on the equipment or the space).

Each of these variables can be modeled to express the relationships between them, similar to the following equation:

$$\text{Minimize} \quad (C_1 R_1 T_1 + C_2 R_2 T_2 + C_n R_n T_n)$$
$$\text{Subject to} \quad D_m = X, D_t = Y, D_n = Z$$

In other words, a linear programming model would attempt to minimize total labor costs (the objective function) by using the inputs of per-hour salary expenses, labor mix by job type, and total transaction times, while using the daily demand estimates as a constraint (i.e., D_m = Patient volume demand on Monday). Many of the popular software packages have built-in algorithmic code and matrix algebra, so users only need to feed the parameters and constraints and the optimized equations are then generated and labor schedules are printed. One of the most popular optimization tools available today is ILOG C-Plex (www.ilog.com) that has been used widely in nearly all industries and applications.

In health care there has been only minimal adoption of optimization techniques to date. Certain studies have reported the use of optimization models to estimate physician schedules in emergency and operating rooms (Carter & Lapierre, 2001). More commonly, nurse rosters have been developed using linear programming (Warner, 1976). Some research confirms that optimization models can save significant operating expense. In one hospital, a reduction of 16% in total labor expenses was achieved through linear program minimization models (Matthews, 2005). There just has not been wide enough deployment of optimization to make a difference yet, but this will change as healthcare practices continue to advance.

There are other more simplistic models for staffing, which are easier to use and faster to deploy. One such approach, often called simulation or activity models, uses simpler relationships between work outputs and labor inputs.

Example

Consider the following example. A receiving department processes 500 packages per day (total demand), and each package takes 7 minutes to process (i.e., time of receipt, scan of bar code, entry into and enterprise resource planning system, etc.). The known constraints are that (1) no employee works overtime, or more than 8 hours per day, and (2) on average, each employee is utilized effectively no more than 90% of the time (which accounts for work interruptions, meetings, breaks, or other unplanned activities). Therefore, eight employees will be needed. This can be calculated in the following steps:

1. Determine the total number of working minutes daily for each employee (8 hours × 90% utilization × 60 minutes = 432 minutes each day).

2. Estimate the total number of output each individual can process (432 hours ÷ 7 minutes for each transaction = 61.7 packages per day).

3. Divide total demand or daily production by the per-person rate (500 ÷ 61.7 = 8.1 employees).

This simple model suggests that staffing based on daily volume of 500 requires approximately 8 employees. If volume was projected to increase the following week to an average of 600, then closer to 10 employees would be required (600 ÷ 61.7). One simulation tool that allows a user to change key variables and assumptions, using known mathematical relationships to estimate the impact on a dependent variable, is **sensitivity analysis**. This is often commonly called "what-if" or scenario analysis.

Most importantly, there has to be alignment between resources and volume. Staffing for average days is never optimal because there will either be too many or too few employees on hand. Similarly, staffing for peaks or valleys creates either labor excesses or shortages. An attempt to match demand with volume is the only way to achieve optimal results.

Optimization and simulation models for generating labor schedules are slightly more complex than the traditional gut feel approach. They require a great deal of data, and they force managers to analyze processes and volumes more thoroughly to generate the appropriate results. They require understanding of cycle times and productivity. All of these help improve processes and reduce costs, so the benefits of using mathematical models are much greater than these risks.

PRODUCTIVITY AND PERFORMANCE SCORECARD

Productivity is just one key of the key metrics that helps define how a department or organization is doing. Performance metrics should focus on all areas of the business, measuring financial results, customer service, competition, and operations. A balanced scorecard, unique to each hospital, is one way to develop a core set of metrics that establish the right ways to ensure progress toward a specific strategy.

While a productivity metric focuses on efficiency, other areas of performance should focus on effectiveness. *Efficiency* measures "doing things right," with minimal resources and waste. **Effectiveness** measures "doing the right things," which relates to strategy and planning. Both efficiency and effectiveness should be measured on a departmental or operational scorecard. A **performance scorecard** is a tool to visualize measurements of key performance indicators for an organization relative to time, targets, or another baseline. A sample scorecard for a generic department is provided in the **Figure 6–2**.

Notice that the operational scorecard in Figure 6–2 has several components. First, it shows a "balanced" view, in that it is not strictly focused on a singular dimension of performance or productivity but attempts to take a comprehensive, holistic view of the function or department (Kaplan & Norton, 1996). Second, the scorecard shows multiple indicators for each category. In general, an operational scorecard should be limited to a handful of key metrics, so as to keep it simple and useful and not overwhelm managers and employees who must use it to translate per-

Category	Key Performance Indicator	Target/ Baseline	Current Period Results	Stoplight Indicator
Operational Focus	Cycle time, procure to pay Cycle Time, room changeover Cost per unit of output (for each key process) Change in productivity ratio (output ÷ inputs) Scheduling Delays/Backlog Supplier performance rating (key vendors)			Green
Customer/ Quality	Safety/Error Rates Customer/Patient satisfaction scores Survey results # of Complaints/Opportunities			Red
Economic	Operating margin Return on capital Days of working capital Days of inventory on hand Days of accounts receivable			Yellow

FIGURE 6–2 Operational Productivity and Performance Scorecard

formance into action. Third, the specific metrics are generic on this scorecard, but each department should define and manage its own customized metrics for each group. Specific Key Performance Indicators, such as number of days of accounts receivable, don't mean anything for one support service, but might for another.

CHAPTER SUMMARY

Managing productivity and performance is important for operational managers to ensure that their operations are becoming more cost effective and efficient over time. Principles of healthcare operations management suggest that the primary goals are to reduce costs, eliminate waste, and ensure that resources are being used efficiently. Productivity management is the ratio of outputs to inputs. Both single- and multiple-factor productivity ratios can be calculated to understand the relationship between outputs and inputs. Labor staffing models should be used to align volume or demand with resources. Staffing models should be calculated mathematically, not with simple heuristics or rules of thumb, employing linear programming algorithms to produce optimal results. Each department and business process can be decomposed into both outputs and inputs so that a periodic performance scorecard can track changes over time. Only by internally measuring and consistently applying these methods over the long term can hospital administrators prove that they have added value and made a positive impact on business operations.

KEY TERMS

benchmarking, capital, capital substitution, comprehensive, consistent, effectiveness, efficiency, input, labor, linear programming, management, measurable, output, performance scorecard, productivity, quantitative, reliable, sensitivity analysis

DISCUSSION QUESTIONS

1. Why is productivity important?
2. What is the difference between productivity and other measures of performance?

3. What is single-factor versus multifactor analysis?

4. What are some common measurement problems?

5. Why should hospitals benchmark?

6. Is a scorecard the only tool used for improving operations?

7. How do staffing models and labor optimization algorithms contribute toward productivity?

8. How can ROI models help the decision-making process?

EXERCISE PROBLEMS

1. Based on the following data, calculate the single-factor productivity ratio using hours of labor for a housekeeping department.

   Number of employees = 100

   Average hourly rate = $5.50

   Total hours worked in September = 15,570

   Total square feet maintained = 190,000

2. In the preceding problem, using sensitivity analysis, if the productivity ratio was 13.1 the previous month, has productivity increased or decreased? By what percentage?

3. Assume that a new piece of equipment could allow 25% of the labor force in question 1 to be eliminated. Using a 173-hour working month for each employee, a total equipment cost of $60,000 (which has a useful life of 3 years), and ignoring the cash flow and time value of money impact, would this be a good use of capital?

REFERENCES

Carter, M. W., and S. D. Lapierre. (2001). Scheduling Emergency Room Physicians. *Healthcare Management Science* 4:347–360.

Godwart, M., and W. Swart. (1994). *An Object Oriented Simulation Model for Determining Labor Requirements at Taco Bell.* Institute of Electrical Engineers Annual Conference Proceedings, Winter 1994.

Kaplan, Robert S., and David P. Norton. (1996). *The Balanced Scorecard: Translating Strategy into Action.* Cambridge, MA: Harvard Business School Publishing.

Matthews, Charles B. (2005). Using Linear Programming to Minimize the Cost of Nurse Personnel. *Journal of Healthcare Finance, 32*(1):37–49.

Swart, W., and L. Donno. (1981). Simulation Modeling Improves Operations, Planning, and Productivity at Fast Food Restaurants. *Interfaces, 11*(6):35–47.

Warner, D. M. (1976). Scheduling Nurse Personnel According to Nurse Preference: A Mathematical Programming Approach. *Operations Research, 24*:824–856.

CHAPTER 7

Project and Change Management

Goals of This Chapter
1. Understand how project management contributes to project success
2. Describe the role that management engineers can play in this process
3. Understand some of the project tools that can be used

Operations management requires that hospitals continuously look for ways to achieve better outcomes. Searching for improved business processes, enhanced staff productivity, and streamlined logistics implies that organizations must continue to change. Only if activities evolve can they improve, and in hospitals there are significant opportunities for improvement. This means that projects will become much more prevalent, as organizations seek to refine and improve operations. However, managing projects in hospitals is complex, given power and political tensions that can exist between business and medical staff. Understanding the role of project management, and using principles of change, managers can positively achieve desired outcomes. The purpose of this chapter is to describe tools and theories of project and change management as well as to discuss the role that internal consulting departments play in such endeavors.

DEFINING PROJECTS

A **project** is an organized effort involving a sequence of activities that are temporarily being performed to achieve a desired outcome. Projects are temporary in that they have both a beginning and an ending, they have objectives that state their purpose and function, and they exist only to achieve a specific outcome or deliverable. A project is distinct from operations in that projects are typically centered on identifying or implementing new or changed business processes, information technology, or other enhancements. Project results typically become operational once the effort has been finalized and deployed.

The Project Management Institute, one of the largest associations devoted to enhancing the body of knowledge for project professionals, defines **project management** as "the application of knowledge, skills, tools, and techniques to a broad range of activities in order to meet the requirements of a particular project" (Project Management Institute, 2004). A **project manager** is the individual who leads the planning and daily activities to achieve the project deliverables.

Some examples of healthcare projects for operations management include the following:

- Deployment of a pharmaceutical ordering and inventory system.
- Implementation of a new picture archiving and communication system.
- Analysis of specific patient-centric business processes.
- Design and construction of a new facility or building.
- Nursing labor optimization.
- Reengineering effort to reduce staffing levels in key areas.
- Startup of a new department, clinic, or operational process.

Although it is difficult to estimate with precision, it is likely that project work in growing hospitals can represent more than one-third of all work effort for managers and professionals. Operational managers are the beneficiary and eventual owner of the changed or new process or system once the project has been completed, so it is important that they are fully involved in managing the project from start to finish. As such, the skills and techniques used to manage projects become extremely important. Even if a skilled facilitator or consultant exists to help support the project, operational managers need to understand the basic concepts and employ the necessary tools to ensure that the project is successful.

POWER STRUGGLES IN HEALTH CARE

Projects require sponsorship to secure financing approval and to ensure commitment of the right people on the project from the outset. One of the problems in hospitals, however, is centered around the well-documented struggles over political power among different factions (Rovin, 2001). Physicians and nurses have historically maintained relationships that are mutually reliant on the other for patient management, yet physicians have clearly dominated the power struggle. Similarly, physician and business leaders clash in certain decision-making processes, where a physician's dominance in the key production process (i.e., clinical care) provides influence and power over others due to his or her medical expertise and control of the customer (i.e., patient). In academic medical centers and teaching hospitals, struggles for control between medical and academic factions are also very common. Therefore, projects that require physician sponsorship or commitment might require additional levels of networking and "selling" to obtain support from key constituents.

In many larger hospitals, though, the power struggle that most commonly exists in business operational projects is tension among managers of different clinical or administrative units. It is not uncommon to have issues of control and influence become more important than the project itself. Tension arises from even the smallest issues, such as whose name appears as sponsor and who leads the project, which can often stall projects indefinitely.

The role of formal versus informal power bases becomes important because, even if an executive sponsors the project, there might be an informal power source (at a "lower" level in the organization) that can influence the approval and direction of the project from the beginning. Leaders of other departments might question the motives of a project, especially if it reaches beyond one department's processes, which creates uncertainty and risk for others. Achieving support, commitment, and buy-in from the outset of any project that is multifunctional or multidisciplinary is required to ensure the project moves forward.

Cooperation and collaboration from all key stakeholders are required. Often this means that project managers need to set up appointments and personally sell the project to others. Education about the project's purpose and charter usually helps remove any uncertainty surrounding projects. Continuous communication also helps reinforce the concept that the project is important and that there are no hidden motives or purpose.

PROJECT SUCCESS

A hospital project is typically sponsored, or supported, by a manager or executive who has the most vested interest in the results or outcomes. A project sponsor ensures that the project manager has all necessary resources and helps eliminate organizational obstacles that might arise. The project sponsor helps recruit the project manager and kick off the project correctly, which helps ensure the project manager gets off to a solid start.

The goal of the project manager is to successfully move the project through all phases, from start to finish, while ultimately achieving the outcomes defined at the onset. A **deliverable** is the tangible outcome that results from the project. Essentially, the deliverable represents the benefits, or the reason a project was initially undertaken. Project deliverables can include successful implementation of a new information system, a report of findings or analyses, a new facility, or a changed process. Deliverables also include customer satisfaction and quality levels, which are expected to increase as a result of the project. Financial or operational performance improvements are also deliverables for many projects. Achieving these expected deliverables represents one component of success in a project.

Project success centers on achieving optimization of four key variables: deliverables, resource investment, scope, and timelines. This is depicted in **Figure 7–1**.

These variables are highly interrelated, and a change in one affects the others. For example, reducing the original amount of resources invested in the project by 50% could obviously affect the completion date of the

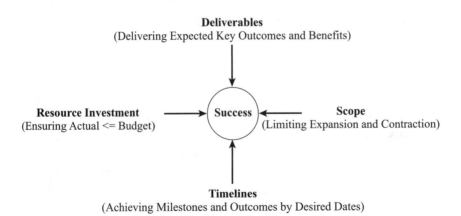

FIGURE 7–1 Defining Project Success

project, which could have a potentially negative impact on overall achievement of the project deliverables. Similarly, a large change in scope in the middle of a project could extend the overall timeline, and a change in deliverables expected could affect scope and resource requirements.

Resource investment represents the budget for financial commitments, as well as staffing and other key resources. This investment level is typically defined up-front, sometimes prior to or during the project planning phase. This is commonly called the *budget*, and it is expected that project managers use project resources efficiently so that the project comes in on or under budget, assuming no changes in scope occur that are outside of their control.

The *scope* represents the boundaries of a project. It limits the types of benefits or deliverables that are being sought, as well as defines which ones are not. Typically, scope is limited by process or organizational boundaries. For example, a project may decide to look at all activities that fall within the diagnostic imaging processes or all activities undertaken by the radiology department.

Timelines represent the critical dates for major milestones. Timelines define the beginning and end point of the project, as well as the sequencing of other activities and milestones along the way. A **milestone** is a key date by which a major project deliverable should be achieved. Timelines are extremely important for projects because they help define the expectations for when activities should occur, when resources will be consumed, and when the project will achieve desired outcomes. Timelines represent significant scheduling efforts, which will be described later.

KEY STAGES OF PROJECT MANAGEMENT

There are four distinct stages in project management: pre-project approval, project organization and definition, project scheduling and design, and project control and management. Each of these stages is critical to achieving the desired outcomes for project success described earlier.

Pre-Project Approval

As described earlier, the key to achieving positive outcomes on a project is to establish reasonable estimates of the benefits and returns of a project and to ensure that the total costs do not exceed these benefits. Some of these benefits may be quantifiable (e.g., increased revenues, increased market share, reduced costs), but many benefits may be qualitative (e.g., higher quality, system end of life).

In many organizations, the process of obtaining approval for the project entails convincing management and investment committees that these benefits will be realized and they are worth the risk. These two concepts—risks and realization—are key to a project's approval. **Risks** are the factors that jeopardize project success or that cause potential impairment or delay. All risks need to be mitigated somehow to achieve the project success and benefits that are expected. A plan outlining the risks and mitigation strategies is a key project deliverable. **Realization** of these benefits is a result of how successful the organization is at mitigating these risks and adapting to changes that arise during the project.

In most hospitals, the project approval phase is quite lengthy. If a project is funded out of normal operating funds, the approval process might be as simple as convincing departmental management of the benefits, approach, and costs. In more complex environments, or where capital funds are being allocated, the approval process might be quite lengthy and could entail several levels of governance, including approvals from local management, the budget department, and separate capital investment committee approvals. In these environments, the use of a structured business case should be used to thoroughly document all aspects of the project. Questions and issues that the business case should fully explore are shown in **Table 7–1**.

Project Organization and Definition

Once approval is obtained, the project enters an early phase called project organization and definition. This phase has also been called analysis, planning, or discovery. In this phase the primary tasks are to document all aspects of the business process, including use of the process engineering tools described earlier. This phase should confirm and refine all of the assumptions listed in the business case and turn the high-level requirements into more detailed specifications. Understanding the specific details, specifications, and requirements for the project is essential, because they can be included in the project only if they are clearly identified and focused.

One of the key aspects of project planning is to identify the work breakdown structure of the project. The **work breakdown structure (WBS)** decomposes project activities into more detailed components to allow for better planning. WBS uses a hierarchy effect to organize tasks,

Table 7–1 Elements of a Business Case

Demographics	• List project sponsor, manager, contact details
Business challenges or needs	• Describe the challenges faced by the process of department
	• Describe issues and causes of problems faced
	• Describe how these opportunities affect performance and contribute to the organization's vision
Business drivers	• Describe the key performance indicators and how the project or technology can affect these indicators
	• Document benchmark figures for comparison against others to show marginal improvement to be gained
Proposed solution	• Document the proposed solution
	• Describe implications on organization, policy, processes, or system architecture
	• Document the risks and how they can be mitigated
Investment	• Define the proposed investment
	• Estimate the total costs, with annual cash flow breakdown
	• Model the return on investment analysis (NPV, IRR, payback)
	• Define recommendations for moving forward
	• List all key assumptions
	• Define the project timelines and key milestones

where the top level is the highest one, and each subsequent level below the top provides more detail for that task above it. Planning typically involves allocating resources and timelines for the highest level tasks, while the next phase (scheduling) focuses on aspects of the more detailed tasks.

This phase requires interviews of key participants, thorough documentation of the process (with aims of identifying bottlenecks and issues), and direct observations and analyses of process outcomes. This phase should be documented thoroughly in a detailed design document that lists the key requirements and specifications. A project plan is also a key output of this process, which shows resource assignments, timelines, and milestones for each task.

Project Scheduling and Design

The project scheduling and design process takes the specifications and maps those against detailed activities and tasks. Project schedules are commonly viewed in Gantt chart form. A **Gantt chart**, named for its founder Henry Gantt, shows activities as blocks or bars over time. It is an intuitive chart used to show resources and time allocations for key tasks, and it supports monitoring of activities during the management phase.

A Gantt chart is very useful; it ensures that all activities are carefully planned for and that the total duration or activity times are considered. The use of a resource field helps isolate which person or department is responsible for the task, and the use of horizontal bars shows project activity over a timeline. A sample Gantt chart is depicted in **Figure 7–2**.

A Gantt chart is often used by managers because it is fairly straightforward to understand and easy to visualize. There really is no sophistication or optimization to arrange the sequence of activities that appear on the Gantt chart, but once they are included, the chart simplifies the management and tracking process.

Two of the more common methods to build sophistication into projects are critical path method (CPM) and program evaluation and review technique (PERT). The **critical path method** is a technique that helps identify the longest path in a project, which therefore makes it the most critical. If delays occur in the longest path, then a delay will occur in the overall project, while a similar delay in a noncritical path does not necessarily cause the project to be delayed. CPM attempts to determine overall time estimates for each activity and then uses predecessor (i.e., which

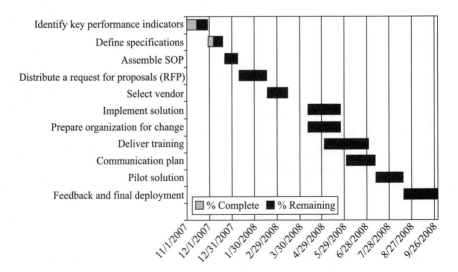

FIGURE 7–2 Scheduling Projects—Gantt Charts

task leads) and successor (i.e., which task follows) relationships for each node (O'Brian & Plotnick, 2005). A *node* is an activity or task and is connected to other nodes via lines or arcs. Using these interdependencies, constraints, and time estimates, it is possible to visually draw various network diagrams, such as a CPM model. Once the network diagram is constructed, it becomes the basis for the Gantt chart. Software tools like Microsoft Project have built-in network diagramming and critical path tools that use the information the project manager provides to build the critical path. A sample network diagram showing concepts of a node, critical path, and interdependencies among activities is shown in **Figure 7–3**.

A **program evaluation and review technique (PERT)** diagram is very similar, except that instead of using only a singular time estimate (e.g., task 1 takes three days), it requires estimates for three cases: a best case, worst case, and most likely case. A best case would assume no delays or issues, while worst case assumes major resource conflicts or delays; the most likely is a conservative estimate somewhere between the worst and the best cases. PERT models use a range of estimates that are more probable and likely. Mathematically, this is calculated as follows, where T_e = expected time, O = optimistic estimate, P = pessimistic or worst case estimate, and M = most likely time duration:

$$T_e = [O + P + 4M] \div 6$$

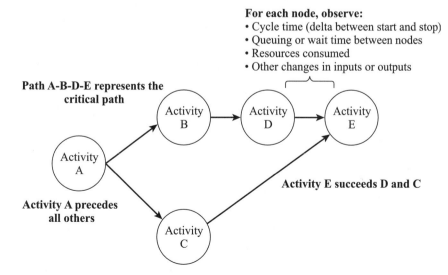

FIGURE 7–3 Nodes in a Network

For example, assume that a task will most likely be completed in 5 days, but optimistically (if all goes well) it could be completed in just 2 days, and worst case it will take 10 days. The PERT calculation to use in the network diagram and Gantt charts would be 5.33 days, or

$$[2 + 10 + (4 \times 5)] \div 6 = (32 \div 6) = 5.33$$

PERT models help simulate ranges of project durations that typically generate more reasonable project timelines. Both CPM and PERT are thoroughly discussed in traditional textbooks, but based on this author's research, they are not employed significantly in practice. They are useful tools, and as the level of sophistication increases in healthcare project management, so too will the use and deployment of advanced network diagrams such as these.

Project Control and Management

Once projects have been approved, defined, and designed, they enter the execution phase and require careful management to ensure tight control over timelines, costs, and scope. Two tools are useful to help improve management. The first is a Gantt chart, as discussed earlier, which helps track projects once they are under way to ensure progress against expectations for timelines. Another tool is a *project dashboard* or *scorecard*, which outlines all key aspects relative to project—budgeted versus actual costs; changes in scope; estimated timelines; earned value to date, if any; project risks; and other updates on project deliverable or progress.

The objective of project management entails finding ways to keep the project team motivated, and the activities on task, to achieve desired outcomes. Use of tracking tools and leading indicators helps managers foresee potential problems or risks before they arise so that prescriptive action can be taken.

CHANGE MANAGEMENT

Well-documented psychological research supports the idea that most people dislike change, or rather, dislike the uncertainty that accompanies change (Landy, 1989). Even change for the better is still change, which can cause both physical and emotional discomfort. Change disrupts people's daily activities, introduces chaos, and generally wreaks havoc for most individuals.

Projects create change. If no change or improvements were necessary, then there would be no value in establishing and managing a project. Because projects are organized and designed to change an existing process, technology, or practice, and because change is generally perceived to be negative, then it is important to minimize the disruptions caused by change.

The formula for overcoming change can be shown mathematically as:

$$Y = f(m,p,a,r)$$

where

Y = successful change management
m = management and leadership skills
p = an operational plan with a vision and strategy
a = alignment of incentives with those that are sponsoring the project and those that are working on and for the project
r = adequate resources.

Without all four components of this equation, change management cannot be successful. Leaving just one of these out creates uncertainty, frustration, or ambiguity for the organization.

- *Management* and leadership help inspire the team and set the direction.
- *Plans* help ensure that the vision can be executed and set strategies for achieving the results.
- *Alignment* of incentives helps keep the project and organization on target.
- *Resources* (such as financial, space, technology, equipment, and personnel) are necessary to ensure that the work can get done and that the strategies are carried out.

One of the best ways to ensure that fear of change does not kill the project is to ensure cooperation and collaboration up-front from all central constituents. This is often called **buy-in**, where sponsors and managers craft a story or vision for their change and then obtain support from others to ensure that no organizational obstacles prevent the project's advancement. A similar concept is the use of **partnering**, or establishing mutually beneficial and cooperative relationships with others, where trust and teamwork help create synergies. Partnering with others in similar roles or adjacent departments can help pool resources and energy to achieve greater project success.

Thinking systematically about the behaviors and expectations that all key stakeholders of change desire is one way to ensure appropriate communication and change management. Understanding the key relationships that need to be nurtured to build trust and support is essential to avoiding potential pitfalls.

Another way to master change is to document and obtain approval for all changes to the plan, project scope, or resource commitments. This change documentation should be supported by a business case, and modifications should be understood relative to their impact on schedule, costs, deliverables, and resource utilization.

Communication about the change is also important. Keeping communication simple and on point (or relevant) is essential. Continuous communication is also necessary. Over-communicating, as long as it follows the key message and helps to reduce ambiguity, is usually much less of a problem than under-communicating.

Besides getting the buy-in of influential people, the participation of all of those affected by the change should be encouraged. Getting people involved and vested in the change helps reduce fears, stimulate positive morale and feedback about the project, and obtain better results. Giving people a "voice" in the change is often more important than the change itself.

A common problem is that managers focus too much on the details when communicating change. Focusing on the high-level or big picture educates people about the purposes of the change and the rationale behind it. Many people are fearful of change when they suspect ulterior motives. If you expect that most people are afraid of the change—possibly because they fear they might lose their jobs or otherwise be less valuable to the organization—then address those fears early and often; you can overcome or minimize the resistance to change by keeping the communication channels open.

RAPID PROTOTYPING

In many hospitals and healthcare organizations, projects consume more resources and take significantly longer than a similar project in other industries. A number of factors make these organizational models more complex; they also create problems for management, because delays and excessive implementation times are two of the major reasons projects fail, have budget overruns, or are delayed significantly.

One of the ways to avoid these issues is to deploy rapid prototyping. **Rapid prototyping** is a concept whereby ideas and solutions can be targeted toward a very small sample to see if the solution improves results prior to wide-scale implementation. Rapid prototyping is commonly used in software development to quickly turn requirements and specifications into a solution, which can then be modified as needed. Iterative and incremental successes in projects help demonstrate success faster and can generate additional ideas for improvement. Rapid prototyping and pilots are similar in that they use small samples and attempt to demonstrate limited success prior to full deployment.

More than anything, rapid prototyping involves two factors: proven methodology and supporting culture. The methodology used to deploy projects must be established and workable to ensure that the project team does not "reinvent the wheel." A methodology that is free from ambiguity is a requirement. But, more importantly, there has to be a supporting culture or environment in the organization that encourages risk taking and the desire for speed and flexibility—while acknowledging the potential for failure. Rapid prototyping will result in some failures, but more can be learned from failures than in many successful projects. The right culture, which supports rapid prototyping, is essential to stimulate the team to deliver—and to discover.

RISKS INVOLVED IN PROJECT MANAGEMENT

It has been suggested that the chance of a complex project surviving and achieving all of the benefits it established early on is around 50% (Lucas, 2006). In other words, one out of every two projects will have issues in some form or fashion that could jeopardize its success. It is crucial that project risks are identified early and that a plan to mitigate these risks is put in place. Any of the following factors can contribute to project failures:

- Long implementation cycles.
- Large dollar commitments.
- New, immature, or innovative technologies.
- Inexperienced employees.
- Lack of project sponsorship or management.
- Lack of formalized documentation or procedures.

- Misuse of tools and techniques for project tracking.
- Lack of training.
- Failure to launch or kick off the project successfully.
- Poor communication.
- Changing priorities or scope of project.
- Lack of financial resources.
- Too many, or too few, people involved in the project.
- Inferior facilitation and coordination in project meetings.
- Organizational politics.
- Lack of preparation or training for new process or system prior to implementation.
- Lack of alignment between departments.
- No pilot or prototype to prove the concept.

These risks can be mitigated if they are considered early on in the project planning phase and then proactively monitored during each of the following phases. Risks should be documented and necessary adjustments made to all Gantt and CPM diagrams.

DEPARTMENTS OF MANAGEMENT ENGINEERING

Many larger hospitals have created a management engineering (ME) department. The objectives of this department are to apply industrial engineering techniques to control costs and improve outcomes (Smalley, 1982). The ME department is often focused on implementing quality management processes, using continuous process improvement techniques, developing operational plans, administering patient satisfaction surveys, performing accreditation, and managing complex projects.

Some of the specific activities that ME departments can undertake, and that are severely lacking in hospitals, include analyzing the productivity and economic impact of information technology, managing performance scorecards and benchmarking processes, and performing advanced process engineering. Rollout of Six Sigma and other continuous process techniques is also high on the list of priorities for most ME departments.

Training and education for management engineers in health care is unfortunately lacking. This text elaborates on the concepts and techniques necessary for management engineers to be successful, because management engineers rely extensively on the operations management discipline. Besides this, there are very few comprehensive, structured training programs that exist—although this is starting to change as universities start to recognize the need for these skills. As this evolves, the more formalized quantitative techniques prevalent in other industries will be adapted to the healthcare profession to provide a toolkit that is relevant to the unique challenges facing healthcare.

Several professional associations exist to support management engineers and to assist with networking and resource sharing. The Healthcare Information and Management Systems Society (HIMSS) is the largest group of professionals, although it focuses primarily on the issue of information technology and to a much lesser role on ME and performance improvement (www.himss.org). Within HIMSS, a task force called Management Engineering–Performance Improvement focuses exclusively on sharing information and building educational tools and programs to advance the performance improvement profession. Another excellent association that represents operations and quantitative management professionals across all industries is the Institute for Operational Research and the Management Sciences; www.informs.org. Similarly, the Society of Health Systems of the Institute of Industrial Engineers (www.shsweb.org) is an excellent resource for management engineers to share information, learn new techniques, and network with other similar-minded professionals.

CHAPTER SUMMARY

A project is an organized effort involving a sequence of activities that are temporarily being performed to achieve a desired outcome. Projects in health care are becoming quite extensive, as technology and process innovation are used to control costs and improve results. More sophisticated management of complex projects is necessary if healthcare projects are to achieve project success. Projects require sponsorship to gain support, and often tension and power struggles ignite that could kill a concept before it is even kicked off.

Projects typically move through four phases. They start with pre-project approval, using business cases and partnering to obtain support and funding for the concept. Projects then get staffed, and a project plan assigns resources to key activities, while requirements and specifications are gathered. Project scheduling and design create network diagrams and paths that are optimized to achieve the desired timelines, while Gantt charts are used to visually track progress against plans. It is important that project managers mitigate all major risks to achieve the success that projects desire, including being on time, within budget, and within scope, while realizing the benefits that were originally expected.

KEY TERMS

buy-in, critical path method (CPM), deliverable, Gantt chart, milestone, partnering, program evaluation and review technique (PERT), project, project management, project manager, rapid prototyping, realization, risks, work breakdown structure (WBS)

DISCUSSION QUESTIONS

1. How does a project relate to day-to-day operations?
2. What defines a successful project?
3. How does a PERT diagram differ from CPM?
4. What are the components of a business case?
5. What are the various stages of project management?
6. If a project is complex, what change management techniques might be necessary?
7. Describe the four key elements necessary to master change.
8. What are some common risks in large, complex projects?
9. What is rapid prototyping?
10. What role does ME play in process improvement and project management?

EXERCISE PROBLEMS

1. Assume that a project has an expected total duration of 25 days, but several optimistic employees feel that it can be completed in as little as 18 days, while others expect it to take nearly 40 days. Using PERT calculation, what is the project duration to be used in project Gantt charts and other tracking tools?

2. If a CPM calculation of project duration was 25 days, how does the PERT calculation in Question 1 compare?

REFERENCES

Landy, Frank J. (1989). *Psychology of Work Behavior*. Pacific Grove, CA: Wadsworth, Inc.

Lucas, Henry C., Jr. (2006). *Information Technology and the Productivity Paradox*. Oxford, UK: Oxford University Press.

O'Brian, James J., and Frederic L. Plotnick. (2005). *CPM in Construction Management*. New York: McGraw-Hill.

Project Management Institute. (2004). *A Guide to the Project Management Body of Knowledge*. 3rd ed. Newton Square, PA: Project Management Institute.

Rovin, Sheldon, Ed. (2001). *Medicine and Business: Bridging the Gap*. Gaithersburg, MD: Aspen Publishers.

Smalley, Harold E. (1982). *Hospital Management Engineering*. Englewood Cliffs, NJ: Prentice-Hall.

CHAPTER 8

Planning for Operational Excellence

Goals of This Chapter
1. Understand the operational planning process
2. Calculate breakeven analyses as part of new program or service development
3. Describe analyses used to define the external environment
4. Describe how operations can benefit from business plans

Creating strategy with a focus on operational excellence requires planning. Rick Page coined the phrase "hope is not a strategy," which implies that the future will become reality only by carefully envisioning it, preparing for it, and then executing it (Page, 2001). Yet many hospitals and healthcare organizations do not carefully plan their operations; and in the absence of a strategy, the results are usually less than stellar. This chapter provides an overview of how to use planning cycles to improve operations.

WHY PLAN?

Organizations plan in order to survive. It is one of the most vital management functions necessary for hospital growth, positioning, and effective execution (Zuckerman, 2005). Operational planning involves mapping the external opportunities and threats with the internal strengths and weaknesses to define strategic alternatives and stake out an appropriate competitive position. The output of business planning is typically a plan that defines the specific functional strategies to employ for each dimension of business strategy.

Planning is a discovery process in which organizations define their markets and assess internal operations. However, the process of planning is more important than the product. A plan is easily discarded or placed on a shelf, and thus may not be that useful. The insights gained from the planning process however help in many ways, as managers think about opportunities, brainstorm new services, or analyze historical performance. The process is important in that it provides the organization with shared concepts about the market, competition, changing technologies, and overall direction. The process allows for mutual discovery of information and should bring consensus among a wide variety of stakeholders. One of the more important results of strategic business planning is alignment among the hospital's administrators about where the hospital is headed and how it is going to get there, such as which product markets to invest in and focus on. This shared vision of future direction and goals is essential for success in turbulent environments.

THE PLANNING PROCESS

Effective operations planning processes have four primary phases: analyze operations and environment, generate strategic alternatives, deploy strategies, and measure and review. **Figure 8–1** presents a summary diagram of the planning process. Each of these stages will be discussed in more detail throughout the chapter.

ANALYZE OPERATIONS AND ENVIRONMENT

The initial phase in the operations planning process is to analyze the internal operations as well as the external environment. There are multiple steps within this phase, starting with the selection process for the planning team members.

Select the Right Team

Prior to beginning the business planning process, critical issues about how to organize the planning efforts have to be addressed. Choices have to be

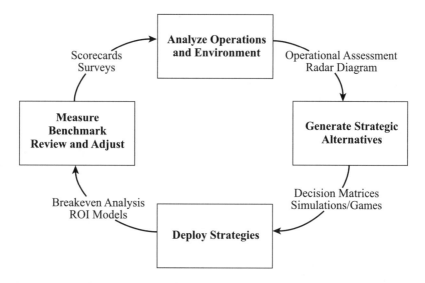

FIGURE 8–1 The Process of Crafting Operations Strategy

made about members of the planning team, representation from internal and external stakeholder groups, facilitation, timing and deliverable dates, and strategic analysis tools.

Choosing the members of the planning team wisely is critical to the success of the planning process. There are two levels of business planning: one at the strategic level and one at the clinic or unit level. For purposes of strategic planning, which involves decisions at the highest levels, hospitals should use key line managers as much as possible. Hospital planning teams might be comprised of the chief executive officer, chief operations officer, chief financial officer, supply chain vice president, chief nursing officer, chief marketing officer, marketing vice president, and other executives responsible for other mission critical functional areas such as specific centers, clinics, as well as the director of strategic planning.

Because hospitals have to satisfy at least multiple stakeholders, it may be prudent to include representatives from several other groups as well. For example, it might make sense to include trustees, vendors, system-level management, patients, or other key participants. As hospitals become more integrated, it will be valuable to have others involved in demand and market scanning activities.

Generally, it is important that planning teams be cross-functional to represent the diverse needs of the entire organization. The composition of the team should be based as much on the skills the participants possess as on position. The team should be comprised of strategic thinkers (i.e., big picture, "out of the box"), who are highly respected and capable of implementing cultural and directional changes within the organization. In addition, the teams must include a mix of more practical and tactical representatives. Having this mix of strategic and tactical thinkers allows the team to be innovative, while at the same time ensuring that the outcomes are realistic and capable of implementation. Most of the time, planning teams should not have more than 10 members to ensure that all participants contribute and are fully engaged in the process.

In almost all situations, because of the broad mix of participants and key topics for discussion, the planning process should be facilitated. The most important role of facilitation is to keep the team moving forward and the process on schedule. Facilitators bring the methodology to the team, provide boundaries for discussions, and ensure that all participants are engaged and active. Facilitators are trained in the use of a variety of techniques to drive sessions, such as brainstorming, flow charting, and force field analysis. Facilitators must have the respect of the planning team members and must be strong enough to bring order and consensus to the process, but insightful and patient enough to promote conversation from all members.

Operations planning should be continuous. Traditional planning models based on an annual frequency are not robust or dynamic enough to respond to the continual challenges of a turbulent industry environment. Instead, the process should be conducted at much shorter intervals, such as every few weeks or months. Permanent staff members who support the process, such as staff from the marketing department or the planning group, should be continually providing new data on markets and competition, and the planning team must come together routinely to evaluate and make adjustments. Additionally, the planning process must have short cycle times (i.e., they must not drag on indefinitely). Typically, if the planning process is frequent enough, the process should consume no more than two to four weeks, although this varies depending on the level of resources committed and the extent of time allocated to planning daily. To ensure that the process is being conducted properly, deliverables and milestones must be established for the process. Dates for each deliverable, such as final analysis of external environment, have to be in place so that the process cycle time can remain condensed.

Planning as a process has been described as more of an art than a science. Regardless, strategies need to be based on real data and information as much as possible. Information comes from using analytical tools and techniques, such as game theory, market research, competitive intelligence, and scenario models. These types of tools ensure that strategies are dynamic and sophisticated and represent an accurate view of the environment.

Sufficient staff and information resources must be devoted to the planning process. Staff resources include those functional groups devoted to capturing and analyzing data for planning purposes, such as the planning and market research groups. Information resources include a variety of published secondary statistical data on the industry markets and needs, as well as internally generated primary data from customers, payers, and other stakeholders. There should also be adequate financial resources allocated to strategic planning to allow participants to conduct benchmarking trips and acquire necessary data and reference materials.

Assess the Current Operational Effectiveness

This step should explore the organization's capabilities. The result of internal analysis should be an identification of the strengths and weaknesses, plus a better understanding of the capabilities and competencies required that allow the industry to compete more effectively. This includes exploring the capacity and demand levels that currently exist, looking for misalignment or other balance issues.

The process of internal analysis includes an exploration of all operating characteristics of the healthcare organization, including a review of current strategies, performance, portfolio, structure, management style, systems, and financial resources. **Radar diagrams** are graphical analyses that show target versus actual performance in key internal areas and identify potential problem areas. To read a radar diagram, look for the differences or gaps that exist between the two lines (one represents actual current performance in each of the criteria, and the other line provides an ideal or expected level). **Figure 8–2** provides a sample radar diagram commonly used for this purpose.

Internal analysis begins with a review of previous and current business strategies. Examining strategic initiatives and priorities provides a sense of

FIGURE 8–2 Analyzing Internal Operations Using Radar Diagrams

whether the current strategy is sufficient to cope with changing competitive pressures. Questions to be addressed include:

- Is the strategy still sufficient?
- Is performance keeping pace with the industry?
- Is the strategy perceived as an industry leader or laggard?
- Do weaknesses exist that competing organizations are exploiting?
- What issues exist that are not covered in the strategy?

Next, determine if the strategy is successful by analyzing historical and current performance in terms of quality and financial outcomes. Specific performance areas to investigate include clinical effectiveness (e.g., patient error rates, safety levels) and operational effectiveness (i.e., customer service levels, supply chain economics, average cost to perform key processes, and financial effectiveness, profitability, and other key ratios). This analysis should include a comparison of performance over time to ensure that performance is improving, but it should also compare the industry's performance with other local competing organizations, as well as others considered to be exceptional organizations. Comparing an organization's performance against others helps provide a clearer picture of strengths and weaknesses that the industry faces.

Additionally, performance analysis helps define the core competency for the organization. A core competency is an internal activity or process that the hospital performs really well relative to all other internal activities. For instance, the industry may be very good at securing research funding or implementing information systems. Performance analysis also helps define distinctive competencies for the industry. A distinctive competency is something the organization does really well relative to other organizations. Understanding both the core and distinctive competencies, in addition to the strengths and weaknesses, helps provide a visual map of how an organization is currently positioned to compete.

Portfolio analysis is used to help hospitals systematically assess their competitive position in each of the service lines they offer. With portfolio analysis, organizations should focus on (1) the current profitability in each service line, (2) the potential for market growth or demand shifts in each service line, and (3) the capability or competencies that the industry has in each service line. Understanding where the service lines stand, both financially and in relation to the competition, will help determine if services should be added, eliminated, or pruned.

Compare Structure and Style

Typically, when reviewing internal influences on an organization, planners should consider the overall organizational structure and resulting management style that has evolved. Decisions on industry support service centralization versus decentralization, the role of a business unit manager in strategic initiatives, and how to measure business unit effectiveness are three critical issues to consider. An assessment as to whether the current structure and style complements or detracts from the strategy to be pursued is vital under this portion of internal analysis.

Use SWOT Analysis

The strengths, capabilities, and competencies of the local healthcare industry can be used to exploit the opportunities available in the market environment, and competitors' weaknesses exposed during the external analysis should become key components of the grand strategy. Weaknesses identified internally within an organization should be fortified or strengthened, either by investing more resources in those areas or eliminating them altogether.

A **SWOT analysis** is a thorough review of an organization's combination of strengths, weaknesses, opportunities, and threats. This analysis generates more questions that have to be addressed to match strategy to situation.

Issues that need to be considered for opportunities include the following: Which strengths exist internally to capitalize on the opportunities in the market? What resources will be required to pursue them? Will the organization have to increase, reduce, or maintain investments into certain product or service lines? Will, or have, any competitors already moved on these opportunities? What can be done to thwart those efforts?

Issues that exist with regard to threats include addressing the following questions: Are these threats real? How can they be mitigated or avoided?

Similarly, when looking at strengths, key questions to address include these: How can the organization's strengths be used to achieve a greater competitive advantage? How can any competitors' service lines or category successes be blocked by building on the strengths identified earlier in the analysis? Should these competencies be built up further by continuing investments, or should resources be invested elsewhere? Will these strengths be enough to achieve an advantage?

Finally, questions that should be addressed with regard to weaknesses include the following: How can competitors be prevented from exploiting the weaknesses identified? Can resources be invested in these areas to convert them into strengths, or at least make them neutral? Will these weaknesses prevent the organization from pursuing certain opportunities?

Assess Management and Information Systems

The planning process should assess the management and information systems in place that support the business strategies. Typically, one of the most important management systems is the pay and reward system used to provide incentives for executives and managers to achieve higher levels of productivity and effectiveness. Other key information systems to evaluate include medical informatics, pharmaceuticals, enterprise resource planning, and reporting and business intelligence systems. Questions to be addressed here include these: Do we have the right systems in place to inform and incentivize managers to make the right decisions? Does the current system enhance organizational effectiveness? Do current policies support organizational direction? Do changes in other systems, such as performance measurement, need to be implemented?

Evaluate Financial Resources

When comparing the internal environment of a hospital, it is extremely important to evaluate both the cost and the financial structure for departments and the overall organization. Because every dollar of resources committed to one service line category has an opportunity cost in terms of what was given up, a cost comparison is important to determine if the level of resources committed to specific service lines is adequate and efficiently employed. Benchmark data from leading organizations about cost-effectiveness and cost structure relative to local competing organizations should be obtained in areas such as total industry volume, market share, consumer demand, and average costs.

Hospital financial position should also be examined thoroughly to ensure that the industry has sufficient funding and is efficiently employing those resources. Benchmark comparisons on debt position, financial returns, working capital, liquidity, and cash management are all important indicators of financial position and help quantify the financial implications of business strategy. Groups such as the International Benchmarking Clearinghouse and industry analysts tends to provide significant venues for benchmarking hospital performance relative to the competition.

Each of the components of internal analysis—strategy analysis, performance analysis, portfolio analysis, analysis of structure and style analysis, and financial resources—helps shape the internal capabilities and competencies that the hospital has as part of its competitive weaponry. The strengths and weaknesses that result from these analyses form the basis for competitive strategy.

Analyze the External Environment

After carefully reviewing all aspects of the internal environment, operations managers should next analyze the external environment. The **external environment** includes all forces external to the industry that potentially influence business strategy. External analysis can be broken down into the four most significant external influences for an organization: customer, competitor, industry, and environment (Thompson & Strickland, 1998).

Strategies have to be based on a thorough analysis of what the organization's current and potential customers want and need. If hospitals are to determine which products to offer and which markets to serve, the changing requirements of the customer have to be defined. In addition to the customers, an analysis of the changes in the major payer's motivation and needs must be explored.

When performing consumer or customer analysis, it is important to examine the major market segments in the industry. A *market segment* would best be defined as a method of targeting specific customers in the market. It is possible to segment customers on the basis of their product needs, such as benefits sought. It is also possible to segment markets on any of the following demographics: geography, lifestyle, sex, age, income, usage levels, size, or application.

Customer analysis should also include a thorough analysis of the changing motivations and consumer behavior of both the purchasers and payers of the industry. Such demographic information helps link demand with overall market characteristics. Answers to a variety of questions could lead to changes in overall strategies:

- What motivates patients to come to this facility?
- Are demographics of the customers changing? How might this affect future demand?
- What attributes of the service are important?
- What valued-added services, options, extras, and components are desirable?
- What objectives do customers (or patients) seek?
- What changes in motivation are occurring or could occur?
- Are customers satisfied?
- Are there any unmet needs?

A thorough analysis of each of these aspects of the external customer analysis will yield useful insight into how to adapt the organization's strategy to better meet the changing needs of the consumers. The customer value-added methodology identifies the clients who add significant value to the hospital, which subsequently drives both customer service and supply chain business rules. This methodology should be implemented at this time. More details on the specific process are provided in Chapter 11.

Competitor Analysis

Competition should be thoroughly understood. As change or turbulence increases and financial returns continue to diminish, competitive pressures will escalate. Analyzing the competition makes your strategy more effective.

Competitive analysis requires the industry to focus on insights that influence strategy. Answers to key questions are required:

- Who are the competitors in these markets?
- How many competitors are there? How concentrated is the market?
- How strong a foothold do they have on the market?
- Why are competitors able to sustain market share?
- Which competitors should be the focus of attention? What are their strengths?
- What plans do competitors have for the short and long term?
- What do the competitors' systems and supply chain networks look like? How effective are they?

Additionally, hospitals must focus on competing organizations individually and in networks. A thorough competitive assessment also includes a description of competitors' size, growth rates, and profitability. The culture of the competition should be examined, as should the competition's economics, including cost structure and margin. Finally, a review of the competitions' past and current strategies is essential to understanding potential future direction.

The success of an organization's strategies likely depends on its competitors' ability to defend their position or build a competitive advantage; thus, it is important to understand the competition's strengths and weaknesses in at least four key areas: product and service innovation, service delivery, marketing, and overall industry management.

Competitors could be strong in innovation if they have highly advanced research and development teams that continually drive new products to the marketplace. If competitors continually introduce new technology into the industry, or have high rates of commercialization or patents, they are obviously quite innovative.

When delivering services, competitors could be strong or weak in terms of service delivery and organization, the service quality level, the extent of integration between competitors, and how easy they are to do business with. By examining customer retention rates, although these are often difficult to find, the strengths and weaknesses of the competition's service delivery becomes more evident.

Extensive competitor analysis includes a review of industry management. Does the competition's management create a specific culture, or does it have loyal employees? Analysis of a competitor's turnover rates, strategic goals, and level of entrepreneurism provides a better picture of the strengths and weaknesses associated with management.

Finally, competitor analysis must focus on marketing programs. Specific insight into the brand or name recognition associated with various organizations is useful for determining the basis of competition. The focus that competing hospitals places on customers may be insightful for finding new markets or exploiting unmet needs. The current breadth and depth of competitors' product lines may highlight opportunities for new markets that might have otherwise been hidden. A review of the advertising and sales or business development strategies also helps determine the future strategic direction for each competitor.

Each of these areas of external competitor analysis is important for finding strengths and weaknesses of competitors. A summary matrix can be used to evaluate the competition's strengths and weaknesses. A competitor's strength assessment matrix should be developed during the planning process by listing each of the key success factors that an industry must have to be successful. The planning team then critically evaluates both the subject hospital and its competing organizations. Weights are assigned to each factor, which are then multiplied by a ranking to obtain a weighted score. Weights must add to 100%. Typically, rankings from 1 to 10 are used, with a 10 indicating a very strong rating. The overall highest total ranking goes to the industry with the strongest competitive advantage—which indicates the industry that represents the most intense rivalry. The matrix is useful for determining competitive position in local industry markets.

Successful strategies recognize competitors' strengths and find a way to mitigate them or reduce their effectiveness. Conversely, successful strategies identify a competitive weakness and exploit that, by building a competitive advantage with that in mind or by building marketing programs that bring these weaknesses to the attention of the market.

Analyze the Industry

The third component of external analysis is to conduct an industry analysis. Hospitals must continually analyze the industry structure and local market dynamics because these ultimately influence industry competitive rivalry. In addition to recognizing general trends occurring in the industry, this analysis helps organizations recognize how local markets are changing.

One of the key outcomes of industry analysis should be definition of the key success factors for the industry. Key success factors are those activities that must be performed well if an organization is to succeed in the industry. For example, one key success factor in the industry is conveniently located industry facility. If an industry is not physically located within the market in the right place, the industry will not succeed. Location is just one of the key success factors. Industry analysis must identify others that are important in the individual local market. Other key success factors might include brand recognition, access to qualified labor, and economies of scale.

Environmental Analysis

The final component of external analysis is to identify changes in the environment that may influence organizations. The environment includes all forces external to the industry that might influence operations. There are four primary components that need to be examined: technological, social, regulatory, and economic.

Technology impacts should address new technologies that might alter productivity, breakthrough technologies that improve quality of patient care or affect service, or technologies that might give the organization an advantage over the competition.

Social factors influence the entire industry, such as demographics or change in average age or mix of patients. Understanding life-cycle trends, changes occurring in the general population, and specific implications for the hospital are all key considerations.

Regulations, laws, statutes, governmental policies, and all other requirements that are mandated or legally enforced affect what hospitals and healthcare organizations deliver and how they deliver it. Regulations requiring additional resources, changes in business process, reductions in reimbursement levels for procedures, or any other changes that are anticipated or known should be identified and their impact carefully assessed.

Finally, it is important to understand the changing economics of the industry, including both macro and micro issues. Macro issues for the industry economics include such grand changes as medical consumer price index changes, unemployment rates, consumer or government spending, interest rates, or currency fluctuations. Macro issues must include an examination of trends in the industry finances and potential issues and opportunities associated with these changes. Micro issues for the industry economics might include how the local city or market is changing in areas such as per capita income.

A great deal of time must be spent analyzing potential and current issues and opportunities arising out of trends and shifts in technology, society, regulations, and economics. Failure to recognize and act on these changes is one of the most probable reasons for organizational failure.

GENERATE STRATEGIC ALTERNATIVES

Once both internal and external analyses are conducted, it will be possible to identify potential strategic alternatives. These alternatives can be prioritized using a combination of several tools, specifically breakeven analysis, decision matrices that use weights and probabilities to assess the most likely or valuable decisions, and simulation tools or games that help improve decision making.

Strategic alternatives in each of the three dimensions need to be explored: overall competitive approach, market orientation, and functional deployment. First, hospitals should have uncovered by this point if they are fundamentally a low-cost service provider (which most hospitals are not) or if they have a strong focus in a select group of product lines (most do not). As a result, the great majority of companies then typically attempt to fall into the broad competitive approach of a differentiation strategy (Trout & Rivkin, 2000). If the overall strategy is one of differentiation, the question of how to differentiate remains. Hospitals must search for a unique competitive position, where they are the premier providers of select products or services, where price competition is low, and where alternative providers are relatively minimal. Differentiation based on brand recognition, location, or types of service lines offered can all form the base of a differentiation strategy.

The next step in developing strategic alternatives is to review the existing operational product line portfolio strategy. Does the current portfolio of product lines make sense under new competitive conditions? Are there distinctive competencies in these service lines that can differentiate the industry from the competition? Should service offerings be removed to free up resources for investment into other service lines? Should partnerships be reevaluated? Is the organization integrated enough to compete with other networks and systems? Each of these questions needs to be answered before proceeding.

The final step in generating alternatives is to address each of the functional deployment strategies (i.e., growth, diversification, pricing, capital investment, and marketing). Do all these strategies support the grand strategy? Do they all make economic sense given the current competitive climate and level of turbulence?

BREAKEVEN ANALYSIS

In many cases, the result of a planning process is identification of a new program or service that is not currently offered (Nauert, 2005). This might include a new support service, new clinical service line, or new medical procedures to extend current programs. All potential additions or extensions of services should be thoroughly reviewed, using feasibility analysis (how likely is this service to succeed?), a competitive analysis (will competition alter the pricing or demand structure?), and internal analysis (does the organization have the expertise and resources to offer this at a high-quality level?). Assuming that the analyses performed support moving forward, a financial technique called breakeven analysis must be performed. A **breakeven analysis** analyzes cost structures and volumes to identify at what point total returns equal total costs. This point of activity, where total revenues equals cost, and thus yields net income of zero, is called the **breakeven point**. A graphical view of the breakeven concept is shown in **Figure 8–3**.

Breakeven analysis typically focuses on how many units (the total quantity) are necessary to be sold or provided to have total revenues cover total costs. Four terms are important to understand for this technique: fixed cost, variable cost, total cost, and price per unit. **Fixed costs** are all the expenses necessary to deliver services, and these costs do not vary with total services provided. For example, if a hospital wants to open a new clinic to provide computed tomography scans, it will, at minimum, need capital equipment to provide these services. All of the initial setup costs for equipment, facilities, and staff are fixed. **Variable costs** are the costs that vary directly with production. In other words, as more services are delivered, additional variable costs will be required—because such costs vary with total quantities delivered. **Total costs** are the sum of both fixed and variable costs. **Price per unit** refers to the fee that will be charged to payers or customers in order to receive the service, and it is typically assumed not to vary. Another key term is contribution margin, which is price less variable cost. Mathematically, the breakeven point can be calculated as follows:

FIGURE 8–3 Breakeven Analysis

$$\text{Revenue} = \text{Cost} \quad\begin{cases} BE = \dfrac{FC}{(P - VC)} = \dfrac{\text{Fixed Costs}}{\text{Price} - \text{Variable}} = \text{Breakeven} \\ \text{Net income} = 0 \end{cases}$$

(handwritten annotations:) Total # of units that need to be sold for NI = Breakeven Point; Fixed Costs ÷ (Price per unit – Variable Costs)

For example, a hospital has decided to offer a new service line (assume it is a new cardiology procedure that has not been offered before). After extensive analysis, the total variable cost to deliver this service (using clinical labor, administrative staff, supplies, and other direct materials) is $220 per procedure. The fixed cost of offering this service involved allocating 50,000 gross square feet of space, installing a new piece of medical equipment, and purchasing a new computer workstation; the fixed cost, then, is $100,000. Based on market analysis, the facility should be able to perform 2,500 procedures annually, and using the standard markup ratio of 25%, the expected price per procedure will be $275. This approximates the reimbursement rate expectations for these procedures from the dominant payer group in the market as well.

Using these figures, the breakeven analysis in quantity is calculated as 1,818 procedures. In other words, the first 1,817 procedures will be performed at a net loss to the hospital; when procedure 1,818 is performed, the new procedure will have broken even. All procedures delivered after this point help increase profits and operating margins for the organization. The breakeven point for this example is calculated as:

$$BE = \frac{FC}{(P - VC)} = \frac{\$100,000}{\$275 - \$220} = 1,818 \text{ units}$$

Using the figures provided, total profits of this new entity would be $37,500 if all assumptions held true. Total revenues are calculated by multiplying per unit price ($275) by the total forecasted volume (2,500), which yields $687,500 in annual revenues. Total costs are calculated by summing the variable costs ($220 × 2,500 = $550,000) and fixed costs ($100,000), which equates to $650,000. Therefore, profits are equal to $37,500 using these assumptions.

This concept of breakeven analysis is a powerful simulation tool that allows managers to play "what-if" and simulate results before they actually occur. For example, holding all assumptions equal, and then varying only one assumption (e.g., reducing total fixed costs by 35% somehow, possibly by using less space or renting equipment), then the total number of procedures to be delivered would be only 1,181 [$65,000 ÷ ($275 − $220)] and total expected profit would be $72,500 [($275 × 2,500) − ($220 × 2,500) − $65,000 = $687,500 − $615,000]. This increases the "time to benefit" by speeding up cost recovery and increasing earning margins. Breakeven analysis is a useful tool when modeling programs, especially when costs and volume structures are dynamic.

Simulating a variety of different activity and cost levels helps managers determine the range of possible outcomes. If feasible, each of the strategic alternatives should be "tested" by using a game theory or scenario analysis technique. **Game theory** is an economic technique whereby the organization attempts to estimate how the competition will respond to its strategies and what the impact on performance will be. Scenarios and simulations are similar in that they help provide structure to "what if" questions that might occur in the future. What if Competitor A opens a new clinic in a nearby market? What impact might that have on market demand? The use of advanced analytical tools to support these types of simulations greatly affects the speed and accuracy of the analysis.

IMPLEMENT, MEASURE, AND REVISE

The boundary between creating strategy and implementing strategy is typically blurred. Strategies are continuously crafted and implemented. Implementation might be done over time in phases or in pilot programs, or all at once. Once such strategies are deployed, they need to be carefully measured and benchmarked to ensure that the strategies are moving the organization in the right direction.

The use of benchmarking programs, as described in Chapter 4, is especially useful in planning environments as well to ensure that strategies achieve desired results relative to the competition. The use of performance scorecards supports continuous monitoring and tracking to assess trends or shifts in performance as a result of the strategies.

Because planning is a continuous process, as well as performance measurement, if strategies are not as successful as planned over the time horizon intended, it will be necessary to revise the plans, reconsider additional strategic alternatives, and continuously adjust based on feedback and results.

CHAPTER SUMMARY

Planning helps a hospital establish operations strategy. By understanding the key elements affecting business operations, hospitals can determine where they want to focus their efforts and how best to use their resources. The result of these plans is a targeted list of initiatives and projects that can be undertaken to drive improved processes and hopefully financial outcomes. There are four key steps to the planning process: analyze operations and environment, generate strategic alternatives, deploy strategies, and measure and adjust. Plans focus on long-term improvements to the healthcare business, which ultimately drive improved financial productivity and operating results. This chapter hopefully laid a framework for beginning the business planning process.

KEY TERMS

breakeven analysis, breakeven point, external environment, fixed costs, game theory, planning, price per unit, radar diagram, SWOT analysis, total costs, variable costs

DISCUSSION QUESTIONS

1. Why should hospitals plan? What result do plans have on operations?

2. What role does a radar diagram or other assessment have in assessing internal operations?

3. What does SWOT stand for?

4. What are the three components of a breakeven analysis?

EXERCISE PROBLEMS

[handwritten annotations:]
$$\frac{1,000,000}{1,500 - (340+160)} = \frac{1,000,000}{1,000} = 1,000$$
FC · Procedure VC · procedure · procedures · medical imaging procedures

1. Lutheran Regional Hospital uses a planning process to define a new radiology service line. The decision matrix gave it a high priority, and administrators want to evaluate its financial feasibility. Estimated fixed costs are $1,000,000, and the estimated net reimbursement level is $1,500 per procedure. Physician and other provider salaries on a direct basis are $340 each procedure, and total operating expenses will add another $160 per procedure. Calculate the breakeven point for this potential new service line.

2. If Lutheran Regional discovered a way to reduce the total initial investment to $600,000, causing the average pricing level to fall to $1,200, and the other assumptions stay the same, how many procedures would be required to break even? *[handwritten:]* $\frac{600,000}{1200-(500)} = \frac{600000}{700} = 857$ procedures

3. Assuming that the hospital feels it can deliver 1,000 procedures conservatively in the first year, which option should be chosen? *Why?*

[handwritten:] Option 2. Lower BE point speeds up cost recovery + increases earning margins.

REFERENCES

Nauert, Roger C. (2005). Strategic Business Planning and Development for Competitive Healthcare Systems. *Journal of Healthcare Finance, 32*(2): 72–94.

Page, Rick. (2001). *Hope Is Not a Strategy.* New York: McGraw-Hill.

Thompson, Arthur A., and A. J. Strickland. (1998). *Strategic Management: Concepts and Cases.* Boston, MA: Irwin McGraw-Hill.

Trout, Jack, and Steve Rivkin. (2000). *Differentiate or Die: Survival in our Era of Killer Competition.* New York: John Wiley & Sons.

Zuckerman, Alan M. (2005). *Healthcare Strategic Planning.* Chicago: American College of Healthcare Executives/Health Administration Press.

CHAPTER 9

Return on Investment Models

Goals of This Chapter
1. Define the complexities and challenges of return on investment (ROI) analysis in health care
2. Understand methods for cost-benefit analysis and ROI
3. Calculate ROI for different scenarios
4. Describe how a formalized capital investment approach can be implemented

Hospitals represent significant opportunities for cost savings and operational efficiencies. This can be achieved by fixing processes, removing cost layers, and increasing the turnover or productivity ratios. One of the most common ways to improve operational efficiency is to use systems and technology to automate processes and to displace capital for labor. This takes careful analysis, however, to ensure that all technology benefits are captured and compared relative to the costs of acquisition and implementation. This chapter details how to analyze ROI for technology and other projects.

LACK OF CAPITAL INVESTMENT MODELS IN HEALTH CARE

Healthcare organizations invest in capital programs for many reasons, but the most common is that it helps to automate, improve, or substitute capital for labor (Lucas, 1999). In many larger hospitals, investment in facilities, equipment, and technology has not always followed the traditional capital investment models used in most other industries. Other industries follow strict financial modeling techniques to clearly identify the expected changes in cost and revenue cash flows associated with the project through formalized discounted cash flows and net present value (NPV) formulas. These models help quantify decisions and allow management to understand the bottom-line impact of its decisions in terms of the net economic value that is being contributed. More sophisticated healthcare organizations also follow ROI models, but they are not significantly deployed throughout the industry.

Return on investment (ROI) is calculated as total amount of profits earned from a project or investment divided by the total cost of that investment. Typically, it looks at the net cash flow impact from revenues and expenses over a specific time period, such as 3 or 5 years, using the concept of the time value of money. Formally, ROI can be defined as follows:

Return on investment =
(Total benefits − Total costs) ÷ (Total investment) × 100

In health care, however, a large number of facility and technology investments are made for reasons not related to financial returns. New clinical technologies might help extend life, provide greater insight into disease that can improve diagnoses, or improve treatment success and morbidity rates. These are all potentially valid clinical outcomes, and after careful analyses, if the total nonfinancial benefit outweighs the costs, they should be considered in the capital budget. Additionally, healthcare organizations tend to rely on the expertise of their leaders, who use heuristics and subjective gut feel to make decisions. Financial considerations have not always been the highest priority.

From an operations management perspective, however, capital budgeting processes must be driven by ROI and financial outcomes. The goal of operations management is to improve efficiency, competitiveness, and operations effectiveness, which require formalized ROI tools.

Unfortunately, because the greatest amount of most hospital's investments are in clinical equipment, facilities, and information technology, the typical hospital has not required ROI projections as part of its decision-making process. In addition, the finance and budgeting departments in the average hospital are usually understaffed and not overly sophisticated. Health care must become more proactive and advanced in its capital processes to accommodate ROI analysis for all capital investments.

THE POLITICS OF CAPITAL INVESTMENT

Hospitals tend to be highly social and political organizations. Physicians hold positions of power, and culture is independent of financial condition. Therefore, capital investment processes tend to have priorities focused on non-value-maximizing attributes. Physicians and other employees with political clout and power tend to dominate investment processes in health care and can influence decisions on technology in areas where they are the most interested or involved, regardless of financial value. Additionally, because physicians often believe that administrators do not understand the value or consequence of their need or their request, there is a general lack of trust in allowing business managers to make critical decisions about capital budgeting.

Prioritizations in the largest hospitals are based to a large degree on qualitative, not quantitative, data, which can be highly subjective. When decisions are qualitative, they do not allow for shared understanding of the criteria used to make such decisions (Weill, Ross, & Ross, 2004). This causes a lack of alignment around importance for different systems. These political investment processes do not generally follow formalized processes and models that help ensure investment in the right areas. This encourages the wrong behavior and eventually leads to deteriorating financial health.

RECOMMENDATIONS FOR IMPLEMENTING A CAPITAL INVESTMENT APPROACH

It is important that hospitals use ROI approaches to capital budgeting. This requires clear, well-established investment guidelines. For example, guidelines might state that X% of the largest NPV projects will be funded during a fiscal year. Or, a guideline might state that any positive NPV project will be viewed favorably, or any projects whose internal rate of return is more than double the cost of capital will be approved. All of these represent guidelines, which help explain the financial priorities to the organization and make the decision criteria clear. There are six key recommendations for incorporating ROI analysis into daily decision-making processes:

1. Define and measure the hospital's true cost of capital.

2. Establish formalized ROI criteria.

3. Align investments to strategy.

4. Eliminate a single annual investment process.

5. Establish an IT portfolio approach.

6. Establish investment committees.

Each of these is described in the rest of this section.

Define and Measure the True Cost of Capital

Many organizations do not measure cost of capital, which makes investments very difficult. The **cost of capital** is the weighted average cost of all funding sources for a hospital, including both debt and equity (Patterson, 1995). The cost of capital sometimes is called the discount or **hurdle rate**, which is the minimum rate of return required on projects. The cost of capital is a very important concept; unfortunately, it is not widely deployed in health care.

The cost of capital refers to the actual cost of money. For example, assume a hospital has no cash, stocks, or any other investments besides loans. This hospital can borrow from a bank, but it has no other sources of capital. The rate that the bank loans money to the hospital then is equal to its cost of capital. If the rate is equal to 6%, this means that if the hospital is to invest $500,000 in a project, it will really cost the organization $530,000 at the end of the first year ($500,000 × 6% interest charge); in other words, it will cost the organization $30,000 to borrow those funds. This cost has to be considered in the ROI equation because the total value or return from the project must now be incremented by this same amount.

Most hospitals, however, borrow money from banks over the short and long term, but they also are major issuers of debt in the form of public bonds. In addition, organizations lease or rent equipment, which has financing charges, and may even use revolving credit through organizational purchasing cards for limited working capital financing. As discussed earlier in Chapter 3, the public for-profit hospital systems issue stock or equity through one of the stock exchanges, and more profitable hospitals tend to finance capital investments using cash or cash equivalents (through retained earnings). All of these represent sources of funds. Each source of funds has its own financing costs associated with it.

To calculate the true cost of capital for a hospital requires that the marginal costs of debt and equity be multiplied by the percentage of the market value that each represents. The comprehensive term for this is weighted average cost of capital (WACC). The formula for calculating WACC is:

$$\text{WACC} = [(w_d K_d (1 - T)) + (w_e K_e)]$$

where

w = weighting factor, or percentage of market value from either debt or capital
K = cost of equity or debt
T = marginal tax rate
d = debt
e = equity, either preferred or common

In other words, WACC is based on the cost of debt in percent multiplied by the proportion of total capital that debt represents, plus the cost of equity in percent multiplied by the proportion of total capital that equity represents. Because most healthcare organizations do not issue stock, they have no associated costs of equity beyond that of the risk-free rate from cash equivalents or other reductions in retained earnings, which is primarily an opportunity cost. Therefore, in most organizations cost of capital is mainly a function of the cost of debt. Cost of debt can then be calculated as the cost of risk-free debt plus a risk premium.

Understanding the true blended cost of capital ensures that projects are not undertaken for purely the initial investment costs, but that they also reflect the financing effects, which can often add between 4% and 15% to a project's total marginal cost. For large hospitals, an 8% to 10% cost of capital is fairly common.

Establish Formalized ROI Criteria

Part of the difficulty in health care is due to the fact that hospitals often do not have a dominant key performance metric for financial outcomes. In other industries, the use of return on invested capital, return on equity, earnings per share, or price-earnings ratios can be used to model financial decisions. In health care, there is still limited translation of the basic measures of profitability, such as operating margin and net income. Because these are limited in their usefulness due to accounting manipulations they are often short-sighted in nature.

Clear guidelines for hospitals should be developed to factor in the cost of capital to drive investment decisions. Prioritization of investments around projects with the highest NPVs or differential between return on capital and the hurdle rate is important if hospitals are to achieve operational excellence.

Align Investments to Strategy

Hospitals also need to align their investments in IT to the hospital's strategies and initiatives (Keen & Digrius, 2002). Understanding the relationship between systems or technology and the hospital's strategy will help clarify the impact on the organization. Technology that is clearly aligned with the strategy should have the higher ranking, all other things being equal.

A hospital must have strategies across all areas of the organization to allow alignment to take place. The use of key performance indicators (KPIs) shows the impact that technology has on a specific KPI, and this can be cascaded back to the hospital's overarching strategy and performance scorecard.

Eliminate a Single Annual Investment Process

In many organizations, capital investments can be made only once per year, at the beginning of a fiscal period. This creates a rush for funding at certain times of the year, such as January or September, which forces decisions among many projects simultaneously. This creates a competitive environment, where managers try to "game" the system rather than simply stating the benefits and facts around the investment. Annual processes discourage creative thinking year round and ultimately do nothing to improve financial results. Instead, revolving or year-round processes should be used so that as new ideas are developed; and as long as they make financial sense, they can be pursued.

Establish an IT Portfolio Approach

When investing in financial instruments, such as mutual funds or stocks, financial planners recommend taking a portfolio approach. A **portfolio** is a collection of investments grouped by different categories that are selected to help ensure a balanced and systematic approach to improving overall outcomes.

An IT portfolio balances the investments in various technologies so that they are not all concentrated around one area. For example, not all investments can be made in business systems that produce financial ROI, and not all investments can be made in clinical technologies with any direct, traceable returns. Similarly, not all capital decisions can be made around a system's end of useful life. Categories for each of the key strategies in IT could be used to create a matrix to graphically represent the portfolio and ensure balanced investments.

Another way to manage the portfolio is across the dimension of *value* versus *risks and complexity*. This suggests that even if the financial return or value is extremely high, complex projects tend to fail faster, and therefore the results may never be seen. The best case is a high-ROI and low-risk project, but those are rare. More than likely, a portfolio will include investments in all of the matrixes of the portfolio. **Figure 9–1** shows a sample portfolio grid.

Establish Investment Committees

The use of an investment steering committee, which is well represented by multiple functions of the hospital, helps to systematically evaluate potential technology or facility investment decisions. Alternatively, steering teams can be used to evaluate priorities for focused areas (e.g., one team for clinical activities, one for financial, one for nursing). Each committee should be encouraged to perform planning in its area to come up with strategic measures or KPIs. For example, is process efficiency the number one goal, or is enhancing revenues? Many times, KPIs are not in place, so

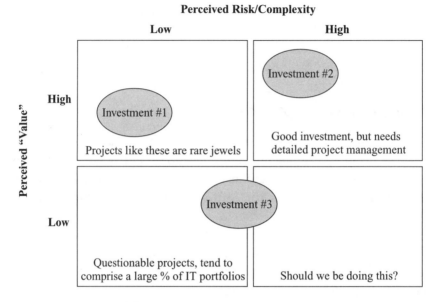

FIGURE 9–1 IT Portfolio Management

there may be a need to first develop strategic criteria for activities that each committee can use for evaluation purposes.

These committees should use departments such as finance or management engineering to help evaluate the business case and ROI analyses being presented for funding. ROI analysis cannot be done well by the department or individual seeking funding, because there is an inherent conflict of interest and biases may exist. The use of other departments helps ensure consistent treatment of cost of capital, and cash flow considerations, and helps provide independence to the process.

No two individuals share the same tolerance for risk or the same risk profile. Therefore, when asked about the level of risk in an IT project, several individuals could rate the same level of risk very differently, simply based on their risk tolerance level. To minimize this bias, committees should use standardized measures of risk and complexity to keep that part of the portfolio as quantitative as possible. For example, ratings can be created based on the number of months for the project's implementation (the greater the time, the greater the risk), total cost, the number of people or departments in the project, or some other quantitative guide that can help model risk fairly and consistently.

These committees should also use some form of expected value analysis, or weighted average ranking tool, for project acceptance. This tool allows the committee to evaluate the proposed IT project against key criteria and scale it based on the level of alignment around hospitalwide strategies and performance goals. Once decisions are made, they can be visually managed on a portfolio dashboard at both the committee and hospital level.

VALIDATING ROI AT MULTIPLE STAGES

A sophisticated capital budgeting process should encourage use of ROI analyses at multiple points in a project's life cycle. This includes pre-implementation, mid-deployment, and post-implementation.

Prior to an investment in new technology, many hospitals use formal or informal executive reviews to analyze the benefits of the investment, even if a formal NPV or discounted cash flow tool is not deployed. In more sophisticated hospitals, steering committee evaluations are used to estimate alignment with hospital strategies and to use quantitative criteria to evaluate and rank IT investments across multiple categories. In the most sophisticated hospitals, the use of business case justifications with extensive ROI models are employed, which are complemented by a portfolio management approach.

While in the middle of deployment or implementation, hospitals should periodically review the project to ensure that no changes have been made—either to the conditions that necessitated the investment or to the underlying assumptions themselves (e.g., change in the cost of capital, change in implementation duration times). Mid-project reviews to assess status and health of the project should be used, and the measurement of earned value recognized to date should be tracked. Earned value allows managers to compare costs incurred on a project against expected benefits of that project at the point of a certain percentage complete.

After the technology has been implemented and in production for a reasonable period of time, there should be formal follow-up reviews to evaluate if the technology is generating the ROIs that were projected during the initial business case. These post-implementation reviews compare expected results against actual results and try to find sources for the variances. For example, if expected results were to save $100,000 in operational expenses per year, but actual results show no savings, then an in-depth gap analysis should be conducted. This gap analysis should consider all of the historical assumptions for the change and identify which assumptions were ignored or invalid, or if other changes mid-project resulted in the error for the initial projections. **Figure 9–2** shows the types of analyses that can be conducted along the project's life cycle.

CALCULATING RETURN ON INVESTMENT

There are three steps to measuring the ROI for a project. These are shown below:

Identify benefits >> Calculate costs>> Model results

Identify Benefits

The first step in the ROI process is to identify and quantify the benefits. A **benefit** is a gain or positive change in an outcome and is often called the **cash inflow** or return. Benefits can be categorized into five areas, shown in descending order for their ability to quantify financial results:

- Those that create revenue enhancements.
- Those that cause reductions in operational expenses.
- Those that improve or expand service lines and levels.
- Those that improve the work environment.
- Those necessary for legal, regulatory, system end of life, or other reasons.

Revenue enhancements are the easiest area to quantify, but they represent a small percentage of total projects for most hospitals. Technology projects that enhance revenue would allow for expansions in revenue-generating areas, higher prices, larger market share, or other ways to exploit new opportunities for top-line revenue growth. For example, if a

PRE-IMPLEMENTATON	DEPLOYMENT	POST-IMPLEMENTATON
• Executive Review of Spending Proposals	• Measurement of Earned Value to Date	• Formal Go-live Review
• Steering Committee Evaluation	• Portfolio Monitoring	• Post-Implementation ROI Review
• Business Case Justification	• Mid-Project Checkup	

FIGURE 9–2 Multiple Points for ROI Analysis in Project Life Cycle

hospital were to develop an online patient referral and admission process, which could potentially attract new patients and new appointments, this could generate greater revenues. Likewise, investments in technologies that improve the brand recognition of the hospital could be seen possibly as ways of increasing revenues.

Most projects, however, focus on reducing costs or expenses (also called cost savings or cost avoidance). Costs are defined here as all incurred costs of an investment, whether they were operationalized or capitalized, direct or indirect. Most IT project investments can be **capitalized**, or recognized as assets on the balance sheet, and spread or depreciate the costs over the time periods in which the benefits will be realized. These costs, however, should be treated the same in the ROI analysis, as shown later in this chapter. Direct expenses are those costs that directly relate to the service being provided and include labor, materials, and other such related costs. Indirect costs include space, utilities, insurance, and other costs that are necessary but are not directly related to the process in question. Reducing costs due to higher productivity, improved reliability, faster cycle times, reduced manual efforts, elimination of duplicate or redundant data and systems, and overall higher efficiencies are benefits under this category.

Another benefit category includes projects that help expand or improve service lines. Improving accuracy, the quality of information provided, the level of care or service given, the access to information, and the ability to deliver more reliable or less variable performance are all areas represented in this benefit category.

Another benefit category is for projects that improve the work environment. These are difficult to measure financially, but they can have positive impacts. For example, ergonomic changes in a production process can allow for higher productivity due to less noise, reduced clutter, and less physical strain. Also, any projects that help generally improve the working conditions for employees can generate benefits in this category.

Finally, benefits derive by being in compliance with laws, regulations, and mandates, as well as having systems that are fully supported and up to date. The cost of noncompliance with these areas could potentially generate penalties and legal problems that could otherwise be avoided. These areas are difficult to quantify, but they are nonetheless important considerations when making investment decisions.

Each of these benefits needs to be summarized. Then, calculation of estimated returns from these benefits should be prepared annually for at least 5 years, unless the technology is estimated to have a useful life less than that. Next, the cash flow impact needs to be detailed for each of the categories, defining all of the key assumptions. Finally, these benefits need to be separated into annual time periods.

Consider this example. Assume a hospital is going to invest in a new technology that will bring in an additional 10 patients per month, as well as eliminate manual processes that would otherwise employ 2 full-time employees. Each employee makes approximately $30,000 annually, not including a 15% benefit package. Each new patient seen generates approximately $500 per quarter in net revenues. Calculate the total annual benefits.

Ten patients generating $2,000 annually ($500 × 4 quarters) is $20,000 in revenue gains. Reduced operating expenses through cost savings are $69,000 (2 × $30,000 × 1.15), if both employees are realigned to other areas. Total benefits to be derived from this technology are $89,000 in the first year. Estimates for benefits in future years have to rely on assumptions for inflation, using the consumer price index as a gauge, as well as other changes that may occur over time. Additionally, the time value of money (using cost of capital) has to be incorporated into more comprehensive analyses, as described later.

Calculate the Costs

It is important to capture all costs associated with the project. Costs represent **cash outflows** for an organization and include six primary areas: labor, hardware, software, implementation support (consulting, training), communications and infrastructure, and miscellaneous.

Labor expenses include the fully burdened personnel expenses associated with salaries, temporary labor, benefits, and training. Labor represents significant costs for most projects, and calculating these accurately at the detailed level allows for a much more comprehensive picture. The use of time and motion studies is encouraged to achieve a very detailed analysis of the actual time and effort associated with the process and/or project being considered. For example, if only 3 hours per day of total labor are connected to a specific process, it would not be accurate to show the costs for an entire employee. Instead, an average, hourly, fully burdened wage rate has to be constructed and multiplied against the actual hours used to estimate labor costs.

Hardware is another major expense area for most projects. Hardware includes all costs to purchase or lease workstations, desktops, printers, fax machines, servers, mainframes, storage devices, memory, and network devices to name just a few. Often, new technology requires investment in new hardware, and a thorough analysis of all hardware requirements and costs must be considered.

Most technology has a software component. Software includes licensing fees, operating systems, and maintenance/support costs, which must be carefully considered. Implementation support includes the cost of any consultants who will be used during the implementation period, as well as training and education costs, travel, internal resources devoted to the project, and any other costs of implementation. Communication and infrastructure fees include the cost of any telecommunications platforms or upgrades or additions to phone or data lines. Finally, a miscellaneous category can be used to capture any other expenses for the project that are not specifically listed in the categories given here.

Once all costs are identified, they need to be summarized by expense category and broken into the respective time period in which the expenses are actually incurred. These costs should be placed in the same spreadsheet as the benefits.

Model the Results

The final step in the ROI calculation is to model or quantify the results. This involves a direct comparison of the expected benefits less the expected costs. As stated earlier, ROI can be defined as total amount of profits or gains earned from a project or investment divided by the total cost of that investment. Again, ROI is expressed mathematically as:

$$\text{ROI} = (\text{Total benefits} - \text{Total costs}) \div (\text{Total investment}) \times 100$$

In simple terms, if a hospital generates \$10 in benefits this year, but will expend \$5 in costs to achieve those benefits, then the net gain will be \$5. Expressed as a percentage, this represents

$$100\% \text{ ROI } (\$10 - \$5)/\$5 \times 100 = 100\%$$

TIME VALUE OF MONEY

If investments were made today, and if the costs and benefits were only accrued today and not in the future, then the preceding method could be used to calculate ROI reasonably well. However, most large projects tend to have **payoffs** (i.e., payback on return) over several years. Some investments in technology usually displace labor or manual effort forever, creating perpetual cost savings. Likewise, **software maintenance** fees (or support payments due to vendors to cover upgrades and enhancements) typically accompany many IT projects and are paid as long as the hospital wishes to remain current and continue to use the software. Capital budgeting is the process of planning asset expenditures over the long term, so a project can be evaluated by estimating the effects of multiple years of cash flows, both inflows and outflows.

As a result, the concept of time value of money is important. **Time value of money** is a financial concept: money received in the present is worth more than the same amount received in the future. Money earns interest, so money received today can theoretically be placed in an investment (e.g., savings account, equities, or bonds) that can generate interest in the interim period, which would make the investment larger in the future. This concept is also referred to as *compound interest theory*, where interest compounds over time. **Interest** is the payment received by those who hold money to forgo current consumption. To calculate the true impact of interest, the use of present value is required. **Present value** of an amount is the value today of a future payment.

Consider this example. A hospital is due to receive revenue from a payer of $50. If it receives this revenue today, it is in fact worth $50. However, if it does not receive this money until next year, the hospital has lost the ability to invest this money and compound the interest. Therefore, $50 next year is worth much less than $50 today. To calculate how much less, it is necessary to understand the present value formula.

The present value formula can be expressed as:

$$\text{PV of } \$1 = [1 \div (1 + i)^n]$$

where,

i = interest rate, or discount rate or cost of capital used by the hospital

p = number of years in the future that the money will be received

Going back to the earlier example, assuming a 10% discount rate (or hospital cost of capital), then $50 received next year will be worth $45. This can be calculated as

$$[\$50 \times (1 \div (1.10)^1)] = \$50 \times 0.909 = \$45$$

Essentially, *today* if the hospital received the money 1 year in the future from the payer, it would essentially be forfeiting or giving up $5 in total returns ($50 = $45).

Alternatively, because money received today can be invested, a dollar received today has greater value in the future. This is called the **future value** of an amount. It can be calculated as:

$$FV \text{ of } \$1 = (1 + i)^n$$

If $50 is received today, that same dollar will be worth $55 next year:

$$[\$50 \times (1 + 0.10)^1] = \$50 \times 1.10 = \$55$$

In other words, in the future, the hospital would be forfeiting not just $5 as found earlier, but actually $10, or 20% of their revenue, to receive the dollar in the future ($55 − $45). This shows the significant impact of the time value of money.

CALCULATING MULTIPLE CASH FLOWS

The preceding examples are fairly easy to calculate, as long as the discount rate or cost of capital to be used in the calculation is known. While discount rate and cost of capital are often used interchangeably, the cost of capital is the actual weighted average cost of a hospital's funding sources, which includes cost of debt (net of tax) and cost of equity. It represents the minimum required return to essentially break even on a project. The discount rate is simply the factor used in preparing present value analyses, and it may be the same as the cost of capital. Many organizations simply use the current interest rate or bond yields as proxies.

When using a stream of cash inflows and outflows, it is wise to use NPV concepts. **Net present value (NPV)** is the difference between the present value of any cash inflows (or benefits) and the present value of cash outflows (or costs), net of taxes. NPV is probably the most commonly used technique for ranking investment proposals and capital projects for most for-profit companies (Shefrin, 2006). Sophisticated hospitals use NPV, but it is not as widely understood and adopted across all hospitals. It is important to use NPV in capital rationing situations because, essentially, NPV measures the amount of economic value that is being added (or removed) from the hospital with each decision.

NPV discounts all after-tax cash flows back to the current year; it could be calculated by using the present value (PV) formula given earlier or by looking up the PV in tables that are commonly available. For example, if $50 were received in years 1, 2, and 3, the PV of those inflows would be $124.33:

$$PV = (\$50 \times 0.909) + (\$50 \times 0.826) + (\$50 \times 0.751)$$
$$= \$45.45 + \$41.32 + \$37.56 = \$124.33$$

Mathematically, NPV can be expressed as follows (Copeland, Koller, & Murrin, 1994):

$$NPV = \sum_{t=0}^{n} \frac{PCF_t}{(1 + k)^t}$$

where

n = number of future cash flow periods
t = time period
k = discount rate
PCF_t = periodic cash flow for period t.

As long as NPV > 0, the project should be accepted because economic value is being contributed to the organization. Exceptions to this include when capital rationing, or limiting of the capital budget, exists, in which case all projects should be ranked from highest to lowest NPV and all projects should be accepted down to the cutoff point, where cumulative investment is equal to total capital budget.

Alternatively, a spreadsheet (such as Microsoft Excel) can be used with a built-in NPV function to provide even quicker analysis over a number of different time periods. A sample ROI analysis spreadsheet is depicted in **Figure 9–3**.

OTHER ROI TECHNIQUES

Besides NPV, two of the more common methods for gauging the returns on projects are payback and internal rate of return (IRR). **Payback** is the number of periods required to complete the return of the original investment and is defined as:

Payback = Initial investment ÷ Expected cash flow each period

Cash Flow Category	Assumptions	2007	2008	2009	2010	2011
BENEFITS						
Reduction in Operational Expenses		$ -	$ -	$ -	$ -	$ -
Increases in Revenue		$ -	$ -	$ -	$ -	$ -
Other benefits	Define and quantify	$ -	$ -	$ -	$ -	$ -
TOTAL BENEFITS		$ -	$ -	$ -	$ -	$ -
EXPENSES						
Capital Investments						
Implementation						
Hardware	(e.g., new server)	$ -	$ -	$ -	$ -	$ -
Software License	(e.g., 10 concurrent)	$ -	$ -	$ -	$ -	$ -
Communication and Infrastructure		$ -	$ -	$ -	$ -	$ -
Consulting, Training, Support						
Labor - Internal and Temporary		$ -	$ -	$ -	$ -	$ -
Total Capital Investment		$ -	$ -	$ -	$ -	$ -
Annual Recurring Costs						
Labor - New Position	(e.g., 1 new FTE)	$ -	$ -	$ -	$ -	$ -
Software Maintenance		$ -	$ -	$ -	$ -	$ -
Server Maintenance		$ -	$ -	$ -	$ -	$ -
Administration Support		$ -	$ -	$ -	$ -	$ -
Total Annual Costs		$ -	$ -	$ -	$ -	$ -
Contingency Budget	(e.g., 15% contingency)	$ -	$ -	$ -	$ -	$ -
TOTAL PROJECT COSTS		$ -	$ -	$ -	$ -	$ -
NET CASH FLOWS		$ -	$ -	$ -	$ -	$ -
Net Present Value, using COC of 10%						
Internal Rate of Return						
Payback Period, # of years						

FIGURE 9-3 ROI Analysis Tool

For example, if a technology upgrade cost $500,000 and each year there was a net positive cash inflow of $50,000, then the payback period would be 10 years ($500,000 ÷ $50,000). The advantage to using the payback method is its simplicity: it is intuitively easy to follow and calculate. The major disadvantage is that cash flows are not typically constant. One way around this is to cumulatively sum each year's cash flows until the total investment is reached. Another major disadvantage is that it ignores the time value of money, as well as any cash flows that might be generated after the end of the payback period.

The other common technique is internal rate of return. **Internal rate of return (IRR)** is a computation in which the NPV of a project is equal to zero. Instead of the discount rate being held constant as in NPV, it becomes the dependent variable that must be solved for by setting NPV to zero and using the variable cash flows. Alternatively, a simple heuristic to determine internal rates of return is to divide 1 by the number of years of payback. For example, 1 divided by 10 years in the previous example suggests this project has a 10% internal rate of return. One major limitation to IRR is that while it provides an intuitive return percentage, it ignores the dollar value of the cash flows and therefore makes it difficult to compare investments of varying sizes.

Example

Bellingham Hospital is about to invest nearly $700,000 over the next 5 years to implement a tracking system that uses both bar code and radio frequency identification technologies; $500,000 will be paid in the first year, and the balance will be evenly split over the next 4 years. These technologies will initially be used to track two types of assets: durable medical equipment (especially infusion pumps) and transportation equipment (such as wheelchairs).

These technologies should help increase the utilization or turns associated with the equipment, which increases effective capacity. Having visibility to where assets are hiding, managers can better position and transport them so that they will not need to purchase as many pieces of equipment in the future. Currently, there is about a 50% utilization rate on both types of assets, suggesting that they are used only half of the time. There will be a projected cost savings of $350,000 annually in cost avoidance of future equipment expenditures for the next 3 years and then a savings of $250,000 for each of the following 2 years. However, there will be a need for one additional full-time employee to manage the systems, which will cost about $50,000 plus 35% benefits. The hospital IT department requires a 5% contingency expense in factoring all ROI analyses.

The hospital is nonprofit and therefore exempt from taxes. The existing financing is approximately 60% debt financing, at a tax-free bond yield of 5%, and 40% equity at 7% (in this example, equity returns are based on a combination of existing cash and long-term marketable securities returns). Using a much-simplified version of the weighted average cost of capital, the COC can be calculated as

$$[(60\% \times 5\%) + (40\% \times 7\%) = 5.8\%$$

Based on this, Bellingham Hospital usually uses a 6% discount or hurdle rate in all calculations. There is also no salvage or residual value left in this technology at the end of the 5-year period, which represents the useful or economic life of these systems.

Is this a good investment for the hospital? Simply looking at the sum of all benefits over 5 years suggests that $1.55 million in benefits will result from a total capital investment of $700,000 and only $287,500 in operating expenses. Using discounted cash flows, with all of the assumptions defined, the first year net cash outflow is <$235,375>, which is comprised of cash outflows of $500,000 for the technology, $57,500 for the fully burdened staff, and $27,875 for the project contingency, for a total outflow of <$585,375>. Cash inflows, or benefits, amount to $350,000 in that first year. In years 2 and 3, there are positive net cash inflows of $237,125 annually. In years 4 and 5, each period had annual inflows of $137,125. At a 6% discount rate, the NPV of this project would amount to $399,000. Any NPV that is greater than zero should be accepted, assuming no capital rationing is in effect, and so this project is indeed a worthwhile financial investment.

CHAPTER SUMMARY

Investments in capital for new facilities, equipment, and technology are often good uses of cash flows if they provide a return at least equal to the costs. Benefits of these investments often include an increase in productivity, displacement of labor, cost avoidance, increased revenue, or other benefits. The costs of capital, however, can be enormous, which can change the economics of the project. It is important to thoroughly understand all aspects of expenses—hardware, software, infrastructure, implementation support, labor, and all other costs to fully model both the cash flow impacts. Careful analysis of the benefits relative to the gains and use of a discounted cash flow approach to measuring inflows and outflows are necessary to gauge the effectiveness of each project. NPV, payback, and IRR are three of the more sophisticated techniques for evaluating capital investments pre-implementation.

KEY TERMS

benefit, capitalized, cash inflow, cash outflows, cost of capital, future value, hurdle rate, interest, internal rate of return (IRR), net present value

(NPV), payback, payoffs, portfolio, present value, return on investment (ROI), software maintenance, time value of money

DISCUSSION QUESTIONS

1. What are some ways that hospitals can avoid qualitative and politically based decision making around technology investments?

2. What are the advantages to taking a portfolio approach to IT?

3. What are the six recommendations for improving capital budgeting processes?

4. Should ROI be analyzed at multiple points during a project's life cycle? Why?

5. How does a hospital calculate its cost of capital? What data sources are necessary?

6. Does the time value of money really affect the long-term financial outcomes for a hospital?

7. What are the limitations to NPV, payback, and IRR?

EXERCISE PROBLEMS

1. Assume that a hospital has steady cash inflows of $10,000 for 3 years and cash outflows of $9,500 for these same periods. At 10% cost of capital, what is the NPV of this project? Should this project be accepted, assuming there are no limits on capital?

2. Assuming that the initial investment of a project is $28,500 in year 0, and that $10,000 in benefits accrued annually, calculate the payback period.

REFERENCES

Copeland, Tom, Tim Koller, and Jack Murrin. (1994). *Valuation: Measuring and Managing the Value of Companies.* New York: John Wiley & Sons.

Keen, Jack M., and Bonnie Digrius. (2002). *Making Technology Investments Profitable: ROI Roadmap to Better Business Cases.* New York: John Wiley & Sons.

Lucas, Henry C. (1999). *Information Technology and the Productivity Paradox.* Oxford, UK: Oxford University Press.

Patterson, Cleveland S. (1995). *The Cost of Capital: Theory and Estimation.* Westport, CT: Quorum Books.

Shefrin, Hersh. (2006). *Behavioral Corporate Finance.* New York: McGraw-Hill.

Weill, Peter, Jeanne Ross, and Jeanne W. Ross. (2004). *IT Governance: How Top Performers Manage IT Decision Rights for Superior Results.* Cambridge, MA: Harvard Business School Publishing.

PART III

Logistics and Supply Chain Management

Part III of this text focuses on one of the key areas in healthcare operations management—logistics and supply chain management. The supply chain consumes somewhere between 20% and 50% of every dollar spent in health care, depending on the type of hospital and the scope of services offered. From an operations management perspective, this area represents huge opportunities for improving service levels, reducing costs, and increasing overall efficiencies.

Chapter 10 is an introduction to supply chain management (SCM) strategy. SCM is defined from a number of different perspectives, and its relevance to health care is explored. An explanation of supply chain management in the service sector is discussed. Details of the three key flows—physical, information, and financial—are explained. Strategies for successful supply chain management, and key capabilities of hospital SCM are documented. A thorough discussion of the evolution of supply chain systems and technology is provided.

Chapter 11 explores the role of purchasing, logistics, and materials management for hospitals. Materials management is typically the department charged with all aspects of procuring, storing, replenishing, and distributing goods and services throughout the hospital. This chapter further describes methodologies for purchasing and "spend analysis" and describes the role that group purchasing organizations play in healthcare materials management.

Chapter 12 is meant to be a primer on inventory management. Accounting and management of inventory is complex in health care for a number of reasons that are explored, and strategies for using inventory to improve operational efficiencies are defined. The basic accounting entries for receiving, issuing, and adjusting inventories based on perpetual and periodic methods are also illustrated.

Chapter 13 discusses the role that products or items play in a healthcare supply chain. The use of item masters for classifying purchasing expenditures (spend) is also discussed. Item masters typically reside in an enterprise resource planning (ERP) system, and their purpose and scope in health care is described. Finally, the product life cycle and its impact on supply utilization are depicted.

Chapter 14 defines the role that collaboration plays in health care. A supply chain is heavily dependent on all parties or players in the chain (such as distributors, manufacturers, retailers, and hospitals), especially as they interact proactively and share plans, pricing, and product information seamlessly. Collaborating effectively eliminates bullwhip effects and promotes cost-efficient supply chain processes.

The final chapter in this part describes pharmacy operations. Pharmacies by their nature are both clinical and operational. Because nearly 75% or more of all pharmacy revenues and expenses are affected by cost of goods sold, and because the primary role is to manage and move drugs to providers or patients so that they can be administered, the operational component of pharmacy administration is quite extensive. Technology and inventory management are two critical elements of operations management for the pharmacy.

CHAPTER 10

Supply Chain Management Strategy

Goals of This Chapter
1. Define supply chain management (SCM)
2. Describe the role of SCM in health care
3. Describe the three key flows
4. Articulate supply chain business strategies
5. Understand the capabilities required for supply chain effectiveness

The term *supply chain* has received considerably more attention in recent years. Television advertisements showing products being moved quickly and efficiently from manufacturer to customer have given companies such as United Parcel Service (UPS) a competitive edge; UPS has moved from a relatively small shipping company to the world's fastest supply chain, using slogans like "What can Brown do for you?" Similarly, television and print ads for computer manufacturers, grocery stores, and even banks have focused on SCM in recent years.

DEFINING SUPPLY CHAINS

But what is a supply chain and how can it help hospitals? The term is often used incorrectly or to only parts of the chain. A **supply chain** can be defined in multiple ways; here are just a few:

> A network of autonomous or semi-autonomous business entities collectively responsible for procurement, manufacturing, and distribution

activities associated with one or more families of related products. (Swaminathan, Smith, & Sadeh, 1996)

A network of facilities that procure raw materials, transform them into intermediate goods and then final products, and deliver the products to customers through a distribution system. (Lee & Billington, 1995)

The management of materials, information, and funds from the initial raw material supplier to the ultimate consumer. (Deloitte Consulting, 1999)

Encompasses the planning and management of all activities involved in sourcing and procurement, conversion, and all logistics management activities. Importantly, it also includes coordination and collaboration with channel partners, which can be suppliers, intermediaries, third-party service providers, and customers. In essence, supply chain management integrates supply and demand management within and across companies. (Council of Supply Chain Management Professionals, 2006)

The key to all definitions of **supply chain management (SCM)** is that it is focused on:

- An end-to-end integration of business process and systems.
- Conversion of goods and services into a deliverable or final "product" that can be consumed or utilized.
- Integrated logistical management of materials, information, and cash.
- Processes that define boundaries and stretch beyond traditional departments, from producers to consumers.

This text often uses the term *logistics* or *business logistics* synonymously with *supply chain management*. There is a slight difference, discussed in the next chapter, but for these purposes the words are intended to mean relatively the same thing.

The primary focus in SCM is to reduce costs through the chain, primarily through reductions in inventory holding costs, and to improve customer satisfaction downstream toward the consumers or users of goods and services. The mission of supply chains has often been characterized as providing the right goods, at the right time, to the right location, at the right price, in the right condition.

In health care, a supply chain includes a number of different parties, including manufacturers, distributors, third-party logistics (3PL) providers, transportation companies, hospital receiving and materials management departments, nursing, and finally the patient. **Figure 10–1** shows a typical healthcare supply chain.

FLOWS IN SUPPLY CHAIN

Three essential resources are depicted in Figure 10–1: information, funds or cash, and goods or services. A supply chain is typically drawn linearly to show product movement from left to right—otherwise referred to as upstream and downstream, where **upstream** is closer to the manufacturer of a good, and **downstream** is closer to final consumption or use. In some other places, supply chains might be depicted as "webs," or circle diagrams, to illustrate the concept that consumer's demand really drives manufacturer production, and thus it is a continuous cycle. Either way, in the illustration in Figure 10–1, goods and services are moving from manufacturers through other organizations (i.e., distributors, retailers, hospitals) and facilities (i.e., plants, warehouses, transportation vehicles) to ultimately end up in use at a hospital.

In exchange for products, cash or financial funds flow the opposite direction. As hospitals receive products, they pay the organization that sold them the goods; similarly, as distributors receive items from manufacturers they pay their invoices as well. Financial flows are depicted by arrows moving right to left because financial flows run directly opposite

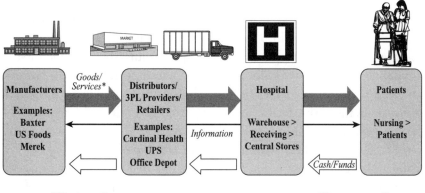

| | "Upstream" Closer to Producer of Goods | | "Downstream" Closer to Consumer of Goods |

"Upstream"
Closer to Producer of Goods

"Downstream"
Closer to Consumer of Goods

*Goods include: Food, Medical supplies, Pharmaceuticals, Linens, Lab supplies, Equipment, Office and other Supplies

FIGURE 10–1 Healthcare Supply Chain

the movement of products (i.e., payments are made in reverse from the sender).

The third vital resource shown in the supply chain is information. Information is every bit as critical as the product itself. Information includes data to address questions such as specific delivery location, items ordered, quantities and price paid, and location of products in the chain. Information is probably the most valuable resource, and systems and technologies are being deployed to exploit information and maximize its potential.

COMPONENTS IN THE CHAIN

There are several key components in the chain, as discussed earlier. Not all products have to pass through each facility, organization, or component of the chain. Some products move from original manufacturer directly to a hospital, others move through intermediaries, and some go through all parties in the chain. All manufacturers, distributors, retailers, and 3PL providers are referred to collectively as vendors. A **vendor** is any party that sells goods to others, irrespective of ownership of assets. The two most dominant players in health care are manufacturers and distributors.

Manufacturers

Manufacturers are companies that produce goods or transform raw materials and components into usable finished products. Typically, they are the beginning of the supply chain when shown linearly. Multiple manufacturers might supply products to other manufacturers as well. For example, a producer of medical infusion pumps might make circuitry, but it purchases the plastic facing and tubing from other firms. Manufacturers can create, extract, fabricate, assemble, or otherwise convert raw or semi-finished goods into more consumable or usable goods.

In health care, manufacturers include firms that produce pharmaceuticals, medical supplies, medical equipment, laboratory and research supplies, office supplies, food products, building maintenance and housekeeping supplies, and much more. In many hospital enterprise resource planning (ERP) systems, the vendor master can list more than 15,000 firms.

As goods are produced, they are logistically moved through one of three stages:

- They can be held in inventory. **Inventory** equals the dollar value of materials that are available for sale, and represents future benefits for the firm. Because there is not always a market available for products immediately, and demand is not always predictable, inventory represents an asset on the balance sheet of the producer until such time as goods are sold and transported to the next stage in the supply chain.
- They can be transported directly to retailers, such as office supplies.
- They can be sold through **distributors**, or intermediaries, that aggregate supply and serve as "middlemen" between the manufacturer and retailers or consumers.

Distributors

Most medical and pharmaceutical supplies are sold through distribution channels. The largest distributors in the medical-surgical supplies business include Cardinal Health (www.cardinal.com), Owens and Minor (www.owens-minor.com), and Medline Industries (www.medline.com). Three of the largest distributors in pharmaceuticals and drug supplies are AmerisourceBergen, Cardinal Health, and McKesson. See the Spotlight on Cardinal Health on page 217. In the food products supply chain, Sysco Foods and U.S. Foodservice are two of the largest. See the **Table 10–1** for a ranking of the top distributors in health care.

Distributors play a very key role in hospital supply chains. There are four primary advantages that distributors offer:

1. They provide access and options to a larger ~~portfolio~~ assortment of products and vendors. Many smaller and specialty vendors would never have an opportunity to introduce new products into the chain without distributors.

2. Distributors aggregate volume and serve as a single point of contact for hundreds or thousands of products; otherwise, a hospital would have to conduct negotiations with hundreds or thousands of different vendors, each of which requires contractual, legal, and administrative resources. This aggregation role simplifies a hospital's purchasing and inventory processes immensely.

Table 10–1 The Largest Healthcare Distributors

Category Rank	Company	*Fortune* 500 Rank (2006)	Estimated Revenues
1	McKesson	16	$80.5 billion
2	Cardinal Health	19	$74.9 billion
3	Amerisource Bergen	27	$54.6 billion
4	Owens & Minor	443	$4.8 billion
5	Henry Schein	445	$4.8 billion
6	Patterson Medical	707	$2.4 billion
7	PSS World Medical	980	$1.5 billion

Source: *Fortune* 500 Rankings, *Fortune*, April 2006.

3. Distributors reduce costs. Using concepts of economies of scale and purchasing leverage, distributors buy in bulk quantities and can often exert significantly more influence on manufacturers than a single hospital could independently. According to some studies, the average transaction cost for purchasing through distributors is only 20% of the cost to purchase directly through manufacturers (HIDA, 2006).

4. Distributors hold inventory in their warehouses and therefore serve as a safety buffer that reduces bullwhip effects on the entire chain. A **bullwhip effect** is the unintended variability of demand and supply that occurs due to the lack of perfect information between parties in the chain (Lee & Billington, 1995). More specifically, they often hold enough inventory of products for their customers to speed up the total order fulfillment cycle time, from initial purchase order through receipt of goods. There is, of course, a cost to holding this inventory, which ultimately is passed on to hospitals, but the offsetting advantage is better response and products available when they are needed. Distributors tend to place their warehouses centrally to accommodate their customers within a reasonable service level, while maintaining maximum efficiencies.

One of the largest professional organizations that represent distributors in the healthcare supply chain is the Health Industry Distributors Association (www.hida.org). This association has more than 208 distributors in its membership, which operates more than 432 distribution cen-

Spotlight on Cardinal Health

Cardinal Health is one of the two largest distributors in the healthcare market, serving both the pharmaceutical and medical-surgical product portfolios. Cardinal Health is the largest company in the state of Ohio (based outside of Columbus in Dublin), and is number 19 on the *Fortune* 500 listing, with nearly $75 billion in 2005 revenues and more than 55,000 employees. Like all distributors, Cardinal Health works on very limited operating margins (Cardinal typically averages around 2%), but it is able to deliver surprisingly strong total returns to shareholders and investors—nearly 15% annually over the past decade.

In a recent interview, Steve Inacker, the Executive Vice President of Global Supplier Services at Cardinal Health, discussed the strategy and future for the distribution business in general and Cardinal Health specifically. Inacker credits Cardinal's success with being able to provide integrated service to providers. "Integration brings together all of Cardinal's services, including technology, products, distribution, consulting, outsourcing, and other services into solutions that offer maximum value by leveraging *scale* and *aggregation*." Key trends he sees continuing include the use of lowest unit of measure and selective outsourcing. "As hospitals continue to have their own margins squeezed, they increasingly are asking what their core competencies are, and the result in many cases is outsourcing of some or all supply functions," Inacker states. The strategy of Cardinal Health is especially focused around customer priorities—which attempt to provide "integrated provider solutions" that will hopefully simplify the relationship with healthcare providers and make Cardinal Health even easier to do business with.

Inacker sees the future of distribution business as ripe for further consolidation, given the large number of regional players and extreme fragmentation in the industry. Further consolidation will support greater purchasing power and higher economies of scale, which should elevate operating margins of the industry.

Cardinal Health is an excellent example of how integration and expertise allows distributors to carve out a vital role in making healthcare more efficient, more integrated, and ultimately more profitable.

Sources: Fortune, 2006; Interview with Steve Inacker, 2006.

ters serving 5,200 hospitals, 159,000 physician offices, and 19,500 long-term care facilities (HIDA, 2006).

BUSINESS PROCESSES IN THE SUPPLY CHAIN

There are four fundamental concerns in business logistics and healthcare supply chains—inventory, distribution, facilities, and customer service—that form the cornerstone of all business processes in SCM. Supply chain strategy is focused on maximizing return on investment, minimizing supply and inventory costs, and improving service levels, so decisions around each of the four cornerstones are crucial to performance outcomes. **Table 10–2** summarizes the four cornerstones of logistics strategy and highlights the types of decisions that fall into each category.

There are many historical processes and practices that have evolved over time to be included in SCM. When people refer to SCM in hospitals, they typically think of supply distribution or inventory management and sometimes purchasing. But SCM is much broader than this and includes a number of different functions. The historical evolution of supply chain includes a focus on the following functions, because they help to manage:

Table 10–2 Hospital Logistics Strategy

Inventory	Facilities
· Acquisition and order process	· Network complexity
· Purchase scheduling	· Number of sourcing points and vendors
· Forecasting right quantities	· Warehouse locations and volume
· Inventory levels	· Space and layout design
· Purchase quantities/lot sizes	· Handling equipment
· Storage decision	· Bin and storage configuration
Distribution	**Customer Service**
· Route and labor scheduling	· Availability of product
· Scanning and replenishment	· Product quality
· Mode selection	· Cycle time
· Equipment	· Key information available
· Expediting	· Overall costs and pricing

- Demand forecasting.
- Purchasing.
- Inventory accounting and management.
- Sourcing and contracting.
- Warehousing.
- Transportation.
- Material handling and safety.
- Distribution planning.
- Order processing and fulfillment.
- Reverse logistics.
- Laundry and linen.
- Central services and sterile processing.
- Replenishment.

Many of these will be discussed in subsequent sections and chapters.

SUPPLY CHAIN STRATEGY FOR HOSPITALS

Because the goal of hospital business logistics strategy is to focus on four cornerstones—inventory, distribution, facilities, and customer service—hospitals must adapt a strategy that is unique to their own situations and environments. For example, a niche specialty hospital that serves only a targeted number of service lines might require a supply chain strategy that is different from an acute care community hospital treating multiple service lines. One might emphasize product quality and availability, while the other might emphasize lower pricing and standardization.

Strategies should be developed around each of the four quadrants, or alternatively around key goals, such as financial, customer service, and suppliers. Financial strategies for hospitals should focus on:

- Creating financial value for all goods and services procured, stored, and distributed.
- Implementing a more collaborative framework for strategic sourcing.
- Optimizing working capital.
- Minimizing unproductive inventories.
- Use of electronic data interchange (EDI) and information technology (IT) to automate and streamline processes.

In areas of customer service, hospitals should focus on:

- Enhancing customer value and service.
- Ensuring timely and accurate requisition and delivery of items.
- Providing useful information systems and reports.
- Proactively developing service-level agreements with major customers that define expectations and performance requirements.

In areas of supplier or vendor management, hospitals should focus on:

- Building partnerships with key vendors through supplier relationship management processes.
- Developing collaborative relationships with key distributors and vendors.
- Establishing service-level expectations and performance requirements for suppliers and systematically monitoring them.
- Expanding EDI transactions with key vendors.
- Continuously striving for improvement in cycle times, costs, and service.

CUSTOMER DEMAND DRIVES SUPPLY CHAINS

In a world where most goods and services are available 24 hours per day via Internet merchants or "e-tailers," competition for the consumer's business is becoming increasingly intense. A proliferation of competitive brick-and-mortar stores and e-businesses is changing the industry structure for virtually all market segments, from consumer goods to energy to transportation. Where competition proliferates, the market increasingly becomes a commodity, driving prices lower. As prices are reduced, manufacturers and retailers are forced to reduce costs—while maintaining product and service quality—in order to equalize profit margins. As downstream retailers cut prices to compete, upstream channel partners are forced to slash margins. This industry dynamic is a sure sign of *commodity economics*, where margins are always under pressure due to undifferentiated competition. As a result, organizations have no other alternative than to continually look for new markets and methods for differentiating themselves from the competition.

So in many respects, the consumer really is becoming king. Consumers are demanding higher quality, better service, streamlined purchasing processes, and shorter lead times (Langabeer & Rose, 2003). Consumers want the products available and delivered immediately, and they want them offered at low prices. This same mentality carries over whether discussing a patient in a hospital or an internal customer department obtaining services from another department.

Because consumers are the focus of a firm's existence, consumer demand should be at the core of a hospital's logistics strategy. Patient demand and acuity should be used first and foremost to synchronize the planning and execution of a demand-driven supply chain, but it also drives strategy. This places immense burdens on the manufacturers, retailers, and distributors in the extended supply chain (i.e., the hospital supply chain plus channel partners external to the firm) to deliver results. Consequently, the supply chain has responded by focusing on improved collaboration through the various chain members to improve the overall supply chain. But this has not been enough.

Traditional SCM has focused on efficiencies, not effectiveness, on today not tomorrow. What is needed to move forward and compete aggressively is for the supply chain to become much more in tune with the marketplace's current and future needs—to become demand driven. Therefore, in many industries the term *demand chain* is replacing *supply chain*.

DEMAND CHAINS

A new term is arising in other industries called demand chain (Ferrari, 2000). Similar to supply chain, it focuses on integrative processes and end-to-end management. But there are a few differences between supply chains and demand chains. **Demand chain** focuses primarily on revenue enhancement as opposed to the traditional supply chain emphasis on cost minimization. The ultimate goal of the demand chain is to satisfy the most profitable markets, while managing service levels for the markets with less profitable demand patterns. For example, demand chains might focus on which pharmaceuticals create the highest value and have the highest prescriptions written from physicians, while a supply chain would focus specifically on replenishment levels and sourcing the items at the best possible price. The difference is primarily philosophical in nature.

Additionally, the supply chain tends to "push" products based on limited knowledge of market versus a "pull" from the consumers based on current demand. This concept of pulling demand from consumers through more targeted demand management processes is critical to reducing inventory levels that are common when products that are less in demand are pushed on the marketplace. The demand chain also blends both strategic and tactical supply chain processes (e.g., it focuses long term on changing demand behaviors but at the same time uses current demand to drive sourcing plans).

The concept of a demand chain is oriented more toward planning and strategy versus being execution or transactional in nature, since the demand chain uses key consumer and market information that is essential to the strategic planning process (Hewitt, 2001). In some respects, the concept of the demand chain is "bigger" than the supply chain, since it incorporates more departments in the hospital—such as marketing, clinical management, nursing, planning, and finance. Although the supply chain has talked about collaboration among parties in the chain, demand actually becomes the focal point for assimilating the extended organization, such as the retailers and distributors outside the company that are vital to the firm's success. Finally, while the supply chain focuses on "facilities," the demand chain focuses more on "markets." This focus on markets is really what both strategic and operational management is all about.

Supply chains emphasize the efficiencies in the production and logistics processes, while demand chain emphasizes effectiveness in the business. Additionally, the demand chain helps improve an organization's processes by:

- Aligning the organization and its extended units around a common plan.
- Improving coordination within the supply chain by using base forecasts and plans, thus reducing common effects of poor coordination in the supply chain such as the bullwhip effect or inventory peaks.
- Allowing marketing and development processes to fully exploit promotional value for products by estimating consumer demand and selecting marketing promotions that are the most effective.

What does all this mean for health care? First, it suggests that if hospital supply chains are to be effective, there must be a philosophical shift away from strict purchasing and replenishing when needed, to using patient volume forecasts to drive the chain. Forecasting and dynamic planning for materials is just one example of this. Second, it suggests a broader role for business logistics professionals, because it will be necessary to use strategic housewide volume indicators (such as patient days or nursing hours) to analyze values, study supply usage trends per area, and suggest process changes to more optimally align SCM resources. Finally, it encourages supply chain executives to step up and assume a leadership role in health care.

PRINCIPLES OF SUPPLY CHAIN MANAGEMENT

There are four key principles of supply chain management: access to information, use of advanced decision support tools, pursuit of supply chain effectiveness, and distributed intelligence.

Access to Information

As the extended supply chain moves to more complete access to patient- and provider-level information, the chain must openly share downstream data. This access to actual information—whether it is through sharing of procedural volume and usage data, bed forecasts, census data, market research, inventory levels, or transactional usage history—is vital to guarding against common effects of poorly communicated supply chains, such as the bullwhip effect.

Use of Advanced Decision Support Tools

The use of sophisticated technology can benefit most of the business processes occurring within the supply chain. Tools such as business intelligence, advanced planning systems, forecasting systems, Internet-based vendor portals, customer relationship management, and market planning systems all support supply chain strategies. As supply chains become more intelligent and require less manual manipulation, there will be a more rapid transition toward decision support systems.

Pursuit of Supply Chain Effectiveness

The supply chains of demand-driven organizations tend to focus on process optimization and overall alignment and effectiveness, rather than on other common metrics such as average costs and staffing headcounts. Supply chain effectiveness requires a focus on all four areas of logistics strategy—not just a single dimension.

Distributed Intelligence

The goal of distributed intelligence is to allow those individuals and supply chain parties most knowledgeable about the patient or market demand to have involvement and insight into the planning processes. This distributed intelligence ensures that all parties are acting on the same information at the same time using the same set of assumptions. Additionally, this creates communication feedback loops for each party in the chain to participate in improving processes and decisions.

STRATEGY AND LOGISTICS CAPABILITIES

As discussed earlier, the supply chain focuses primarily on the flow of goods, information, and funds through the distribution channel and a network of facilities. Thus, an effective supply chain strategy is one that is focused on optimizing the positioning of facilities, rationalizing and streamlining the network, and continually improving the manufacturing and logistics business processes that move products to the market (Fisher, 1997; Gattorna, 1998). A supply chain strategy must emphasize three key performance metrics: improving speed to market, minimizing throughput and total transaction costs, while simultaneously improving customer satisfaction levels.

A collaborative supply chain strategy should be developed with each of the key participants in the extended supply chain. All parties in the supply chain have the same goals and interests (i.e., improving total margins); however, it is often difficult to arrive at a consensual strategy that maximizes the total chain's performance. Suboptimization in the chain occurs more often than not, due to incomplete sharing of information between the parties, lack of true collaborative technologies, and an unwillingness to expose key business data such as prices and margins.

To achieve collaboration, the supply chain must focus on the key strategic capabilities that it seeks to develop. The five most important capabilities that supply chains should develop include:

- *Speed* or time to bring products from design to market, and from the supply chain through the demand chain.

- *Consistency* in product and service quality in all items and locations.
- *Acuity* of patient and provider demand preferences and usage patterns.
- *Agility* in the flexible sourcing and responsive distribution and logistical processes.
- *Innovativeness* in product conception and delivery (Stern & Stalk, 1998).

As hospitals continue to emphasize a supply chain strategy that is built on these capabilities and is geared toward emphasizing alignment and responsiveness through the network, the supply chain strategy will continue to build demand-driven organizations.

EFFICIENT VERSUS RESPONSIVE SCM STRATEGY

There are two philosophies in SCM for hospitals: responsive (also called just in time) and efficiency (or supply to stock). This choice of strategy reflects a continuum, with both strategies dichotomously positioned (Chopra & Meindl, 2001). Very responsive chains have resources ready to use at all times. The term **just in time (JIT)** is a concept that was inherited from the Japanese and their quality programs; it means a stockless environment where materials and resources are received when they are needed for consumption. This is also commonly referred to as *lean marketing*. In principle, this implies that just as a nurse is ready to pick up an item to dispense to a patient, the material arrives on site and is placed in the right location just prior to usage. In essence, JIT implies *stockless*; however, in reality, some degree of safety stock must always exist to guard against shortages and **stockouts** (where inventory is 0 when demand is greater than 1). Most hospitals compensate with a purchasing and inventory policy whereby replenishment is designed to reach a minimum level that might approximate 24 hours or more of supply.

On the opposite dichotomy is an efficient chain, which tends to buy in bulk and have fewer quantities on hand, emphasizing lower total costs. **Supply to stock (STS)** is a philosophy whereby larger quantities of materials are purchased and placed into an inventory location for storage and distribution. Typically, items are purchased in bulk quantities to take advantage of pricing discounts and economies of scale; the items are then broken down into smaller units of measure for storage internally, either in a hospital-owned warehouse or central stores. **Economies of scale** are synergies or reductions in total costs due to purchase or production of larger quantities. STS, by definition, implies higher stock levels and greater need for careful inventory management and accounting (see Chapter 12).

JIT requires a more *flexible* and *responsive* supply chain. It is more responsive because, as items are issued or consumed, they must be replenished. To make this happen, the supply chain has to be quick, responsive, and integrated between the hospital and all vendors.

STS, or bulk, is more *efficient* and probably *cost effective* in the long term. STS requires manufacturers and distributors to focus on more economical production runs; requires hospitals to own finished goods inventories; and encourages hospitals to purchase in economical sizes, for both shipments and purchase quantities.

JIT is often called lowest unit of measure. **Lowest unit of measure (LUM)** describes the process whereby hospitals purchase and store items strictly in the unit in which they will ultimately be consumed. For example, if a hospital purchases a pallet-load filled with boxes of gloves, but gloves are ultimately dispensed and possibly charged to patients by each one used, the lowest unit of measure is "each." Although LUM and JIT are often used interchangeably, they are *not* synonymous.

JIT, as the more responsive strategy, requires hospitals to be able to quickly change over between items. If a specific type of catheter is being used today, but tomorrow it could be phased out, then a JIT environment requires quick response. **Quick response** is a process in which lead times are minimized, rapid processing of orders occurs, and changes in demand and business requirements are instantly communicated over the supply chain via collaborative information systems (Boyson & Corsi, 2001). In other words, quick response allows hospitals to, among other things:

- Update the item master with new items, cost, and attributes.
- Contact the vendors and distributors to procure new items.
- Change bar codes and bins in all inventory locations.
- Change pricing in the charge description master.

Distributors play a vital role in providing flexibility and quick response, in that they have instant access to a broad portfolio of products and therefore reduce the transition time between changeovers. **Table 10–3** provides a summary of the characteristics common in both JIT and STS environments.

JIT is very difficult in a rapidly changing environment and requires good information systems, collaboration with vendors, higher-level personnel, and more flexible business processes (Cox & Blackstone, 1990). It is often accompanied by premium pricing and higher transportation rates from vendors to accommodate such rapid response.

The impact on purchasing is that JIT typically results in a smaller number of line items on an individual purchase order, while STS might have many more lines and quantities per purchase order. When looking at productivity metrics for the purchasing department, the choice of JIT versus STS must be understood because the choice influences output ratios.

The impact on inventory and replenishment is quite evident. STS requires a significantly higher investment in inventory levels, which requires high cash outlays and higher working capital prior to material usage or consumption (Sanderson, 1985). JIT capitalizes lower inventories, but requires premiums for supply expenses, because JIT is usually associated with a premium somewhere between 5% and 15% higher costs.

The relationship between *service* and *efficiency* is a well-documented trade-off (Bowersox, Closs, & Cooper, 2002). A supply chain can be

---

Table 10–3 JIT versus STS

Supply to Stock/Bulk (STS)	· Economical purchase sizes
	· Use of Economic Order Quantity
	· Higher levels of inventory
	· Higher number of items per order
	· Fewer, lengthy orders
	· Lower costs
Just In Time (Quick Response)	· Rapid product change-outs
	· Rapid order fulfillment processes
	· Integrated information systems
	· Short lead times
	· More collaborative supply chain
	· Smaller more frequent orders
	· Premium prices

highly efficient, but it might be too slow to respond to nursing's and other providers' changing needs and requirements. On the other hand, a very responsive and flexible chain might provide excellent service, but there definitely is a premium in terms of total long-run costs.

As is evident, total long-run costs increase as service levels and responsiveness increase. Similarly, as inventory levels increase, so too do total expenses. The total cost behaves similarly to other U-shaped curves, where an optimal point can be determined in this trade-off between service and efficiency. Service and responsiveness come at a cost. **Figure 10–2** presents the cost behaviors that are implicit in logistics.

REVERSE LOGISTICS

There has not been significant research to provide exposure to the true costs of reverse logistics in health care. **Reverse logistics** is the process and methods by which hospitals reverse the physical flow of goods, returning them back internally to the originating department or all the way back the chain to distributors and suppliers. Typically, products are reversed because they are the wrong product, they have expired, they are overflow, or for some other reason. The standard flow of products is normally better defined because it is the norm, but in some cases goods moving the reverse direction can be quite substantial. In other industries, reverse logistics can make up as much as 25% of total supply chain costs.

In some areas of the business, such as pharmaceuticals, products are commonly distributed from the bulk pharmacy distribution area to nursing units in lowest units of measure, only to find that the patients have been discharged or moved. These items are then returned back to the primary location, and they then have to be received back into the system,

FIGURE 10–2 Cost Behaviors in Logistics

credits provided to the patients electronic medical record, and inventory restocked to inventory shelves. Expired drugs are another common problem; some manufacturers or distributors accept the product back upon expiration, so this requires reverse logistics processes and systems.

In other cases, inaccurate products are received and must be returned back to distributors and manufacturers. A purchase order might request one product, but another one was erroneously picked or substituted. In these cases, staging areas must be assigned, return goods authorization forms must be completed, credit memos must be applied, and careful monitoring of all accounts must occur to ensure successful completion of the transaction. Reverse logistics requires greater effort typically than normal logistics because it is the exception and, thus, no standards exist.

Hospitals are not designed to handle reverse logistics very well. While it is the exception, it may involve a significant percentage of total transactions. Reverse logistics needs to be carefully analyzed in much the same way as traditional product flows. Mapping the return process flow for key vendor groups, setting standards for length of time items can sit in staging, defining cost thresholds at which reverse logistics fails to make economic sense, establishing physical inventory locations, and systematizing the entire transaction are necessary to treat reverse logistics properly.

SUPPLY CHAIN SYSTEMS

The healthcare supply chain is complex. It is characterized by multiple vendors, large and powerful distributors, and a disintegrated network of products and partners loosely held together by manual and people-intensive processes. Supply chain information systems are required to better manage the flow of supplies or products, information, funds, and services from all parties in the chain: from manufacturers to distributors to the point of care and consumption. This is especially difficult in healthcare supply chains relative to more technology-intense industries like consumer goods or retail environments. As supplies move downstream toward hospitals and clinics, the quality and robustness of accompanying management and information systems used to manage these products deteriorate significantly. Technology that provides advanced planning, synchronization, and collaboration upstream at the large supply manufacturers and distributors is rarely in use at even the world's larger and more sophisticated hospitals.

Technology to better plan and manage the acquisition and replenishment of key resources (e.g., pharmaceuticals, supplies, equipment) in hospitals today is severely lacking relative to other industries. Driven by continual cost pressures and other operational constraints, the supply chain represents one of the largest opportunities for cost savings and value creation in the healthcare enterprise—if only there were a comprehensive roadmap to help get hospitals there. Data suggest that hospitals create an evolutionary path for supply chain technologies, implementing better business practices and more advanced technologies to increase vendor collaboration, optimize pricing and sourcing efforts, and improve prediction of required order quantities and inventory levels.

When most hospital executives talk about technology, most commonly they are referring to clinical decision support, medical informatics, or electronic records (Ball et al., 1995). A wide range of technologies and systems is developing that bring advanced decision support to the forefront of healthcare practice in the "front office" (i.e., the point of care or place at which care is provided to patients) (Kreider & Haselton, 1997). In the "back office" (representing the administrative and financial functions), there has been only minimal progress. There is continued deployment of hospital resource systems, but it tends to focus primarily on those business processes generally more visible and seen as "strategic," such as human resources or financial management.

Although most of these hospital systems have procurement, inventory, and distribution capabilities, they are fairly rudimentary in scope and function—providing mainly transactional and limited reporting capabilities. This limited capability needs to be expanded to take a wider, strategic perspective on the clinical supply chain. As stated earlier, supply chain management is defined as the planning, organizing, and controlling of functions inside and outside a company that enable the chain to make products and provide services to the customer. All of the parties in the clinical chain (patients, providers, materials department, vendors, distributors, and manufacturers) need to work together to create a chain that is effective, although in reality each is fighting to carve out a profit margin for its respective components.

The focus on the entire chain, from suppliers through delivery of care, is a relatively new concept in hospitals, and it represents a departure from the normal materials management perspective of managing internal, discrete business functions separately. It does represent major opportunities for cost savings and margin enhancements, however, as other industries have learned over the past decade. Optimizing the supply chain is very important, because pharmaceutical supply and materials expenses consume approximately 25% of hospital expenditures in most organizations. When accounting for all supply chain expenses—including the administrative cost of procuring, receiving, and administering the supply chain—total supply chain expenses can account for nearly one-third of all hospital expenses. Because hospitals have tackled a number of quick fixes that have generated savings (i.e., the "low-hanging fruit"), clinical supply chains are now primed to begin the transformation that most other consumer-based industries have undergone during the past 20 years.

This area, known as *supply chain management technology,* has yet to receive significant attention in hospitals. In the healthcare industry, supply chain technology has been widely used with medical supply manufacturers and with large distributors, but it has yet to trickle down the chain into hospitals and the point of care. Outside of health care, in industries such as manufacturing, automotive, and retail, there has been significant deployment of SCM systems. Hospitals, however, have not significantly adopted the majority of these technologies, and so they remain very limited in scope and sophistication relative to virtually every other industry. A meta-search of healthcare information systems material published in the past decade shows very little coverage of supply chain systems, their importance, or their future. Where supply chain technology topics were covered, they were discussed in generic ways with their most common functions of automating inventory control, purchasing, and receiving. In advanced texts on SCM and technology, there is almost never any mention of the hospital industry in cases or context.

Regardless of the current state of hospital supply chain technology, the direction is clear but the pace of change is not. While the hospital industry definitely has unique intricacies and challenges, the basic requirements remain the same in all industries. The need for predicting the right location, the right price, the right time, and the right products is consistent across all industries, which suggests that hospital SCM systems will evolve as they have in the consumer-driven and manufacturing industries. The only unknown is the timing of when individual hospitals will begin to evolve, which will partially be based on each organization's financial condition and the vision of its materials management leadership team.

EVOLUTION OF SUPPLY CHAIN TECHNOLOGY

Consumer-driven industries have led the effort to develop and deploy enterprise systems and associated supply chain technologies (Blackwell & Wexner, 1997). Historically, the scope of enterprise systems has focused on automating specific transactions, such as order processing and invoice generation. The initial spotlight on automation during the 1960s through the 1980s was the period when IT was regarded as primarily a means to reduce costs and improve operational efficiencies. This early focus on internal activities, efficiencies, and execution resulted in some early success in terms of cost minimization. When ERP systems were first introduced, they were seen as the way to handle large volumes of hospital data in terms of sales transactions, materials masters, and other manufacturing and sales data required to manage the entire business.

Since then, there has been a gradual shift away from execution toward planning processes, and new processes and technology were developed for material requirements planning (now termed manufacturing resource planning, or MRP), which began the shift toward better planning of the production and inventory requirements necessary to manage logistical operations (now called supply chains). The continued evolution toward MRP was an extension of this focus on planning. Today, there is a much broader focus on using the Internet and e-solutions to extend the breadth and connectivity of information (Kuglin & Rosenbaum, 2001; Martin, 1999).

During the 1990s, SCM technology began focusing on planning and effectiveness versus execution and efficiency (Lowson, King, & Hunter, 1999). Business process reengineering and total quality management helped force a "process" view of the hospital; companies were urged to start looking not only at inputs, but at outputs as well and the process used to link the two. Advanced planning systems were the first to focus on areas such as production scheduling, demand forecasting, capacity planning, and network optimization. Customer relationship management emerged and began capturing all customer data in one location to improve call center management, sales force automation, and marketing automation (Blattberg & Neslin, 1990). Now that the operational and tactical processes are addressed, SCM technology can start focusing more on what the software industry calls demand-based systems (predictive modeling, data mining, and business intelligence). These systems continue the evolution of more strategic planning solutions for SCM optimization, because they help focus firms on effectiveness and margin enhancement.

Hospitals cannot simply transition or evolve from manual, paper-based supply chain processes into a fully automated organization. The best approaches favor phased-in or evolutionary processes, which build on a solid foundation and continue to improve. **Figure 10–3** shows a theoretical evolutionary model of development for hospital supply chain technology. Directionally, SCM technologies focus more on becoming strategic and enhancing planning and effectiveness (i.e., moving up the y-axis of this model) and less on the more tactical processes of automation and efficiency. On the x-axis, hospital technology generally moves through three phases as they become more strategic.

Most hospitals, including the largest and most advanced, are only in Phase 1 of development on this evolutionary model. During this stage, there is a strong emphasis on automating the business key processes and

FIGURE 10–3 Evolution of SCM Systems

transactions. Ensuring that procurement staff are using electronic requisitions and purchase orders and ensuring that electronic order entry is being used for supply requests from floors are examples of this focus on transaction automation. In many hospitals, paper requisitions remain the norm, but this is problematic for maturing supply chain technologies. The switch to electronic forms is a necessary step to create transaction history, which is a requirement for organizations as they move to subsequent phases and need to rely on this information for analysis and intelligence. Also in Phase 1, hospitals explore limited use of EDI with key vendors or distributors. Typically, this means that of the most common EDI transaction sets, only one or two are commonly in use (e.g., EDI 850 for purchase orders). Additionally, there is a general lack of trust between hospital staff and key vendors and distributors during this early phase of development, so technology strategy is not focused on building collaboration or using electronic commerce to bridge processes. Finally, the overall technology is focused around managing and minimizing supply costs, which produces a strategy around centralization and automation. While Phase 1 produces stable results in the supply chain, there are no stellar performers.

During Phase 2, there is a significant amount of transaction history that has been captured—typically upward of 2 to 3 years. Hospitals that have reached this phase wish to put such data to use in creative ways, replacing manual, people-intensive processes with more intelligent system processes. Using advanced analytical systems, such as forecasting and predictive modeling, supply chains can make more intelligent replenishment decisions, optimize inventory levels, analyze spending patterns in key categories, and track performance metrics in significantly greater detail. Hospitals also begin to value collaboration with key suppliers and distributors and expand the use of EDI for more than one or two transaction sets. Typically, EDI progression in Phase 2 supports several transactions, such as EDI 840 (request for quotation), EDI 843 (response to a request for quote), EDI 850 (purchase order), EDI 855 (purchase order acknowledgement), EDI 856 (advanced shipment notice), EDI 870 (order status report), and EDI 810 (electronic invoice). Additionally, hospital supply chains in this phase start to explore the use of broader e-commerce tools, such as e-Procurement or other Web technologies. The initial use of XML in collaborative planning and forecasting processes, for example, and Internet-enabled e-procurement and online catalogs for suppliers are ways in which hospitals can move beyond EDI toward more scalable, flexible Internet technology (Cross, 2000). Overall, the technology strategy in this phase focuses hospital management systems on optimization.

As hospitals progress to Phase 3 in this model, there is a much higher concentration on collaboration and integration—both of internal business processes and with external parties in the supply chain. While during the first two phases the supply chains tend to be inward looking at supply costs and efficiencies, during this phase there is a heightened focus on alignment with the revenue cycle. Ensuring seamless integration of supply chain and revenue cycle is vital during this phase to obtain higher effectiveness. Tracking a supply's history into the chain, ultimately ending at consumption or point of use to a specific patient, is important to aligning revenue and supply processes as well as reducing system redundancies.

In Phase 3, hospitals and suppliers become integrated through systematic processes and technology. For example, consider an environment in which a facility's patient acuity or procedural case mix changes. Analytics would automatically suggest different buying and replenishment plans, and key suppliers would be instantly alerted to this change. Plans are adjusted, causing fewer inventories to be held in the chain, thus reducing expenses and ensuring strong collaboration with all parties. While such systems seem distant, they are in use today in many food and beverage and other consumer goods industries.

Technology used during this phase helps support many advanced decisions that are today seen as unpredictable. For example, a hospital will have an instant ability to determine how many items to purchase, how and where it should store the product, key timings in the chain, which vendor it should use, what the patient chargeable price should be, and what the overall financial margin impact will be on the chain. Most of these questions go unanswered in most hospitals that remain in the first two phases.

Potential obstacles that stand in the way of the development and delivery of this integrated SCM system are numerous and well documented. There are literally dozens, including lack of financial resources, lack of physician sponsorship, too many competing interests, low prioritization from chief information officers and staffs, and lack of leadership and vision from SCM. But the two most significant, yet manageable, are trust and discipline. The most obvious of these roadblocks is trust—trust internally among the various functions in the hospital, but more than that, trust that allows the hospital to share information openly with external vendors and distributors. The movement toward e-procurement and other Internet-enabled processes linking multiple parties requires significant trust with key business partners. Hospital supply chain managers have historically lacked this trust. Additionally, lack of disciplined strategic thinking in materials management has limited SCM technology deployment. The lack of disciplined thought to build a technology plan, to build required business cases, to explore new technologies and bring them into health care, and to take a disciplined approach to implementing and following through has contributed to the quality and robustness chasm that exists between hospital SCM technology and those of other industries.

As previously stated, most of the 6,000 hospitals in the United States today are sitting in a Phase 1 of this evolutionary model. Many hospitals have not focused their limited IT resources toward the supply chain, but that will begin to change as hospitals start using their supply chains as a competitive tool.

RECOMMENDATIONS FOR SUPPLY CHAIN MANAGEMENT TECHNOLOGY

Hospitals significantly lag behind other industries in the deployment of advanced management systems to drive supply chain optimization. Hospitals must begin to value the supply chain as a potential tool for competitive advantage and focus on management systems in this area if they are to catch up or make progress. Second, hospitals need to shift their internal information systems technology strategy to focus more resources and vision toward the supply chain. Chief information officers and their staffs must become more engaged in defining SCM business processes and performance metrics and align the SCM technology strategy and respective roadmap accordingly. Third, an integrated portfolio of management systems will have to be deployed to achieve the vision of an optimal SCM system, because it is highly probable that a single vendor will not be able to provide advanced functionality in each of the areas specific to the hospital industry. This integrated approach requires prioritization of functionality and establishment of a single supply chain technology strategy, knowing which areas will add the highest value for each individual hospital. Finally, this integrated SCM system must focus on collaboration, optimization, planning, and effectiveness. Opportunities exist for significant cost reductions and revenue enhancements, as they do in other non-healthcare industries, if they are pursued ambitiously and with vision and discipline. If executed appropriately, based on experiences from implementations in multiple industries, hospitals can expect significant improvements in performance, such as a 15% to 20% decrease in inventories, several percentage point improvement in revenues, 10% reduction in returns, and significant declines in cost of goods sold.

CHAPTER SUMMARY

The supply chain is a key component of operations management. SCM entails the integrated management of resources, finances, and information among the various parties that produce, distribute, sell, and consume. Hospital SCM needs to consider the role of information and intelligence in a number of key processes from procurement to inventory management. Supply chain strategy should be built around four key cornerstones: inventory, distribution, facilities, and customer service. Responsive supply chains are quicker, more agile, and react faster to different patient and provider needs, but they come at premium pricing. Efficient supply chains are more cost effective but are typically slower in responding, require greater in-house labor and storage space, and provide lower levels of customer service. The concept of JIT helps improve speed and cycle time and has a definite role in many hospital supply chains. Technology has now evolved substantially for supply chains in other industries, and gradually hospitals are beginning to adopt these technologies and incorporate them into daily operations. These technologies will make health care significantly more operationally effective.

KEY TERMS

bullwhip effect, demand chain, distributors, downstream, economies of scale, inventory, just in time (JIT), lowest unit of measure (LUM), manufacturers, quick response, reverse logistics, stockouts, supply chain, supply chain management (SCM), supply to stock (STS), upstream, vendor

DISCUSSION QUESTIONS

1. What does *integrated* mean when used in the definition of SCM?

2. What is the primary focus of supply chain?

3. There are four cornerstones to logistics and supply chain. Describe them and give the key components of each.

4. What does *upstream* mean?

5. Name three reasons distributors add value to a hospital's supply chain network.

6. Demand should be aligned with supply to optimize the chain. What does demand mean for health care?

7. A stockout is common when supplies are distributed throughout all areas of the hospital. What are some ways to reduce stockouts?

8. Are the concepts of LUM and JIT the same? Why or why not?

9. What role does reverse logistics play in SCM?

REFERENCES

Ball, Marion J., Donald W. Simborg, James W. Albright, and Judith V. Douglas. (1995). *Healthcare Information Management Systems*. New York: Springer-Verlag.

Blackwell, Roger, and Les Wexner. (1997). *From Mind to Market: Reinventing the Retail Supply Chain*. New York: Harper Collins.

Blattberg, Robert C., and Scott A. Neslin. (1990). *Sales Promotion: Concepts, Methods, and Strategies*. Englewood Cliffs, NJ: Prentice Hall.

Bowersox, Donald J., David J. Closs, and M. Bixby Cooper. (2002). *Supply Chain Logistics Management*. New York: McGraw-Hill.

Boyson, Sandor, and Thomas Corsi. (2001). The Real-Time Supply Chain. *Supply Chain Management Review*, 5(1), January/February: 44–50.

Chopra, Sunil, and Peter Meindl. (2001). *Supply Chain Management: Strategy, Planning, and Operation*. Englewood Cliffs, NJ: Prentice-Hall.

Council of Supply Chain Management Professionals. (2006). Supply Chain Management/Logistics Definitions.

Cox, James F., and John H. Blackstone. (1990). *APICS Dictionary*, 9th ed. Alexandria, VA: APICS.

Cross, G. (2000). How e-Business is Transforming Supply Chain Management. *Journal of Business Strategy*, March–April: 36–39.

Deloitte Consulting. (1999). *Energizing the Supply Chain*. Research Report.

Ferrari, Robert. (2000). *The Report on Supply Chain Management: Demand Planning and Management Will Leverage the Web.* AMR Research Report.

Fisher, Marshall. (1997). What Is the Right Supply Chain for Your Product? *Harvard Business Review,* March–April: 105–116.

Fortune. (2006). Fortune 500 Listing. April 17, 2006.

Gattorna, John, ed. (1998). *Strategic Supply Chain Alignment: Best Practice in Supply Chain Management.* Hampshire, UK: Gower Publishing.

Hewitt, Fred. (2001). After Supply Chains, Think Demand Pipelines. *Supply Chain Management Review, 5*(3): 28–38.

HIDA. (2006). *HIDA Fact Sheet.* Alexandria, VA: Health Industry Distributors Association.

Inacker, Steve (2006). Interview conducted via telephone by Jim Langabeer on December 14, 2006.

Kreider, Nancy A., and Becky J. Haselton. (1997). *The Systems Challenge: Getting the Clinical Information Support You Need to Improve Patient Care.* Chicago: American Hospital Association.

Kuglin, Fred A., and Barbara A. Rosenbaum. (2001). *The Supply Chain Network @ Internet Speed: Preparing Your Company for the E-Commerce Revolution.* New York: AMACOM.

Langabeer, James R., and Jeff Rose. (2003). *Creating Demand Driven Supply Chains.* Oxford, UK: Spiro Publishing.

Lee, Hau L., and Corey Billington. (1995). The Evolution of Supply-Chain-Management Models and Practice at Hewlett-Packard. *Interfaces* (INFORMS), *25*(5), September–October: 42–63.

Lowson, Bob, Russell King, and Alan Hunter. (1999). *Quick Response: Managing the Supply Chain to Meet Consumer Demand.* New York: John Wiley & Sons.

Martin, Chuck. (1999). *Net Future: The Seven Cybertrends That Will Drive Your Business, Create New Wealth, and Define Your Future.* New York: McGraw-Hill.

Sanderson, Edward. (1985). *Effective Hospital Materiel Management.* Rockville, MD: Aspen Publishers.

Stern, Carl W., and George Stalk. (1998). *Perspectives on Strategy from the Boston Consulting Group.* New York: John Wiley & Sons.

Swaminathan, Janyashankar M., Stephen F. Smith, and Norman M. Sadeh. (1996). *A Multi-Agent Framework for Modeling Supply Chain Dynamics.* Technical Report, The Robotics Institute, Carnegie Mellon University.

CHAPTER 11

Purchasing and Materials Management

Goals of This Chapter
1. Describe materials management
2. Understand the impact that facility design has on logistics
3. Describe the basic approach to cost minimization or optimization models
4. Describe the basic purchasing methodology
5. Understand the role of group purchasing organizations
6. Describe key elements of customer service and service level agreements

---

In health care, departments called "Materials Management" are responsible for directing the supply chain. Materials managers control significant resources. Total expenditures, or spending, can total nearly 50% of a hospital's budget. Sourcing methodologies and value analysis can help health care create financial value. Materials management organizations are usually large and have a broad scope of responsibilities; many of these roles are discussed in this chapter.

MATERIALS MANAGEMENT ORGANIZATION

In hospitals, the common name for departments that focus on acquiring, storing, distributing, and replenishing materials and supplies is materials management. Other names include distribution, central stores, purchasing, patient supply, receiving, inventory, procurement, acquisition, and many more. In recent years, larger hospitals and systems have started to name departments either supply chain management or logistics, a positive trend that will continue, but this currently is the exception—most hospitals refer to their operational support department as materials management.

The basic mission of healthcare materials management is to direct and control the movement of goods in an efficient manner through the hospital. In health care, materials management performs supply and resource logistics. Logistics management is "that part of supply chain management that plans, implements, and controls the efficient, effective forward and reverse flow and storage of goods, services and related information between the point of origin and the point of consumption in order to meet customers' requirements" (Council of Supply Chain Management Professionals [CSCMP], 2006). Logistics management includes inbound and outbound transportation management, fleet management, warehousing, materials handling, order fulfillment, logistics network design, inventory management, supply/demand planning, and management of third-party logistics services providers (CSCMP, 2006).

Materials management directs the healthcare supply chain by coordinating the flow of goods from manufacturers, through distributors, through hospital receiving docks, to the point of ultimate use or consumption. Centralized coordination of the chain relieves clinical departments and nursing from the intricacies involved in ordering products, negotiating and managing vendors, and performing other nonclinical tasks.

The name **materials management** means different things at each hospital. Ordinarily, in most community hospitals, it is an umbrella department that includes many other functions:

- Purchasing.
- Inventory management.
- Supply distribution and replenishment.
- Central stores and warehousing.
- Revenue charge capture for supplies and equipment.
- Sterile processing.
- Laundry and linen operations.
- Mail and courier services.
- Patient transportation.

In smaller hospitals, these functions can be performed by a handful of people, but in larger ones, materials management can encompass hundreds of employees. A fairly typical organizational structure for large hospitals is depicted in **Figure 11–1**.

To successfully manage hospital supply chains, there has to be a solid foundation of skills around customer service, logistics, human resources, finance, and business analysis. Unfortunately, many times the succession to management is the result of tenure, not academic or formal preparation. One of the major problems today is the lack of specialized skills and preparation that would prepare administrators to better manage the supply chain.

In other industries, it is a job prerequisite that logistics professionals receive undergraduate or graduate degrees in logistics and supply chain management. Schools such as the University of Tennessee, Michigan State University, Massachusetts Institute of Technology, and Arizona State University all have well-established programs that teach the fundamentals of what hospital supply chain executives need to know, from inventory optimization to customer service. In health care, such job prerequisites are not common, although they should be.

CULTURE OF MATERIALS MANAGEMENT

In many hospitals, materials management departments are considered very tactical and relatively unimportant, much like housekeeping or plant

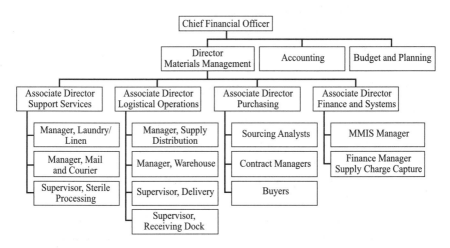

FIGURE 11–1 Materials Management Organizational Structure

maintenance. There are similarities: the nature of the activities in these departments is actually quite operational, they have an impact on downstream departments and patient satisfaction, they are labor-intensive processes, and many times they draw from the same labor talent pool. But, the comparisons should stop there. Materials management has significant influence over expenditures of millions of dollars (Kowalski-Dickow Associates, 1997). It requires complex accounting to manage inventories and revenues associated with medical supplies. Materials management departments are also quite large in terms of number of employees, size of operating budget, and overall scale and complexity. In short, materials management is a challenging and complex environment.

Historically, the culture of most materials management departments, however, is poor. Salaries are often lower than in other areas, and despite the challenging tasks, these professionals receive very little publicity or recognition for their efforts. Materials management is typically housed in basements, giving materials managers a "basement mentality," but it might also be housed in a remote warehouse location, adding to the feeling of remoteness or isolation. Finally, most chiefs or directors over materials management were not (until recently) high-ranking hospital officers. They typically report to a chief financial officer or other vice president who does not have the operational appreciation for their efforts.

This is starting to change. With significantly more technology being deployed in materials, the level and type of professionals who find themselves in materials management are starting to positively shift the hospital culture. Certification might help as well. The Association for Healthcare Resource and Materials Management (AHRMM) offers the Certified Materials & Resource Professional certification, which helps provide specialized knowledge about healthcare logistics. As materials managers are viewed more as professionals, equal to those in accounting or patient care, the culture and image of the department will continue to improve.

REVENUE GENERATION IN MATERIALS MANAGEMENT

The materials management department can be organized as either a cost center or a profit center. This is dependent on a number of factors such as the reimbursement strategy of the hospital overall, the significance of the level of potential supply revenue as a percentage of total revenues, and the role that service lines or business units play throughout the hospital. Some hospitals choose to have all revenues roll up to departments or service lines, such as the operating room or cardiology. In this case, all professional services (i.e., physician fees, room charges, and drugs and supplies) would be credited to that department.

In a great majority of hospitals, however, materials management departments serve as profit centers and are responsible not only for managing inventories but also for generating revenues. A **profit center** is a business unit in which managers have the responsibility and authority to make decisions that affect both revenues and expenses.

In this case, a different skill mix of employees is required because revenue management requires a number of skills that do not exist in traditional procurement and inventory functions. These skills include pricing, sensitivity analysis, some "marketing" efforts, ability to understand product life cycles and patterns, as well as an understanding of medical reimbursement programs.

Most hospital supplies today are billed to payers using a **healthcare common procedure coding system (HCPCS)**, which is a coding system that allows uniform coding and reporting of medical supplies, durable medical equipment, pharmaceuticals, and procedures (American Medical Association, 2001). **Durable medical equipment (DME)** is equipment that is used repeatedly for multiple patients, is used for a medical necessity, is appropriate for use outside of the hospital, and is not of beneficial use to patients if or when they return to good health.

HCPCS is Level II of a three-level coding system. Level I is called **current procedural terminology (CPT)** and was developed by the American Medical Association for reporting services performed by providers. CPT has been in existence for nearly 40 years and continues to be modified and improved. Prior to this uniform code, each payer had its own standards, and hospitals were responsible for managing thousands of codes for each payer. HCPCS is officially required for Medicare and Medicaid reimbursement but is used for many other commercial payers and managed care organizations because of its simplicity and its widespread adoption.

Level II of the system is the HCPCS, and it is used primarily for medical supplies and pharmaceuticals, as well as DME. HCPCS uses a 5-digit, alphanumeric code, with the first digit being alphabetic followed by four numbers. For example, C1753 is a specific type of catheter (intravascular ultrasound) that can be used for outpatient services only, and A4570 is a splint. In these examples, the first alpha digit, A, defines the supply as a medical and surgical category, and the C tells the user it is a temporary outpatient code.

HCPCS is a very complex coding system for the following reasons:

1. Many of these codes appear nearly identical, and it takes careful examination to determine which ones can be used for specific types of patients.

2. There is regional variation to these codes; in some regions a code might be reimbursable, and in others it may not.

3. The codes are constantly changing. New codes are added, and old ones are changed and deleted all the time. Updates and careful analysis are required on a continuous basis.

There are multiple, critical questions for materials departments to address if they are responsible for generating revenues, including:

- Which items are **chargeable** or reimbursable? In other words, which items can be separately billed to patients in addition to other hospital professional and provider charges?
- How can these items be tagged appropriately in the purchasing and inventory system, as well as the Charge Description Master (CDM)?
- How can a systematic process to review all charges be built and integrated? How can minimal lost charges be ensured?
- Which items are included in procedural or room charges and should not be charged separately?
- Under which conditions are they chargeable?
- What pricing levels, or markup strategy, should be used?
- What is the process for entering the item in all systems (enterprise resource planning (ERP), CDM)?

Based on the answers to each of these questions, it is highly advisable that materials and logistics professionals partner with their counterparts in finance and reimbursement to help build processes and procedures to address these questions uniformly, especially since reimbursement has both legal and regulatory impacts.

In general, a markup formula will have to be applied for each supply that is introduced into the hospital. **Markup** is the difference between the invoice cost and the price charged to patients and is used to cover the reasonable costs of doing business; markup is typically expressed as a percentage. Markup ratios on supplies and drugs are normally set to cover costs plus a reasonable return or profit margin. However, because a hospital's overall pricing strategy is also reflective of losses that occur in some parts of the business, and because those losses must be offset in other areas, supply markup ratios can range anywhere from 10% to 300%, depending on the pricing strategy for hospitals, the geographic location, and other factors. There is no single acceptable markup percentage. Markup ratios need to be created comprehensively by understanding required profit levels, analyzing historical deduction rates, and modeling supply usage patterns. Again, the distinction between gross charges and the net revenue collected must be well understood. Hospitals can charge $10.00 to all payers for a $0.50 item, but they may only collect $1.00 from each payer. In this case, while $10.00 is the gross patient revenue, the net patient revenue is only $1.00. Selecting a pricing markup strategy that does not artificially inflate gross revenues, and subsequently have huge deductions, is a more practical and effective strategy.

The act of issuing or dispensing items to patients generates revenue. Typically the inventory flow is as follows:

Materials >> Nursing unit supply room
>> Exam or treatment room >> Patient

In this flow, the material exchanges custody at the nursing supply room, which is then relocated (when required) to the examination or treatment room, and then finally issued to patients. When this issue occurs, it is documented in the medical record, whether in paper or electronic form. The **medical record** is the formal, auditable account and history of a patient's encounter in the hospital, including description of illnesses, procedures performed, supplies provided, notes, and discharge procedures.

In many hospitals, the use of a removable "sticker," which essentially is a bar-coded tag identifying the type of supply, is removed and placed on a manual charge form that can then be keyed into the patient billing system, when collected. This manual process of using stickers is quite common, even though it is quite inefficient and time-consuming, and places the burden of charging on nurses.

Alternatively, the use of automated technologies or **point-of-use (POU) systems** can help streamline this process. A POU system is similar to a vending machine in that it allows automation to drive replenishment, charging, and inventory calculations. Two of the most common POU systems in place today are provided by Cardinal Health's Pyxis and Omnicell.

All charges are applied against the patient as issued or administered, which generates revenue, assuming of course that the hospital's pricing policy bills supplies separately and does not embed them in the overall procedure codes for the diagnosis-related group or CPT. Based on this revenue, proper inventory management must be used to track actual cost of goods sold so that a realistic estimate of operating margins from supplies can be calculated. Accounting for inventory and supplies is described in Chapter 12.

OPTIMIZING FACILITY LAYOUT AND DESIGN

Ideally, hospitals should be designed with supply and logistics operations in mind. In the retail business, stores are laid out and designed with one goal—moving customers through aisles in a particular fashion to ensure high traffic flow, extended routes through multiple aisles, and higher receipts per customer. In hospitals, the design goal should be moving patients and resources efficiently through the units and floors to minimize wait and transport times. The fact that the average hospital is several decades old, and that in the design process there is usually a higher focus on nursing and clinical space layout than operational efficiency, creates logistics problems.

Operations management must spearhead efforts during facility expansion and construction phases to raise visibility of the importance of layout and its impact on operational efficiencies. There are five important principles for improving productivity and efficiency in hospital logistics.

Keep Distribution Cycle Times and Productivity in Mind

Analyze the length of time it will take to move staff, supplies, and other resources from point A to point B. Analyze the staffing/productivity levels of one design over another. Time and motion studies should be used to observe movement patterns, volumes, distance traveled, and costs incurred. The productivity impact from different scenarios should also be modeled using scenario analysis.

Separate Patient Traffic Flows from Staff

The Disney model developed at Disneyland and Disney World does not allow guests to see back-office operations. Disney has high guest satisfaction levels, which should be a primary driver for hospitals as well. This model should be applied significantly more in health care, where patient and staff traffic flows are separated. Unfortunately, in most hospitals, patients routinely vie for space in hallways and elevators with replenishment carts and personnel, creating crowded corridors, confusion, and delays. Use of separate elevators and especially dedicated supply or resource corridors is essential to improving patient satisfaction and operational efficiency.

Focus on the Interdepartmental Process Flows on Each Floor

Consider work flow and movement around each unit and floor. Ensure that costs and utilization are fully understood during the design process. Creating a matrix of interdepartmental movements and activities ensures that interactions, staging points, volumes, and trigger points are all documented and considered.

Use a Hub-and-Spoke Model

A hub-and-spoke model will centralize space and supplies, similar to airline distribution models. Placement of procedural carts, key resources (e.g., medical supplies, linen, and DME), and geographic proximity to patient examination or treatment rooms need to be carefully understood to minimize total number of trips, total distance traveled, and total overall cost.

Use Optimization to Minimize Costs

It is important to balance the two competing sides of the service/cost equation. On the *service* side, there is a need for higher utilization, better access, higher patient satisfaction, facility flexibility, and improved staff morale. For example, wider walkways allow faster throughput and generally easier access. On the *cost* side of the equation, there are design and construction costs and constraints. Increased walkways are costly, and they reduce the revenue that can be gained if the same space were used for beds or treatment rooms. Both sides of the equation (improved flow and handling), with costs and space constraints, are important and need to be considered when designing floor layouts. Focusing strictly on clinical needs, without carefully analyzing the operational impact, results in higher operational expenses in future years.

Optimization is a mathematical approach to solving a problem in which an optimal (or best) solution can be reached given the constraints and parameters defined. Optimization is typically used to maximize a dependent variable (such as revenues or profits), or minimize outputs (such as costs or resource usage).

A sample floor layout needs to be built for optimal results, using a number of important parameters and considerations such as space constraints, distance, and costs. A sample floor layout is depicted in **Figure 11–2**.

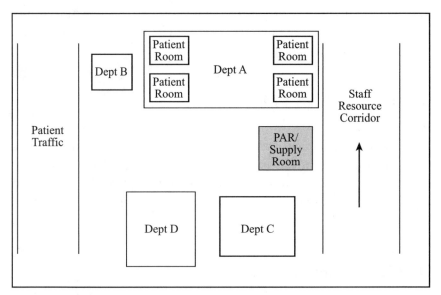

Considerations:
- Location of key resources (line, supplies) centrally located using the cost minimization model
- When movement occurs most frequently between areas, the areas should be placed contiguous
- Distance traveled between all points fully documented and minimized
- Patient satisfactioin and staff interaction
- Space capacity constraints
- Productivity of employees
- Cost, design, and operational space utilization

FIGURE 11–2 Layout Impacts Costs and Throughput

COST MINIMIZATION MODELS

It is important to construct analytical models that provide various scenarios and show operational impacts on overall utilization, costs, and cycle times. There are several process-oriented mathematical and optimization models that can be used to help build optimal designs for operational efficiencies. Software such as ARENA (www.arenasimulation.com) and ProSim (www.prosim.net) offer simulation tools that can help solve these types of problems.

Other models can be constructed that focus on queuing and staging supplies and patients to better understand human and product traffic flows. One such model has been used to model patient movements between floors and units in hospitals (Heizer & Render, 2004). A general assignment or cost minimization model can be expressed as:

$$\sum_{i=1}^{n} \sum_{j=1}^{n} X_{ij} C_{ij}$$

where

n = total number of departments in the model
i, j = specific individual departments
X_{ij} = number of patients moving between each of the departments
C_{ij} = distance traveled, or cost incurred

Using models such as these to help manage layout decisions has proven to minimize costs in layout decision-making processes. To apply this cost minimization model, it will be necessary to construct a matrix showing product movement, and associated volumes and costs, from department i to department j. Using simple matrix algebra, it is possible to solve for a number of different combinations and select the one with the lowest overall cost.

Use of this cost minimization model is fairly straightforward. Consider this example. Look back at Figure 11–2, which has four departments on the floor. A hospital wishes to optimize the positioning of these departments, based on minimizing costs of logistics (which would include reducing cycle time, because the longer it takes to get from one location to the next, the greater the labor effort). The general process for solving this problem requires six steps:

1. Determine the maximum number of potential layout options that exist (i.e., number of observations times [N] times $N - 1$, until

$N = 1$. This is calculated as the factorial of n, or $n!$, which is the product of the number n with all the other numbers less than n. In this example, there are 24 potential layout options (i.e., 4!, or $4 \times 3 \times 2 \times 1 = 24$).

2. Estimate the total traffic flow between each of the units or departments. For example, observe or estimate the number of times a patient or staff member moves from department A to department B.

3. Construct a matrix diagram that shows each of the four locations in a table (see **Table 11–1**), and place the count from step 2 in the appropriate matrix.

4. Estimate the costs for contiguous and noncontiguous placements. This would require a detailed analysis of how long it takes to move between each location, multiplied by an average salary rate for the type of employee performing the task. For this example and to keep things simple, assume $10 for the following nodes (A→B, B→C, C→D are considered adjacent for these purposes for their close proximity, while all other nodes are not considered adjacent and therefore cost $20 each move because it takes more steps for distance traveled, which requires greater labor. For instance, in **Figure 11–3**, departments A and B are contiguous, while A and D are not.

5. Using a network diagram, model the current results. In this case, the total current costs are $2,350 and would be calculated as follows:

   a. A → B = 10 moves, and since this is considered adjacent, it costs $10 per move. Total costs then are $100.

   b. A → C = 50 moves × $20 = $1,000

   c. A → D = 20 × $20 = $400

Table 11–1 Cost Minimization Layout Model 1

	Department A	Department B	Department C	Department D
Department A	—	10	50	20
Department B	—	—	30	40
Department C	—	—	—	15
Department D	—	—	—	—

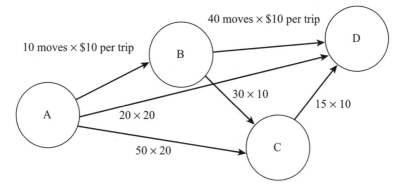

FIGURE 11–3 Cost Minimization Layout Model 2: Construct Node Diagrams and Assess Costs

> d. B → C = 30 × $10 = $300
>
> e. B → D = 40 × $10 = $400
>
> f. C → D = 15 × $10 = $150

6. Iteratively, reposition the locations to achieve improved results. For example, it is clear that the highest volume movements occur between locations A → C and B → D. If these two locations could be placed contiguously, swapping, for instance, the lower movement areas such as A → B, then total costs can be minimized. The use of sensitivity analysis or repeated iterative calculations can help identify more optimal cases. For instance, if C is positioned in the place of B in this layout, it could change the diagram and reduce total costs to $1,950. This comprehensive modeling process can be seen in **Figure 11–4**.

The uses of a general assignment or cost optimization model are limitless. They can be used to determine the order in which nursing floors or units are resupplied, to position nursing stations, to locate par linen and supply rooms, to install pharmacy dispensing cabinets, or to improve process layout for all departments relative to those in newer buildings.

PURCHASING

The purchasing function represents a significant source of potential financial value for hospitals. The primary role of purchasing is threefold:

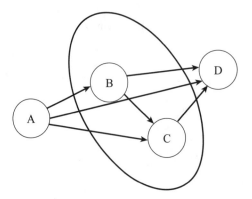

$$\sum_{i=1}^{n} \sum_{j=1}^{n} X_{ij} C_{ij}$$

Total Current Costs = $2,350
After Simulations = $1,950
Repositioning C & B saves $400

FIGURE 11–4 Cost Minimization Layout Model 3: Apply Minimization Formula and Simulate

1. To find sources of supply for various types of goods and services that the hospital requires.

2. To manage the sourcing process for soliciting vendors and obtaining competitive responses.

3. To engage in purchase contracts that minimize total costs over the long term.

The purchasing process or methodology is shown in **Figure 11–5**.

In many hospitals, however, purchasing is seen as an administrative function, processing purchase orders (POs) and pushing paperwork. Manual POs, those that are paper based and require routing from one department to another, do not help change this perspective, so it is important that purchasing departments transform themselves into more automated, value-focused functions.

In hospitals, the purchasing department does not develop product needs or specifications, but it does document them and provide detailed assessment of those specifications. For instance, the need for a new medical device is based on physician preference or procedure, but documenting these specifications to allow sourcing analysts to study the market, find vendors, and solicit pricing information is a core function.

Competitive bidding is a formalized process that engages multiple vendors simultaneously, which ensures a competitive marketplace, improves economics, and possibly lowers total cost of ownership. Competitive bidding also ensures that a contract is not entered into without exploring all

Special Focus on:
• Internal controls and audit trails
• Ensuring ethical purchasing practices
• Creating long-term financial value, through economies of scale and standardization
• Reducing order fulfillment cycle time

FIGURE 11–5 Standard Purchasing Methodology

options. Bidding works on the "perfect competition" theory, which suggests that rationality, free flow of information, and a competitive marketplace with multiple suppliers will reward those firms that offer the best products at the best prices. Bidding documents include a request for proposal, a request for information, and a request for quotation, which are all fairly standard in hospitals to ensure vendor access, transparency in the purchasing process, and competition.

As the competitive bids are reviewed, it is advisable to utilize an evaluation scorecard. A **scorecard** is an evaluation tool that lists the key attributes or decision criteria and applies a quantitative approach to evaluating responses. Having all internal parties, or those individuals primarily affected by the decision, rate each vendor in a number of areas ensures collaboration and feedback from multiple sources. It also ensures that the process is fair, competitive, and focused on multiple criteria and not solely price. A sample evaluation scorecard is shown in **Figure 11–6**.

Once the requirements are defined and supplier research and competitive bidding is completed, negotiations are conducted with the vendors that are most competitive. A thorough valuation analysis should be conducted at this point to examine baseline costs, given current pricing and quantities, and compare these with the competitive responses. Negotiations conclude with contract management, where legal terms and conditions and all performance and service levels are defined. It is also important to consider *price protection*, or price escalation, for future periods.

Defining and including service-level expectations into contracts for each vendor are also necessary to continuously improve performance (Lambert, 1999). Excluding these performance expectations creates problems

			-------- Competitive Options- ------		
	Decision Criteria	**Weight**	**Supplier #1**	**Supplier #2**	**Supplier #3**
1	Proximity of regional warehouse	10%			
2	Total annual costs	20%			
3	Perceived product or service quality	30%			
4	Meets all product requirements	20%			
5	Number of referenceable customers	5%			
6	Product ease of use	10%			
7	Expected ability to meet service standards	5%			
	Average				

Instructions:
• Evaluate each vendor against all criteria
• Use a 5 or 10 point rating schedule
• Multiply rating times weight
• Sum results

FIGURE 11–6 Supplier Evaluation Scorecard

because both parties are more focused on execution post-contract, and many vendors adhere to only the most minimal service levels required to keep them in good contractual standing. Buyers have the most leverage prior to the initial award and contract. Defining minimal performance, penalty clauses for inferior performance, and even performance rewards or gain-sharing for exceptional service should be part of all major vendor agreements. During the sourcing and contracting phase, it is important to remember the cost-quality relationship and ensure that the right vendor is selected to create an optimal balance between lowest price and best service. This is sometimes called best value.

In many cases, the use of bundled contracts can be explored. Some of the larger medical supply vendors have dozens of product lines and hundreds of items. Handling each of these items separately, with different competitive bidding events, can be cumbersome.

Once contracts are finalized and the executive and legal approvals are obtained, contracts must be administered. This includes ensuring that the vendor's products are updated in the hospital's item master of the ERP or materials management information system. Current prices and all vendor details (e.g., bank account information, addresses) must be input as well in the accounts payable and ordering systems.

At this point, requests or requisitions from user departments can be taken for purchases. A central processing group is typically assigned to convert requisitions into completed POs. This represents the transaction order processing phase of purchasing.

PURCHASING INTERNAL CONTROLS

There are several inherent risks in the hospital purchasing process. First, there are a limited number of vendors in certain vendor categories, which creates a lack of perfect competition. These environments introduce ethical dilemmas where vendors might offer gifts, trips, and other potentially negative inducements to purchasing agents. Developing policies and procedures that limit gifts and encourage ethical behaviors will reduce bribery and other negative outcomes.

Second, there is a definite need to maintain a complete audit trail or history for all vendor negotiations, PO transactions, and pricing adjustments (e.g., rebates, credits, discounts). The key concern is that an unethical buyer might agree to purchase from a specific vendor without going through a competitive process or, more commonly, to pay a fictitious vendor (i.e., one that does not exist but is artificially created by the buyer to redirect funds to itself or to other people working in concert with the buyer). There have been multiple audits in which rogue purchasing agents have been found to fabricate companies and in which they have managed to direct purchases and payments to themselves.

Historically, one of the most basic ways of limiting this is to ensure a **three-way match**, meaning the three key documents in the procure-to-pay process are performed by different individuals, therefore segregating duties and responsibilities. These documents include:

Purchase order >> Receipt or proof of delivery >> Invoice

If a PO is generated by one person, and the confirmation of the receipt is by a second individual, and then payment by a third party, unethical behavior would require participation or collusion by at least three individuals—making it that much more difficult to commit fraud or theft. A continuous review process of vendors and items purchased, as well as careful examination of vendor masters for incomplete and suspicious information, is essential to improving internal controls.

One of the problems with the use of a three-way match is that it is manual, requires storage and movement of lots of paper, and is generally slow. Technology has matured greatly over the past 20 years, which has significantly automated this process. As hospitals continue to use further automation and electronic commerce in operations, such as electronic data interchange (EDI), automated routing from vendors to hospitals will completely eliminate redundant paperwork and forms. While automation is great, it does require different internal controls and policies because paper trails are eliminated. Hospitals using two- and three-part carbon forms, which can be detached and routed through various departments, are decades behind in streamlining their operations for efficiency. Creating sampling techniques that pull transactions for auditing either randomly or through exception-based management will be required because files storing the combined forms will no longer exist in paper format.

SPEND OR VALUE ANALYSIS

Once an item, its classification, its phase in a life cycle, and its usage patterns are understood, what happens with all the data? First, simple spend analysis could be performed. **Spend analysis** is an in-depth, comprehensive analysis of a hospital's expenditures (primarily routine operating expenses) focused on what, how, and with whom an organization spends dollars. Typically, spend analyses focus on which vendors are being paid, how many transactions or POs are being issued, which commodity types and item categories are purchased, the types of items most commonly used, and how items are used to identify opportunities for cost savings and improved contractual negotiation. Understanding the source of spending allows procurement managers to selectively isolate contracts and vendors that can create financial value for the hospital. Spend or value analysis typically involves three steps, as shown in **Figure 11–7**. The three phases in this figure represent the process for getting started in spend analysis processes: automate, analyze and forecast, and measure and reinforce.

Automate

Automating items is the first phase, and there are multiple steps:

- Automate all item master data and ensure that there is limited use of manual, paper-based purchase requisitions and orders.

Measure and Reinforce

• Process only automated transactions
• Use data as basis for vendor negotiations
• Use data to change operating unit behavior
• Encourage buying patterns compliant with favorable contracts and vendors
• Continually measure and communicate results

Automate

• Automate all item master data
• Capture item attributes
• Classify all items using UNSPSC
• Establish process for ongoing new item introductions and phase-outs
• Use exception analyses to spot outliers

Analyze and Forecast

• Analyze vendor/classification/commodity
• Identify trends and changes
• Identify opportunities for leveraging purchasing quantities and scale
• Identify opportunities for item standardization
• Understand cost and margin impacts
• Estimate future price increases
• Use intelligence to predict shifts in volumes and pricing
• Report insight to hospital executives

FIGURE 11–7 Value/Spend Analysis

- Capture and add all item attributes in the required database field in the ERP (more details on item master fields will be discussed in Chapter 13).
- Institute a formalized item classification system, such as the United Nations Standard Products and Services Code (UNSPSC) or a similar scheme, and ensure its full use and rollout across all items and PO transactions.
- Establish a process for ongoing new-item introductions and phase-outs so that as new items are introduced, they also are automated and classified appropriately.
- Use exception analyses to spot outliers and act appropriately.

Analyze and Forecast

The second phase focuses on analyzing and forecasting. There will be a need for analytical skills during this phase: using tools—such as spreadsheets, databases, online financial analyses, comparison and benchmarking tools—to understand spending and cost behaviors. At a minimum, this phase involves the following tasks:

- Analyze transactional spending data across a number of attributes and levels, such as spending by vendor, a certain family or segment classification, and commodity type.
- Challenge the concept of physician preference behavior. The concept of **physician preferences** in this context reflects a situation in which a provider chooses established vendors and known products, based on existing comfort level and a possible reluctance to change. These preferences do not always represent the best value or economical choice. The introduction of additional vendors and products encourages collaboration with clinical staff, offers a broader portfolio, and instills discipline in the spending processes.
- Identify trends and changes over time, such as a shift in usage from one vendor to another or from one item to another. Look for exceptions and large spending categories that are not actively covered with negotiated contracts.
- Identify opportunities for leveraging purchasing quantities and scale. Ensure that all high-volume areas have contracts, either through the group purchasing organization (GPO) procedure or a direct contract negotiated with a vendor internally. Identify areas where the last contract review date was greater than 12 months.
- Identify opportunities to review pricing against any published benchmarks, if available. Ensure full leverage of existing GPO contracts.
- Identify opportunities for item standardization. Find areas where small orders frequently ordered from a low-volume vendor might be able to move toward one of the more strategic vendors.
- Understand cost and margin impacts from all analyses and recommendations.
- Estimate future price increases, if known, to model in spend analyses and budget preparations for the following periods.
- Use intelligence to predict shifts in volumes and pricing.
- Report insight to hospital executives.

Measure and Reinforce

The last phase of the spend analysis process involves measuring and reinforcing. This phase ensures that all analyses and recommendations—for vendor or item changes, future contract negotiations, standardization, and other purchasing practices—are systematically measured and buying behaviors are reinforced. This phase requires that hospital materials managers:

- Process only automated transactions. Eliminating manual, paper-based forms is one of the first steps to ensuring that the sourcing opportunities analyzed become a reality.
- Use data as the basis for vendor negotiations. Continually measure performance and transactional usage data with vendors at all meetings. Create service-level agreements on pricing, usage, supply fill rates, and other performance areas to ensure that vendors uphold their end of the deal and that spend savings are realized.
- Use data to change operating unit behavior as well. Presenting requesting departments with data supporting recommendations and analyses for operational savings will be necessary to ensure that requestors commit and follow-through with desired purchasing behaviors.
- Encourage buying patterns compliant with favorable contracts and vendors.
- Continually measure and communicate results to all parties.

Spend analyses are very useful tools for generating operational efficiencies in the hospital. They must be used as part of a comprehensive toolkit, however, if operational managers are to succeed in the mission of reducing costs, eliminating inefficiencies, improving productivity, and shrinking overall process cycle times.

GROUP PURCHASING ORGANIZATIONS

A **group purchasing organization (GPO)** is a collaborative arrangement in which multiple parties unite for the purpose of increasing their collective bargaining power with vendors. If a hospital purchases 1,000 oxygen tanks per year from a vendor, it might be able to purchase each item for $65; however, if 20 hospitals collectively contract with the same vendor, they might be able to buy it for $40 or less. GPOs are similar in concept to unions, which collectively bargain and determine ground rules for employees.

GPOs can change the competitive dynamics of a marketplace by encouraging suppliers to reduce costs to secure additional business. GPOs are avid proponents of the competitive bidding process, where multiple vendors are given the same opportunity and business requirements but may offer a variety of different cost-quality combinations in an attempt to win the business. In doing so, GPOs have been known to drive down collective costs of many items, especially in the commodity product lines that have many suppliers and limited buyers. They work less well in places where only a handful of vendors offer differentiated, specialized, highly expensive, and customized products, like in the medical technology category. A GPO collectively sources, negotiates, and contracts with vendors to achieve economies of scale and lower total costs for its members.

GPOs offer their members a portfolio of products that their member hospitals utilize. **Penetration** represents the percentage of usage or purchases against a specific contract. The higher the penetration, the more likely the supplier will continue to offer attractive prices to the GPO for future periods. Lower penetration rates represent three potential issues for GPOs:

1. They have a sourced product that is not well received or desired by their member hospitals.

2. They made poor vendor selections, and their members are not interested in obtaining goods and services from those vendors.

3. The hospital could directly negotiate better local rates than the GPO.

Most GPOs claim they can reduce supply costs by 1% to 15%, although this is difficult to confirm and measure.

GPOs are viewed by the supplier community as a collaborative partner or customer, and as a competitor. Obviously, any organized attempt to reduce pricing and exert greater influence is not typically welcomed by powerful suppliers. Less mature companies, or those that might have difficulty gaining market share without an introduction by a large GPO, would, however, find GPOs quite appealing because they offer a faster potential growth strategy. Although there has not been any conclusive academic research about GPO economics, evidence suggests that many suppliers view GPOs as one of many entrances to hospitals, and therefore they selectively choose which products to offer to the GPO and which ones to retain for direct sales to hospitals.

Many suppliers use the GPO channel to market loss leaders and gain entry into an organization so that they can offer exposure and opportunity to sell other more profitable products. A **loss leader** is an item that is sold by a vendor at a loss to attract customers to buy other premium items. Loss leaders are usually very early-stage or late-stage items, have poor growth prospects under normal conditions, or might not otherwise sell well. Loss leaders allow suppliers to protect pricing for their premium products by not disclosing prices or destroying price points through a competitive bidding process, while still showing some participation on a GPO's contract lists. This will help them get into the door of most hospital purchasing departments, where they can then directly attempt to sell other higher-margin products.

The largest GPOs in the U.S. healthcare market are Premier, Novation, and MedAssets:

- *Premier Inc.,* www.premierinc.com. Based in North Carolina with nearly $30 billion in member purchases, Premier is generally considered to be the largest and possibly most successful GPO, with a very positive growth rate over the last few years.
- *Novation,* www.novationco.com. Based in Texas with more than $25 billion in purchases and 2,500 members of the University HealthSystem Consortium and the VHA, Novation represents many of the largest, academic teaching hospitals in addition to VHA hospitals.
- *MedAssets,* www.medassets.com. Based in Georgia with nearly $12 billion in volume, MedAssets is a large and growing competitor in the GPO arena.

Collectively, the top 10 GPOs account for nearly $100 billion in purchasing volume (Modern Healthcare, 2005).

TRENDS IN HOSPITAL PURCHASING

There are several trends developing in most healthcare facilities, including smaller, value-focused teams; implementation of e-procurement and electronic commerce systems; standardization; and postponement.

Purchasing teams are getting smaller, more focused, and more analytical. With expected annual GPO savings representing anywhere from 1% to 15%, many administrators are questioning the role of large, extensive purchasing organizations internal to the hospital when GPOs can serve the sourcing, negotiating, contracting, and performance monitoring functions for hospitals for seemingly less money. Designing smaller, more focused purchasing teams that help manage the vendor community, administer and participate in the GPO contracting process, and use advanced analytics to perform value analysis are the new roles of purchasing professionals.

Another key trend is the continued use of EDI; automated requisitioning and supply chain systems are reducing cycle time and streamlining the procurement process. Electronic procurement systems are being used to streamline the purchasing process and offer punch-out capabilities to supplier product lines, in addition to standard electronic commerce functionality. E-commerce typically focuses on improving the level of EDI penetration rates, while simplifying the purchasing system's ease of use. This translates into higher productivity levels and significantly reduced staffing.

Standardization drives another trend in health care—value focus. Aggregating purchase volumes from multiple departments, and standardizing them around the same goods and services, allows purchasing departments to source higher quantities and volumes, which helps drive efficiencies into operations. Focusing on value is primarily visible through two structural mechanisms: the spend analysis process, which was described earlier, and the use of what many hospitals call the "clinical supply evaluation committee," or *materials use evaluation*. This group is an ad-hoc interdisciplinary team of physicians, nurses, materials managers, and administrators who assemble to evaluate the introduction of new materials into the supply chain. The role of these groups should be threefold, but rarely do they perform all three functions well.

- The first objective is to control access of vendors' products into the organization, which allows some standardization over the types of items used by physicians and in procedures.
- The second objective is to evaluate the economic impact of these new-item introductions into the organization. If surgery begins using a new medical surgical supply, what will this do to overall surgery costs? The role of this committee should be to explore the economic impact and determine if the improved outcomes or clinical efficacy are greater than the increased product costs, if any.
- The third objective of this group is to communicate findings and analyses to all units and floors about the product changes so that it is not left solely to purchasing and materials managers.

Typical problems that many people see with these committees is that they tend to make easy decisions (i.e., adopt a new product) but not address the implementation of that decision or address the more difficult questions (e.g., eliminate the older product, standardize usage among all units, and decide not to adopt products where costs are greater than proposed benefits).

Postponement is another emerging trend. **Postponement** refers to making decisions about purchasing until the latest possible point in the process, which reduces inventory levels and encourages rapid response on the part of vendors. Postponement is especially useful in reducing transactional purchasing costs because they can be aggregated and submitted only when necessary. Also, losses from stale or obsolete inventory decrease because purchases will not be made until the latest possible time. Postponement is a concept related to quick response and just in time.

Internal value processes will move purchasing from order takers to internal consultants. Using principles of aggregation and standardization, purchasing professionals can help large departments such as the operating room and radiology understand their consumption patterns and change utilization behaviors. This type of role is significantly different from that of a traditional purchasing agent and requires different skills and techniques.

RESOURCES FOR MATERIALS PROFESSIONALS

Very few resources are dedicated to materials and supply chain management for health care. The American Hospital Association maintains the AHRMM, which is an association that facilitates knowledge transfer and networking among materials managers in health care. AHRMM provides education, publications, and conferences as resources for materials managers. Another group, the American Society for Healthcare Central Service Professionals, is more focused on central supply and sterile processing, but it is another good resource for education and networking. Both groups are governed by the American Hospital Association.

Outside the healthcare industry, other professional associations exist that offer knowledge and networking for supply chain management in general, and these associations can provide materials managers with a large group of organizations with which to network and affiliate with. While the products and networks in health care might be different, a supply chain is a supply chain. Individuals who want to learn about inventory management, transportation, supply distribution, network management, and purchasing have a whole list of professional associations available to them, even though most of these are quite foreign to the typical hospital manager. Many of these have very respectable journal publications; have professional certifications that emphasize tools, concepts, and techniques; and have a wide multi-industry focus. Here is a list of well-known and respected professional associations:

- American Society of Transportation & Logistics (www.astl.org)
- Association for Healthcare Resource and Materials Management (www.ahrmm.org)
- American Society for Healthcare Central Service Professionals (www.ashcsp.org)
- The Association for Operations Management (www.apics.org)
- Council of Supply Chain Management Professionals (www.cscmp.org)
- Institute for Supply Management (www.ism.ws)
- Institute of Management Accountants (www.imanet.org)
- Materials Handling & Management Society (www.mhia.org)
- International Warehouse Logistics Association (www.iwla.org)

CUSTOMER SERVICE IN MATERIALS MANAGEMENT

Customer service can generically be defined as the means by which a provider attempts to keep customers happy and loyal, while differentiating itself from others (Wayland & Cole, 1997). Since materials management is a service provider, it needs to be especially focused on customer service levels and trends in performance.

Materials management and the supply chain serve two major groups of customers—those internal to the organization and those external. Internal customers include nurses, technicians on the floors and units, physicians, and other healthcare providers. Any department that orders, receives, or uses goods and services is a customer. External customers include hospital patients and their families and friends. Patients are very important, but they are usually customers of nursing or unit personnel and only indirectly served by materials management. While external, vendors represent a different type of stakeholder and are not necessarily customers. Similarly, employees in the chain are important, but they are different than customers. Customers represent buyers or consumers of goods.

Internal customers are very demanding on materials management. The key for nursing and other clinical divisions is product availability and service reliability. If products are available when needed, with minimal paperwork and effort, clinical departments are usually satisfied. As items become out of stock or unavailable, or if the process to procure and receive these items is bureaucratic and lengthy, then customer service will be considered poor.

When designing a materials management customer service program, it is essential to focus on those factors that are most important in supply chain management, namely, reliability (accuracy), speed (responsiveness, timeliness), customer acuity (intelligence, foresight about customer needs), and accountability (Boyson & Corsi, 2001). Materials management departments should focus their efforts on process and system improvements with these outcomes in mind.

An essential aspect of customer service is a proactive system that records and triages process breakdowns as they occur. A complaint or issue tracking system, with resolution processes, will help managers not only record problems but analyze sources of these problems. By understanding the sources of variability in the outcomes (i.e., reliability, speed, etc.), then the outcomes can be measured and improved.

Another essential aspect of customer care is to document performance-level expectations with end users through a service-level agreement. A **service-level agreement (SLA)** is a formal agreement that clearly communicates the types of services to be offered, performance expectations, hours services are provided, inputs or resources to be committed, and payments if any. An SLA allows for history to be kept about new service lines or commitments.

For example, if an operating room department creates a new program where they open for surgical cases 2 hours earlier than before, there will be a significant downstream impact on materials management. Employees' schedules might have to change, vendor delivery schedules might be affected, increased usage and storage of supplies might be required, and more resources will be consumed. Any time a new program is created, or as existing ones change, an opportunity is created for a lack of clarity about the actual customer needs and business requirements. During these times, service-level satisfaction typically dips, as customers get frustrated with the inability for materials to respond appropriately. If an SLA were created in advance, the exact inputs and outputs would have been discussed openly and agreed to, which would minimize the margin of error.

In addition to SLAs, customer surveys and other monitoring tools should be used to remain connected to the customer's pulse and satisfaction. Interviews with key customers should be conducted periodically to establish benchmarks in each of the performance areas. Critical areas of surveys and interviews would be cost, quality, cycle time, and interactions with personnel, in addition to reliability, responsiveness, and accountability. Most complaints about service in hospitals can be categorized as a late delivery, missing or unfilled items, or damaged or expired products. These three areas represent the significant majority of customer issues.

A performance scorecard should be created and monitored to track customer service performance over time. The specific metrics could include:

1. Number of telephone calls coming into the department.
2. The volume of complaints and concerns.
3. Product availability (or "on-shelf" fill rate percentages versus out-of-stocks).
4. On-time deliveries.
5. Total order cycle time.
6. Delivered cost.

A scorecard should be created using these metrics on a continuous basis (i.e., monthly, quarterly) and disseminated to employees, managers, and customers. This scorecard should define future plans and strategies because it highlights gaps and deficiencies in current performance.

LAUNDRY AND LINEN

In some of the smaller hospitals, laundry operations are considered part of materials management. In most larger hospitals, though, laundry management is a separate function and requires hundreds of employees processing millions of pounds of laundry per year. Either way, laundry and linen management is essential to the proper operation of a hospital. Without clean linens, hospitals would not be able to offer the same high-quality care environment that patients expect and that is required by regulations and quality guidelines.

Laundry operations can either be managed internally or outsourced. Surveys suggest that 50% of all hospitals outsource their laundry processing to third parties or engage in "cooperatives" with other hospitals to process their laundry (Hospital and Health Networks, 2001).

Laundry operations are subject to strict quality control guidelines, due to the high risk of disease transmission from patient to patient. The Centers for Disease Control and Prevention and the Joint Commission on Accreditation of Healthcare Organizations are two groups that have created guidelines for proper handling of laundry. There are several specific guidelines governing design and construction of new hospital laundries or operations of existing ones, including the following (Healthcare Purchasing News, 2004):

- U.S. Department of Health and Human Services. "Guidelines for Construction and Equipment of Hospital and Medical Facilities"
- Office of Health and Safety, Centers for Disease Control and Prevention. "Guidelines for Laundry in Healthcare Facilities"

These guidelines primarily emphasize the control of infection and reduction of disease transmission. Some specific recommendations include the use of hot water (greater than 160°F for most linens for periods equal to or greater than 25 minutes) or the use of specific chemicals if lower-temperature washing is used. Safe handling of linens require that transportation methods and devices should not contaminate clean linens and that soiled linen collection needs to be in bags that are leak-resistant (Centers for Disease Control and Prevention, 2002).

Laundry management is defined as the process of collecting, processing (washing, drying, assembling, staging), transporting, and replenishing linens during the linen life cycle, from acquisition to final ragout or disposition. **Linens** are fabrics used for healthcare purposes and include scrubs, pillows and cases, sheets, blankets, towels, lab coats, rags, and protective gear and gowns. Some of the largest linen or textile manufacturers specific for health care include Standard Textile Company Inc. (www.standardtextile.com) and Medline Industries (www.medline.com).

In larger hospitals, collecting **soiled** (i.e., dirty or used) **linen** is usually performed by the housekeeping, laundry, or materials management department on a prearranged pickup schedule. In smaller hospitals, nursing collects the linens and uses automated chutes to move linens back to lower floors of the hospital to be picked up by laundry personnel. Either way, the movement of soiled linens is a resource-intensive, manual process. Soiled linen weighs approximately 10% more than clean linen, and carts full of linen can weigh several hundred pounds or more.

Most laundry operations use par levels to manage inventories of clean linens on each floor or unit, very similar to the concepts used for medical supplies or pharmaceuticals. A **par** is an inventory location that holds a specific product mix with minimum quantities that will cover the unit for a predetermined number of hours or days and defines what type and how many linen items are required for each location. In many hospitals, a par refers to either a physical location (e.g., the par in pediatrics) or inventory levels and mix (e.g., the par for sheets is 20). Pars exist for medical supplies and pharmaceuticals, as well as for linens. Smaller hospitals might have a dozen or fewer pars, while larger hospitals can have several hundred pars. A typical par will have a breakdown of items required for the period (e.g., 12 towels, 15 sheets, and 20 rags).

Pars can be replenished by use of either exchange or bulk replenishment carts. **Exchange carts** are large steel structures, and new items on a cart are swapped entirely for the existing cart. In this replenishment process, one cart is always redundant and is used solely to provide fast exchange of all items on the par. **Bulk replenishment** occurs when items are simply augmented to the existing cart. If 10 towels are on the par, but only 3 exist, 7 more would be added from bulk stock. Neither exchange nor bulk replenishment is necessarily better. They both have advantages and disadvantages that must be considered. Bulk is often much more economical for washing but less efficient for replenishment, while an exchange cart is faster and usually has higher service levels. A careful analysis of the economics and service levels for each should be conducted for each location.

Laundry is processed or cleaned at a production facility that uses commercial laundry equipment. One of the major pieces of equipment is a tunnel washer, which is a modular machine where batches of linen move through phases or modules during the process. Tunnel washers are typically called *continuous batch washers* because they operate as a production process. Washers are some of the more expensive pieces of equipment and can process 1,000 pounds or more of linen per hour.

In addition to washers, hospital laundries must have commercial dryers, extractors, ironers, folders, etc. Other technology, such as conveyor belts, help push linen through the assembly-line production process, as shown below:

**Sort >> Wash/extract >> Dry >>Iron or fold
>> Assembly >> Transportation**

The cost of new laundries must factor in the capital equipment as well as the land and building costs. Total costs, then, can be $10 to$20 million for new laundry facility construction (Dukenews, 2001).

The total cost of laundry and linen for a hospital is a component of four factors:

- Acquisition and replacement cost of linens.
- Cost of processing (washing, drying, folding).
- Cost of collecting and distributing linens.
- Consumption and utilization patterns.

Together, these four components significantly add to the cost structure for a hospital. In many larger hospitals, total costs can amount to several millions of dollars annually. On an adjusted, per-patient per-day basis, the total cost of linen can range from $5 to $15, which is quite significant. More common metrics are recorded on a per-pound basis and typically range from $0.35 to $0.50, based on overall economies of scale and other efficiencies.

To continually improve service levels to nursing, while reducing laundry and linen expenses, requires careful oversight. Laundry operations need to focus on managing nursing utilization patterns to ensure that the right linens are being used for the right task and that excessive amounts are not being used for any one task. **Utilization** refers to the usage patterns of linens; thus, linen use must be carefully monitored to ensure stable or declining utilization over time. Managing staff productivity for distribution and collections is also important, which requires careful scheduling and monitoring of employees during routes. The use of automation and work flow (including chutes, belts, and automated guided vehicles) can also reduce labor expenses, so their use should be encouraged when cost effective. Finally, ensuring that the right levels of inventory are on-hand at all times (i.e., not too many, not too few) is extremely important, so the use of economic order quantities, safety stock calculations, and proper replenishment practices covered in subsequent Chapter 12 are extremely relevant for laundry management. Excessive safety inventory is evident when linens are stockpiled in nursing supply or patient treatment rooms, and this results in excessive costs to the linen system.

CHAPTER SUMMARY

The materials management organization in large hospitals plays a very key role in operations management. Materials management typically includes oversight of purchasing, strategic sourcing, inventory replenishment, laundry and linen, patient transportation, and sterile processing, in addition to revenue responsibilities for medical supplies and equipment. A comprehensive purchasing process focuses on the use of GPOs and strategic sourcing methodologies to lower total costs and increase financial value. Internal controls are important in this process because materials management has a fiduciary responsibility to prevent loss, reduce waste, and provide sound oversight to the use of operating funds. The management of laundry and linen is just one of the areas with large customer and patient impacts in a hospital, and it should be managed appropriately.

KEY TERMS

bulk replenishment, chargeable, competitive bidding, current procedural terminology (CPT), customer service, durable medical equipment (DME), exchange carts, group purchasing organization (GPO), healthcare common procedure coding system (HCPCS), laundry management, linens, loss leader, markup, materials management, medical record, optimization, par, penetration, physician preferences, point-of-use (POU) systems, postponement, profit center, scorecard, service-level agreement (SLA), soiled linen, spend analysis, three-way match, utilization

DISCUSSION QUESTIONS

1. What role does materials management play in health care?
2. What are the key functions and processes?

3. How does the layout of a hospital floor or unit affect operational efficiency?

4. Discuss the concept of cost minimization models. When can they be applied, and what are the steps to follow when using them?

5. What is a GPO? What value can it bring?

6. Why does a hospital need both a GPO and a purchasing department?

7. What types of technologies are involved in laundry management?

REFERENCES

American Medical Association. (2001). *Healthcare Common Procedure Coding System, 2002.* Atlanta: AMA/Ingenix Publishing Group.

Boyson, Sandor, and Thomas Corsi. (2001). The Real-Time Supply Chain. *Supply Chain Management Review, 5*(1), January/February: 44–50.

Centers for Disease Control and Prevention, Office of Health and Safety. (2002). *Guidelines for Laundry in Healthcare Facilities.*

Council of Supply Chain Management Professionals. (2006). *Supply Chain Management/Logistics Definitions.*

Dukenews. (2001). *New Facility Takes Laundry High-Tech.* www.Dukenews. Duke.edu.

Healthcare Purchasing News. (2004). OSHA Guidelines for Laundry in Healthcare Facilities, August.

Heizer, Jay, and Barry Render. (2004). *Operations Management,* 7th ed. Englewood Cliffs, NJ: Prentice Hall.

Hospital and Health Networks. (2001). Contract Management Survey.

Housley, Charles E. (1983). *Hospital Purchasing: Focus on Effectiveness.* Frederick, MD: Aspen Publishers.

Kowalski-Dickow Associates, Inc. (1997). *Managing Hospital Materials Management.* Chicago: American Society for Healthcare Materials Management.

Lambert, D. (1999). *Strategic Logistics Management.* New York: McGraw-Hill.

Modern Healthcare. (2005). 2005 Group Purchasing Survey, *Modern Healthcare,* August 15, 2005.

Wayland, Robert E., and Paul M. Cole. (1997). *Customer Connections.* Boston: Harvard Business School Press.

CHAPTER 12

Inventory Management and Accounting

Goals of This Chapter
1. Define inventory
2. Understand the pros and cons of maintaining inventory
3. Understand the difference between perpetual and periodic methods
4. Explain common accounting entries for inventory management
5. Calculate common inventory ratios

Inventory is a complicated subject in most industries, and it is even less understood in health care. Inventory represents acquisition and storage of materials that will not be consumed today (and thus have some value in the future) and that will be used within the normal operating cycle. It is therefore treated financially as a current asset, and proper treatment requires capitalizing it and recording a value on the balance sheet.

However in most hospitals, inventory is geographically dispersed and of relatively small financial value in disaggregated form (i.e., hospital inventory usually sits in treatment and exam rooms, surgical suites, and supply closets). When aggregated, however, these supplies can represent millions or even tens of millions of dollars for most hospitals. This chapter discusses the basics of inventory accounting and management in health care.

INVENTORY AND
ITS ROLE IN HEALTH CARE

Inventory can be defined from an accounting or an operations perspective. From an accounting definition, **Inventory** includes those assets that are used to generate revenue and that will be converted to cash in the short term. They are assets (e.g., supplies) that are held for sale. In the case of hospitals, medical supplies and pharmaceuticals are directly or indirectly charged back to patients—through direct charges through healthcare common procedure coding system (HCPCS) or other procedural charges—or they are reimbursed as part of per-diem, room, or other service procedure codes. This depends on the specific hospital, the types of services they typically receive reimbursement for, and the specific payer mix. Regardless, most medical supplies and drugs are reimbursed either directly or indirectly, and therefore they represent costs incurred that will deliver future benefits.

From an operations perspective, inventory represents a margin of safety to protect the business from unpredictable levels of demand. Without inventory, hospitals could purchase just enough products to sustain normal operations, but if one more incremental unit was used or consumed, then the entire supply chain would be thrown in chaos with stockouts, reduced service levels, and a potential inability to fully treat a patient. In operations terms, inventory is a buffer against demand variability.

Operationally, inventory serves a multitude of other functions:

- Inventory improves customer service by making products available immediately.
- Inventory allows for economies of scale, as it encourages aggregation of production, purchase, and transportation to achieve reduced costs.
- Inventory allows for batching of orders, which creates purchasing scale. Larger orders usually are associated with pricing discounts.
- Inventory takes advantage of pricing discounts for large quantities. For most manufacturers and distributors, it is significantly easier to work in larger volumes or batches than in smaller quantities (e.g., "each" or individuals). Because manufacturers produce in large batches, and distributors receive quantity discounts for buying in volume, they are often able to pass significant savings on to hospitals if they can purchase in larger volumes. Unfortunately, many hospitals have very little warehouse or storage space and have to work on a just-in-time (JIT) basis.

- Inventory allows for transport economies from larger shipment sizes. Smaller orders have a very high transportation cost, especially relative to the unit cost. For example, assume a $2 surgical procedure kit was ordered and shipped with transportation costs of $3 minimum for overnight delivery. The transportation cost, then, is 150% of the product cost. Assume 10 items could be purchased and shipped using this same $3 minimum shipping (weight of 10 items falls under the weight restrictions), then shipping costs per unit would be only 15% of the total cost (i.e., $3 ÷ 10 items = $0.30 per item; $0.30 ÷ $2 = 15%).
- Inventory hedges against price changes. If a supply cost is increasing at a greater rate than the average consumer price inflation of 3%, it is sometimes beneficial to hold larger volumes of inventory to hedge the risk of rising prices.
- Inventory allows purchasing to take place under most favorable price terms.
- Inventory protects against uncertainties in demand and lead times.
- Inventory helps accurately report financials, because the timing of the supply expense must be associated with the period in which revenues are generated. If material is not actually used and patients have not been charged, then it is proper not to expense it. Therefore, inventory serves a valuable financial purpose.
- Inventory protects against demand volatility. When demand is less than certain, or variable, inventory helps protect against this variability. For instance, if 100 packs of bandages are used fairly consistently, but a large incident might create demand for another 50, inventory would help provide some measure of protection or margin of safety to keep operations running when demand levels and lead times cannot be known for sure.
- Inventory provides buffers against tragic events and other disruptions in supply. When the major hurricanes of 2005 hit the Gulf Coast, supply lines were essentially cut off completely—highways were jammed and many vendors and distributors were closed down. In the event that a hospital was forced to continue operations, it likely did so because of inventories that were built up prior to the storm.

Thus, there are many positive reasons a hospital would want to hold inventory, but there are also some negative and financial reasons not to do so. The biggest reason not to hold excessive inventories is that they consume cash and capital resources that might be put to better use elsewhere. Inventories represent prepaid supplies; if a hospital does not need an item for some period in the future, the most optimal case is that that item is not procured or delivered until as close to point of need or consumption as possible. This is called *postponement*, which is one of the trends described in Chapter 11. For example, if a hospital paid for $1 million of pharmaceutical supplies 2 weeks earlier than they were needed, at a 5% cost of capital or interest forfeited that could have been invested elsewhere, the hospital forfeited $1,923 unnecessarily. This does not even include the additional holding cost (i.e., cost of storage and handling of the items while at the hospital).

Of course, this is not always possible, as discussed earlier. But from a cash flow perspective, the timing of the receipt and payment of goods should be as late as possible to allow cash to be invested in other higher-returning areas, such as new buildings, investments, or other capital programs.

Another reason not to hold inventories is they often hide problems. Inventory serves as a buffer, and as such, operational problems that exist might go unnoticed for many periods. For example, if a nursing unit forgets to accurately record supply usage or administration against a patient's medical records in a timely manner, then there could be potential for lost charges. If hospitals do not build inventory, it is much easier to discover this; otherwise, days or weeks worth of inventory sits onsite and might only be discovered during periodic cycle counts. Also, in systems that are not working properly, lower utilization rates, slow cycle times, and otherwise unproductive processes are often masked by inventory.

THE COSTS OF SUPPLIES AND INVENTORY

The purchase costs of pharmaceuticals and medical supplies are anywhere from 13% to 17% of a hospital's total operation expenses, based on the size of the organization (Healthcare Financial Management Association, 2005). But this is only a small part of the total supply cost. Most hospitals are nonprofit and therefore prepare financials differently than a public firm would (especially in the manufacturing or retail industries); calculating the true cost of goods sold is not ordinarily performed. If it were, the cost of converting or transforming these products into revenue would include all salaries for time spent by nursing and materials personnel moving supplies toward point of consumption, inventories, logistics, information technology, and other associated carrying expenses. Based on this author's previous research, the true cost of supplies is somewhere between 25% and 35% of total operating expenses.

In smaller organizations, supply costs can range from $3.2 million for a hospital with a $25 million annual expense budget, to $170 million for a $1 billion organization. Add the costs of materials management departments, the salaries of technicians and nursing staff who touch supplies, warehouse and other facility expenses, the cost of systems time, and finally the expense for managing these items, and total costs only get bigger.

Since most hospitals are nonprofit and do not necessarily follow **generally accepted accounting principles (GAAP)** to accurately record expenses and inventory values (GAAP represents the accounting principles required for use by public companies), there is little consistency in how supplies are expensed and inventory is capitalized. A few findings from this author's research of published hospital annual reports and Medicare cost reports for nonprofits suggest that these accounting practices are not used correctly in most cases. For instance, most published financials for hospitals tend to show a very small inventory balance and lump supply expenses under a large group called operational expenses. Very little detail below this is publicly available. Where the data are available, they are inconsistent with actual practice and should be approached with caution.

The best way to understand the true costs of inventory and supplies, in an environment that is probably more cost-conscious and that is required to use GAAP accounting, is to examine the publicly traded, for-profit hospital systems. Examining the inventory balances of several of the largest for-profit hospital chains shows the following patterns:

- Average inventory for medium-size hospitals is around $3 million to $4 million per hospital.
- Inventory represents approximately 5% to 15% of current assets.
- Investments in inventory constitute about 2% to 4% of total assets and net revenues.
- Inventory represents the largest portion of working capital requirements.

The bottom line is that inventories are a significant investment for hospitals and should be treated accordingly.

DIFFERENCES BETWEEN SUPPLY EXPENSE AND INVENTORY

So what is the difference between supply and inventory, and is there really a distinction between the two? The answer is yes—but the distinction can be described in just two words: timing and chargeable.

Timing represents the difference between when a supply is purchased and when it is consumed. If it is purchased and consumed in the same period, it is treated as a supply expense and is presented on the income statement with all other expenses. If it is purchased in one period but not used as of the end of that period, then it is shown on the balance sheet as capitalized inventory.

Chargeable means that if the purpose of the material is to charge it back, directly or indirectly (through room or procedure rates) to patients, and if it is not consumed by the end of the period, it is held as inventory. If an item has no role in reimbursement (e.g., office supplies for administrative purposes), then the cost of those items, whether or not they are used in that period, is probably expensed. (Note: if there is a significant amount of monies represented, these could be capitalized as prepaid assets, but they would not be considered "inventory.")

IMPACT OF TIMING ON EXPENSES

Consider this example. A large hospital purchases $5 million of pharmaceuticals in preparation for a category 4 storm that is heading toward the city. The distributor delivers 1,200 totes, which are put in a back room just in case. The date is July 29. The hospital continues operations; fortunately the storm never reaches the city, and all operations continue as normal. The general ledger officially closes for the month, and the hospital finds itself with a $3 million loss. This is fairly standard treatment for most hospitals.

The quality and maturity of information systems used in most healthcare settings for managing supplies, inventory, and the supply chain are generally quite poor. In retail, manufacturing, and consumer goods industries, sophisticated enterprise resource planning (ERP) tools are used to manage the movement of goods through all parts of the organization with extreme precision. In health care, however, most of the larger hospitals and systems use some form of ERP, but the configurations were not originally set up to bring the hospital systems up to the same level.

The hospital described earlier did not use or consume the $5 million of drugs purchased in the period in question. An entry should have been made to record this as inventory because it is prepaying a future expense and it is used for items generating revenue. If the hospital had booked this as inventory, the net effect on expenses would have been significant and the hospital would have shown a $2 million profit for the period. Current assets would have increased by $5 million, and more than likely accounts payable (i.e., a short-term liability) would have increased by the same amount. The net effect on cash flow would remain unchanged.

This is not an accounting scheme or game; it represents matching expenses to the appropriate period in which the revenue was incurred. Because the hospital did not use or charge a patient for the pharmaceuticals, the expense should not be recorded, and the future benefit of the current asset should be offset by an expense at a future date.

IMPORTANT FACTS ABOUT INVENTORY

Inventory on most hospitals' books is severely undervalued. If all hospitals complied with GAAP and Financial Accounting Standards Board pronouncements, there would be a much broader emphasis on comprehensively counting and valuing hospital inventories. For this reason however, benchmark comparisons about inventory levels with most hospitals will not yield fruitful results due to the undervaluation and lack of consistency in treating supply expense versus inventory.

The cost of inventory is directly related to the hospital's case mix index. Therefore, a hospital that has more intense, complicated, and resource-intensive procedures will likely see a higher percentage of its operating budget being spent on supplies and inventory. A **case mix index** is calculated based on classification schemes such as diagnosis-related groups.

The larger the hospital, in terms of beds and procedures performed, the higher the associated supply expenses. Inventory, however, reflects efficiency in utilization and in planning and may not be directly related. A hospital that employs quantitative planning and inventory techniques and attempts to model inventory using economic order quantities (EOQs) or forecasting practices would probably have less inventory than a similar hospital, even though current-period supply expenses might be comparable.

It is very difficult to explore utilization of supplies and inventory on a per-procedure basis, especially in larger hospitals, given the state of information systems. Implementing an activity-based costing approach to service-line management in clinical settings would be highly advantageous to track actual quantities of items utilized relative to patient reimbursements.

In most industries there are three classifications of inventory: raw materials, work in process, and finished goods. Most hospitals deal with only finished goods inventory, which refers to items that are complete and ready for sale (i.e., there is no conversion or manufacturing that must be done to make them usable).

There are two other types of inventory. **Consignment out** reflects the hospital's inventory that is placed elsewhere for sale. This type of consignment might be where a hospital provides certain supplies to other facilities or even retail stores for them to resell. Consignment-out inventory needs to be recorded on the hospital's books. The opposite of this, **consignment in**, measures somebody else's inventory (i.e., some type of vendor, either the manufacturer or the distributor) that is being held or stored on the hospital's facility at no charge until sold. Examples of this are stents and other expensive cardiology or operating room supplies, where a vendor will place them onsite until they are consumed. At the point of usage, the vendor is paid, expenses are increased, and the vendor's inventory is decreased. The hospital does not own the inventory, so it does not include it on its balance sheet.

CRITERIA FOR INVENTORY

To capitalize the value of materials on the balance sheet, there have to be criteria that determine materiality (i.e., what dollar threshold should be placed on inventory that is capitalized versus expensed) and what makes inventory unique to each hospital. Without criteria in place, and without complying with GAAP accounting requirements, organizations would just immediately expense all items that were purchased, which of course does not properly reflect timing and matching principles in accounting (Bragg, 2006).

Criteria should be defined so that each department and location purchasing and storing materials would check the following:

- Are the items held for sale to patients directly (i.e., through HCPCS codes) or indirectly (i.e., through bundled hospital room or procedure charges)?

- Are the items consumable?
- Are they greater than the dollar amount defined as "material" to the hospital? (This must be defined based on the size and unique situation of each hospital because no standard material threshold exists.)
- Are the materials owned by the institution and not leased, rented, or otherwise consigned to the hospital?
- Are the materials used in permanent and ongoing service lines? (That is, they are not to be used in a special one-time situation.)

The capitalization criteria defined should be consistent across all areas of the hospital and should identify each unit, floor, and nursing station that holds inventory and then apply the criteria comprehensively. Any inventories that meet this test should be physically counted, valued, and recorded in the general ledger on the balance sheet (this assumes, of course, that the items are not already in a perpetual inventory system, which will be discussed later).

VALUATION METHODS

One of the most important decisions to be made in inventory management is the choice of accounting valuation methods. **Valuation** is an assessment of the financial value of an asset (Muller, 2002). This is an important decision and has broad financial impacts, but in the healthcare industry it is not well understood even by accountants—especially if they do not come from other, more inventory-intensive industries.

Accounting Research Bulletin 43, Chapter 4, is the official pronouncement with the highest level authority in GAAP, and it lays out the inventory pricing conventions. There are a multitude of valuation methods in use, but the three most common are: first in, first out (FIFO); last in, first out (LIFO), and weighted average. Other less common methods are dollar-value LIFO, retail method, specific identification (used for high dollar items, such as airplanes, where specific units are recorded) and moving average. Choosing a method can have different effects on the financial statements, especially if prices are continually changing.

First in, first out (FIFO) is probably the most common valuation method in health care. It assumes that the first unit purchased is the first unit sold, and therefore the units that are remaining in inventory are the last units purchased. For example, if a hospital purchases two expense items at a cost of $1,000 per case and sells only one of these in the period, the supply expense would equal $1,000 and an additional $1,000 would be added to the inventory balance. But if the first unit cost $1,000 and the second one cost $1,500, then FIFO valuation would report the same level of expenses but $1,500 would be added to inventory, because the first one purchased was the first one utilized. In an environment in which prices are rising, FIFO expenses the lower-costing items, which therefore causes net income to be higher than other methods (this will be discussed in more detail later).

Under **last in, first out (LIFO)**, the premise is that the last unit purchased is the first unit sold. Alternatively, the oldest item in the inventory would be the first item purchased. This method assumes that sales are made from the most recently acquired units and that ending inventory is comprised of the oldest available goods. This method is generally problematic in health care in that it does not reflect the true physical flow of goods, where most medical supplies and drugs have expiration dates that require earlier products to be sold first. It does have an advantage in that it matches the most current cost against current revenues, but the balance sheet appears undervalued relative to current market or replacement costs. Using the earlier example of two items, one purchased for $1,000 and the other for $1,500, suggests that expenses on the income statement would be higher this period, and ending inventories would increment by $1,000. The net result is that net income would be lower using this method in this period, as long as quantities remain constant or increase.

Another common valuation method used in health care is weighted average. **Weighted average** assumes that the cost should reflect the averages of all items purchased over time. In the earlier example, the two items total to $2,500; therefore, the weighted average for each item is $1,250. This amount would be expensed in the current period, and the same amount would increment inventories. The net impact on the financial statements would be lower net income than FIFO but higher than LIFO.

Most hospitals choose to use either FIFO or weighted average for their valuation methods. Most information systems can support either of these, and it is acceptable to use a combination of several methods, as long as it can be supported. The most important thing is to select one of these methods and stick with it. This consistency principle is important so that comparisons can be made over time.

LOWER OF COST OR MARKET

Regardless of the method of inventory costing chosen, the value has to follow the "conservative" principle of accounting, which states inventory should be valued at the **lower of cost or market or LCM**. The complexity in this is to understand what is meant by "cost". Determining market cost is a little complex, as described below, but market typically refers to the current replacement cost or cost to purchase a new unit.

The first step is to determine the market cost. Hospitals should use the concept of a "ceiling" and "floor." A *ceiling* is the upper limit, defined as selling price minus all cost to sell the items, which also is called the **net realizable value**. Next, look at the *floor*, which is defined as the ceiling minus the normal expected profit margin. The result is two numbers, a ceiling and a floor, and the market price will fall somewhere in that range. Now, compare the current replacement costs for that item to the range. In general, hospitals use the replacement cost if the replacement cost fits between the ceiling and the floor. If the replacement cost is below the floor, use the floor. The second step is to compare the historical cost to the market figure calculated earlier. Hospitals report the lower (or more conservative) of the two figures.

Consider this example. A drug is purchased for $200, which reflects the original purchase cost. The average markup is 30% on this type of item, and therefore the sales price is $260. Additional selling costs are estimated at 10% of cost on all pharmaceuticals, and so the net realizable value is

$$(\$200 \times 1.3) - (\$200 \times 0.10) = \$240$$

Thus, $240 is the ceiling price. The floor is defined as the ceiling less normal profit margin which is $60 in this example, or ($260 − $60) = $200. The current replacement cost for that same item is $225. Because this replacement cost falls inside the relevant range, the replacement cost of $225 will be used for inventory valuation purposes.

In practice, most hospitals have thousands of items to manage, so it is impossible to calculate an LCM on each item. The principle is important but, in practice, very difficult to manage without good systems. The real distinction that most hospitals make is whether to book at historical cost or replacement cost (which is captured in the earlier discussion of LIFO, FIFO, and weighted average).

PERIODIC VERSUS PERPETUAL SYSTEMS

Another choice to be made with regard to inventory is whether to manage items on a periodic or a perpetual basis. Periodic inventory in general is easier to manage. **Periodic inventory** does not keep a running record of items that are sold or purchased, so a real-time balance of inventory on hand is never available. Periodic inventory relies heavily on physical counting and observation of goods because no system is used to track balances.

Perpetual inventory, on the other hand, keeps a running record of the inventory balance on hand at all times. Perpetual inventory is very common in retail and manufacturing industries, where precision around inventory is very important. In health care, it is used less, although the trend is to incorporate more perpetual systems throughout hospitals.

In central stores and the warehouse, perpetual systems are commonly used. They can be used here for several reasons:

1. A person usually works the location and is responsible for closely guarding the inventory.

2. A system at this point can be used to enter requisitions from units (or issues against inventory) as well as receipts or additions to inventory.

3. They are usually smaller, more controlled environments where all ins and outs can be monitored.

Perpetual systems can best be used in situations involving a small number of locations with a high dollar unit value, whereas periodic systems are often used in situations that are low cost and high volume. In decentralized storage areas of the hospital (sometimes referred to as a par or supply room), there is typically no centralized control or monitoring of supplies coming in and out. Multiple people over several shifts come in and out of these areas to retrieve items for patients, and in these cases a perpetual system is not necessarily appropriate or cost effective (the use of supply automation that enables perpetual monitoring even in decentralized locations is discussed later).

In a periodic inventory, a physical count is taken at least once at the end of the fiscal period. Receipts or purchases from vendors are typically incremented to separate purchases or expense accounts. A physical count of inventory at the end of the next period yields a figure, and the difference between the beginning and the ending inventory is adjusted to find the true **cost of goods sold (COGS)**. COGS becomes the supply expense for the period, which reflects actual usage of items, or the delta between beginning and ending period positions. Alternatively, items could be expensed as procured, and then an adjustment is made for any differences at the end of the period. When using periodic inventory, the ending inventory in units is multiplied by the FIFO or weighted average values to determine an inventory balance.

A perpetual inventory system, however, recalculates based on each transaction occurrence. If beginning inventory is 5, and 3 items are purchased the next month, the total goods available for sale is 8. Subtract the issues to patients or floors to get the ending inventory balance. Automated ERPs and materials management information systems allow for real-time entry of receipts as supplies come through the dock and issues as they are charged out to patients or units.

The real advantage to a perpetual system is that it provides valuable information about supply expenses and inventory values throughout the year. If a hospital is only interested in end-of-year financial positions, then either method will yield the same result, but because most hospitals are encouraging sound financial practices and continuous performance measurements, intra-period balances are extremely important. In addition, this same perpetual information will drive improved inventory replenishment plans, because transaction histories are associated with the actual months in which they occurred—which is vital to predicting demand and generating usage forecasts for the future.

Another advantage to perpetual systems is that they help materials managers avoid excessive inventory levels throughout the year. Working capital, the net current resources necessary to sustain operations, should be held as minimally as possible so that investments in more productive assets can be made. Inventory is one of the key components driving increases in working capital, so a more detailed, real-time understanding of inventory will lower working capital requirements.

Perpetual inventory systems also allow for the use of automated replenishment versus manual ordering and replenishment processes. Obviously, automated replenishment is less people-intense, more efficient, and less expensive in the long run, but it is also faster and ensures fewer stockouts (i.e., having zero items on a shelf when one is needed). Two ways these perpetual systems can automate the replenishment process are:

- Forecasting an order based on transactional usage history, which will generate an automatic order based on previous consumption patterns.
- Using predetermined minimum and maximum (min-max) levels. This is discussed in more detail later, but basically if current inventory falls below the minimum required on hand, an automated order is placed for the difference between the minimum and the current quantity.

At most hospitals there will be a combination of both perpetual and periodic systems. Although the perpetual system is preferred, given that the cost does not exceed the benefits derived, it is often not practical in all locations. For that reason, an understanding of the accounting treatment for both periodic and perpetual inventory is important. Under either scenario, periodic physical inventory counts have to be conducted to verify the accuracy of the book records.

ACCOUNTING ENTRIES FOR SUPPLY AND INVENTORY

Accounting treatment is different depending on whether the hospital or department is working in the perpetual or the periodic environment. Starting first with perpetual inventories, the basic calculation of inventory is:

$$BI + P - COGS = EI$$

where,

BI = beginning inventory, in units and dollar value
P = cost of the units purchased
$COGS$ = the cost of goods sold for issues to departments and patients
EI = ending inventory

For example, assume that there is $500,000 in beginning inventory on January 1. Inventory has a debit balance on the balance sheet and reads $500,000 under current assets. (Note: Debits will be referred to using the abbreviation "DR," while credits will be "CR.") During January there were total purchases of $1,000,000. The entry to record, assuming that the invoice was not paid immediately from a cash account, would be:

DR inventory	$1,000,000
CR accounts payable	$1,000,000

In other words, a liability is created, and there is an offsetting asset for the same amount. Assume that there were sales or issues of $1,750,000 for charges to be reimbursed by payers for supplies that were given to the nursing units or floors for direct dispensing to patients. The entry to record this would be:

DR accounts receivable	$1,750,000
CR revenue	$1,750,000

When the actual payment is made to the manufacturer or distributor, based on the contractual invoice terms, an entry would be made to reduce cash and to reduce the liability, as follows:

DR accounts payable	$1,000,000
CR cash	$1,000,000

Next, an entry will have to be made to record the cost or expense of the items that were sold. Using FIFO and ensuring the LCM, the hospital determined that $900,000 in inventory expenses was consumed. The entry would be:

DR supply expense (COGS)	$900,000
CR inventory	$900,000

The net impact of this is shown in **Table 12–1**. Thus, the net impact is a $100,000 increase in inventories on the balance sheet. The impact on the income statement, for these transactions only, shows a positive operating margin of $850,000 (or $1,750,000 in sales less $900,000 in COGS).

Under periodic inventory accounting, the treatment is somewhat different. Beginning inventory stays the same, at $500,000, but instead of booking the items purchased into inventory, they are recorded to a separate, temporary purchases or expense account that will be closed at the

Table 12–1 Inventory Accounting

INVENTORY			
Beginning Inventory	$500,000		
		$900,000	Issues/COG
Purchases	$1,000,000		
Ending Inventory	$600,000		

end of each period. Inventory maintains the same balance until the end of the period, when it would be physically counted again. If the count reveals only $400,000 worth of inventory on hand, the calculation would be made as follows, assuming the same level of sales:

Beginning. inventory	$ 500,000
+ Purchases	$1,000,000
− COGS	XX
= Ending inventory	$400,000

Solving for the COGs shows that it would have to be $1,100,000. The transactions would be as follows:

DR purchases	$1,000,000
CR accounts payable	$1,000,000

Notice that these purchases are not recorded into inventory as under the perpetual method. Also, the entry to record the revenue and accounts receivable would remain the same:

DR accounts receivable	$1,750,000
CR revenue	$1,750,000

The entry to record the payment to the vendor is the same as the previous entry for perpetual:

DR accounts payable	$1,000,000
CR cash	$1,000,000

Since beginning inventory ($500,000) plus purchases ($1,000,000) equals cost of goods available for sale of $1,500,000 and the ending inventory was observed and counted to be $400,000, the COGS would be $1,100,000 as shown earlier. The entry then has to be made to net out the temporary purchases account and book this to COGS.

DR COGS/supply expense	$1,100,000
CR purchases	$1,000,000
CR inventory	$100,000

This brings the inventory account down to $400,000 as counted, closes out the purchasing account, and moves all COGS to a supply expense.

The net impact on the financial statements using periodic accounting methods is net operating margin of $650,000, versus $850,000 in the earlier example. This is just coincidental, however, because both methods will yield the same results over time, assuming that perpetual is capturing all transactions and that periodic counts are conducted.

In addition, under both the periodic and perpetual methods, there will have to be entries made to reflect any adjustments to inventory. Adjustments are made when a comparison of the general ledger to actual observed quantities shows material variances. For example, if a cycle count was performed in a perpetual environment, and the count showed $100,000 worth of items but the general ledger reported $122,000, an adjusting journal entry would have to be made to record an additional $22,000 of expense. This adjustment would be called **shrinkage** or loss, which can arise as a result of any number of reasons:

- Failure to charge out properly to patients as they were dispensed or utilized.
- Misplacement or overuse of drugs or supplies.
- Items that have passed the expiration date or are obsolete and therefore have no value.
- Loss due to theft.
- Pricing or value decreases.
- Any other general loss.

To accommodate for this shrinkage, another journal entry would have to be made to credit inventory and to debit supplies.

INVENTORY ERRORS

Hospital supplies are dispersed geographically and decentralized throughout the hospital in multiple rooms, closets, and other storage areas. A physical count of the inventory results in a figure being recorded on the balance sheet as inventory. It is quite common to have errors in the counts, to have pricing discrepancies due to a large item master and complex pricing structure, or to overlook certain pockets of supply, which might understate or overstate the balance sheet.

One concern already stated is the effect that inventory errors have on reported earnings, especially as inventory does play a role in determining current-period operating margins. For tax-exempt or nonprofit organizations, the relative size of earnings may not matter, but in for-profit hospitals, there has to be careful consideration of the inventory effects on earnings. Here are a couple of facts to keep in mind about inventory:

- Overstating EI leads to understating COGS and therefore overstating gross operating margin.
- Understanding EI overstates COGS and therefore understates gross margins.
- The EI of one period becomes the beginning inventory of the next period.
- An error in one period carries over to the next period, having the opposite effect on gross margin.

Inventory errors generally "correct" themselves at the end of the second period. This is one of the positive facts about inventory: eventually, all errors self-correct over time. So, if inventory is not counted one year, resulting in undervalued inventory and higher supply expense on the income statement, it will be caught and fixed in the second year when an additional count discovers the error and makes an adjustment. So, by the third period, all inventory errors have self-corrected. This is not the case for most other line items on the balance sheet.

INVENTORY RATIOS

It is important to track inventory ratios and statistics over time, to gauge the health of the business, to monitor utilization, to look for trends, and to ensure internal controls. The key is to look for consistency of the ratios, and if a ratio is far outside of the normal range or published benchmarks, then additional research and analysis can be conducted.

One of the key ratios that is used in hospitals is *days of inventory on hand,* which alternatively can be called days of supply or DIO. This metric measures the amount of inventory on hand relative to an average daily usage. The calculation can be made for either quantities or dollar values, assuming pricing is relatively stable. The calculation for days of supply is:

DIO = Total number of units on hand ÷ Average daily usage

For example, if there were 1,000 syringes on hand, and on an average day

100 were utilized, there would be 10 days of supply on hand. This is simple enough when looking at each item, but when there are thousands of items and a materials manager wants to measure the portfolio as a whole, it requires conversion to currency. In that case, the calculation would be *Annual Supply Exp* total dollar value of inventory on hand divided by average daily COGS. From the earlier example, assume an average usage or COGS of $1,000,000 monthly in a 30-day month and an average inventory of $450,000 [($500,000 + $400,000) ÷ 2]. It is possible to calculate this ratio using just EI values as well, but average inventory is more common. In this case:

$$DIO = \$450,000 \div \$33,334 = 13.5 \text{ days}$$

Another useful metric for inventory management is *inventory turnover*. This metric is often used to measure liquidity, because it shows how efficiently the organization is turning or converting supplies into cash. The metric basically is similar to the earlier definition of days of supply, but it provides another way of looking at it. The calculation of inventory turnover is:

$$\text{Inventory turnover} = [\text{Cost of goods sold} \div \text{Average inventory}]$$

In the earlier example, COGS was $1,000,000 and average inventory value was $450,000, so the inventory turnover is 2.22.

Another useful metric is *gross margin percentage*. This ratio allows tracking of the relative importance of supply cost on a hospital's supply revenue; alternatively, it can estimate the gross markup on supplies. This figure differs from the actual markup used in the Charge Description Master, of course, which is based on gross revenues and purchase cost, not actual usage or COGS. The definition for gross margin percentage is:

$$\text{Gross margin percentage} = [(\text{Net supply revenue} - \text{COGS}) \div \text{Net supply revenue}]$$

Assume a hospital generated $500,000 net in supply revenue (i.e., gross revenues less contractual adjustment and discounts for the supplies, assuming that the entire net amount is collectible), and cost of goods was $210,000. The gross margin percentage would be calculated as 58%:

$$[(\$500,000 - \$210,000) \div \$500,000] = \$290,000 \div \$500,000 = 58\%$$

If materials management departments fully charge for all hospital supplies, another useful metric is *return on inventory*. This metric basically examines the net income effect of inventory and is calculated as:

$$\text{Return on inventory} = \text{Net income} \div \text{Inventory}$$

If net income (or operating margin, after subtracting labor, supplies, and other costs from net revenues) is $50,000 and the total inventory balance at the end of the period is $500,000, then the return on inventory would be 10%. Analyzing this figure over time helps managers find useful patterns and remain focused on supply profitability.

Finally, a shrinkage calculation can be performed. Shrinkage can exist for a multitude of reasons, including theft, lack of internal controls, date expiration of supplies or drugs, and many other factors as explained earlier. Shrinkage or loss calculations can be defined in terms of percentage of total inventories. For example, shrinkage percentage would be calculated as:

$$\text{Shrinkage} = [(\text{Total book value} - \text{Observed value}) \div \text{Inventory}]$$

OTHER INVENTORY CALCULATIONS

There are a number of other important inventory calculations that can be used to monitor asset utilization and improve operational efficiencies. These analytical calculations include safety stock, customer service levels, EOQ, and cycle inventory.

Safety Stock

The basic purpose of **safety stock** is to carry additional inventory to satisfy unexpected demand (i.e., demand that exceeds the amount expected to be used, or forecasted). This unexpected demand or variability can be predicted using the calculated standard errors from the forecast and incorporating them into a final version of a forecast. For instance, if the demand plan showed 12 units being sold in a specific department in a certain period, and the actual demand was 15, a shortage or stockout would have occurred. To counter the effects of demand variability in the planning process, safety stock calculations are used to counter the uncertainty in the supply chain. Although there are multiple ways to calculate safety stock, here is the most common way, using service levels as the parameter (it is also possible to use fill rates and replenishment policies to calculate safety inventory):

$$\text{Safety stock} = sz(p)$$

where

s = standard deviation of a sample of errors from the sales and forecast history

p = desired customer service levels

$z(p)$ = z-value or number of standard deviations from the mean on a normal distribution curve for a specific service level. The higher the z-value, the lower the risk of stocking out.

Thus, safety stock builds in previous forecast errors and the desired service levels to create inventory buffers.

Customer Service Level

The customer service level is a measure of the probability that product will be available when the internal customer demands it. It can be measured in multiple ways, including product fill rates or stockout percentages, but here is the most common method.

$$\text{Customer service level} = (Q - (E(z))/100$$

where

Q = order quantity

$E(z)$ = expected number of units short

z = number of standard deviations of safety stock.

$E(z)$ can either be calculated with an equation that examines annual demand, orders placed, and orders short, or it can be estimated. For example, suppose monthly demand is 100 units and standard deviation is 10 units. If there is half a standard deviation, or $z = 0.5$, then using a z-value table finds that $z = 0.198$. Therefore, to solve for customer service level:

$$\{100 - [(0.198)(10)] \div 100\} = 98\%$$

Alternatively, and to maintain simplicity, fill rates are used to measure customer service level. Fill rate is the percentage of orders that are filled completely and accurately. Mathematically, fill rates are calculated as:

$$\text{Fill rate} = \frac{R}{O}$$

where

R = number of purchase orders or lines actually replenished
O = the total number of orders requested or submitted

Economic Order Quantity

The **economic order quantity (EOQ)** is one of the most basic calculations used to help firms improve the balancing between demand and supply. EOQ affects the lot sizes, which represent the average size in units that a firm should procure at a given time to take advantage of economies of scale. Since many hospitals use a JIT basis of replenishment and have no inventory outside of the distributor, this formula may not be useful for them. For hospitals that own their own inventory or buy in bulk, and break down and distribute that inventory to the nursing units and floors when required, this formula will be useful. Using the EOQ formula, hospitals can define the optimal amount of inventory to reduce overall inventory carrying costs, reduce working capital, while maintaining adequate service levels. The formula is as follows:

$$\text{EOQ} = \sqrt{\frac{2(\text{Annual Usage}) \times (\text{Order Cost})}{(\text{Annual Carrying Cost})}}$$

where the annual supply usage is in units, the order cost (i.e., purchase or setup costs) is the total costs each time an item is ordered, and the annual carrying cost is the total cost of keeping inventory on hand (e.g., warehouse or storage costs, taxes, insurance, etc). Carrying cost is usually stated as a percentage of the total dollar amount spent on products.

In reality, the EOQ is extremely valuable, but it is rarely used in practice because of the difficulties in implementing it and capturing the required data elements. It works best when demand is fairly stable or certain and when quantity discounts are minimized.

Cycle Inventory

The calculation of **cycle inventory** is used to manage the effects of lot sizes that cannot be matched precisely to actual demand (e.g., if a hospital needs to produce 100 units to balance demand with supply but the required lot size is 200, the difference—averaged over time—is the cycle inventory). The calculation is fairly straightforward as follows:

$$\text{Cycle inventory} = (\text{Lot size} \div 2)$$

LIMITATIONS OF INVENTORY RATIOS

There are four limitations to the use of inventory ratios in health care. First, all ratios are meaningless unless they are tracked and measured over time. An inventory ratio equal to 2.2, without understanding the context and specific department, is meaningless by itself. This ratio must have points of comparison, such as looking at other departments of similar scope and structure. Most importantly, it has to be tracked consistently over time to see if the metric is improving, stable, or declining.

Second, there have to be average values and standard deviations that are expected for each metric. Tracking the ratio monthly relative to the average and minimum-maximum standard deviations provides very useful information that allows application of exception management and looks for red alerts and potential problems.

Third, ratios have to be tracked relative to other hospitals in the industry. A 2.2 turnover ratio in the healthcare industry means nothing by itself. Attempting to benchmark turns in health care against other industries is irrelevant. Average turns in the publishing business might be 50, while the grocery industry might be 20, because the industry has expected demand variability that drives unique inventory behaviors.

Fourth and most important, if inventory is not consistently and comprehensively measured in each location, it is impossible to produce valuable statistics. Comparison of inventory benchmarks is fairly impractical in the nonprofit hospital structure at this time, given the variety of different treatments that inventories and supplies are given. If one hospital expenses all of its items as purchased and does not count any inventory except possibly what is stored in a central warehouse, then the inventory would be significantly undervalued and the COGS would appear overstated. A ratio for this type of hospital cannot be compared equitably against a hospital that comprehensively values inventory for all locations. The key is to select the benchmark hospitals carefully—probably from the for-profit hospital sector that is more methodical about the use of generally accepted accounting principles and proper valuation techniques.

INVENTORY POLICIES AND PROCEDURES

A hospital needs to have a policy in place to ensure that it is comprehensively and completely valuing and managing its inventories. At a minimum, all of the components described earlier need to be in this policy (e.g., valuation method), but the policy should contain all of the following as well:

- *Inventory capitalization criteria.* This policy should focus on which inventories to **capitalize** (to hold as an asset on the balance sheet), thresholds for "materiality," and general expense versus capitalization procedures.
- *Scope and purpose of inventory.* This policy should detail the extent of coverage and the role of internal auditing in inventory management and should generally provide the framework for concepts of inventory accounting.
- *Periodic versus perpetual.* This section, if not detailed in other policies, should focus on the method of accounting for inventories— either perpetual or periodic—and discuss which is appropriate, preferred, and allowable.
- *Definition of supply versus inventory.* This policy is probably a subset of a policy listed earlier, but it should clearly define when to expense supplies versus capitalize them.
- *Inventory reporting requirements.* This policy should describe the timing and nature of management reporting, as well as define acceptable metrics and baselines.
- *Instructions for cycle counts.* This policy should provide details around cycle counts, if used in a perpetual or periodic method, and describe how they should be administered, what precount instructions are required, what level of documentation is acceptable, and how to report timelines back to the general ledger.
- *Instructions for other periodic physical inventory counts.* This policy is the same as that defined earlier, only for other more comprehensive periodic counts, such as the end of the fiscal year.

- *Treatment of obsolete inventory.* This policy should clearly define how to account for obsolete inventories. **Obsolete** means that the useful life of the product has expired. This policy should establish which accounting treatments will be given, how to physically dispose of inventory, and instructions for reverse flow logistics.
- *Calculation of period end inventories.* This policy describes how the final accounting entry will be determined for a fiscal period, given the observed inventory count plus adding all receipts and netting all issues out.
- *Management of consignment inventories.* This policy should describe physical location of consignment inventories, procedures for notes or entries into non–general ledger systems, and general segregation of owned versus consigned inventories.
- *Use of systems, RFID, and bar codes.* This policy should lay foundations for deployment of systems that meet key criteria of automation; use standard coding technologies; and allow for real-time, perpetual management of inventories.
- *Receiving of materials into inventory.* This policy governs how materials are systematically received into a hospital resource system and describes the accounting entries necessary to increment inventory, plus how to track and manage inventory once it has been received.
- *Treating shrinkage and suspected inventory losses.* This policy discusses the accounting entries necessary to support shrinkage and loss, and also describes the documentation required in the event of theft. Loss prevention procedures should also be documented here.
- *Inventory measurements and metrics.* This policy sets the required inventory calculations that must be managed by each inventory location, including a description of the metric, a definition, and acceptable data sources.
- *Approved inventory valuation methods.* This policy outlines which of the generally accepted accounting procedures are allowable for each hospital, whether they are LIFO, FIFO, weighted average, retail method, or some other method.
- *Inventory records retention.* This policy governs the retention period (i.e., length of time a document must be maintained by regulatory bodies) for inventory records, including systems transaction history.
- *Internal pricing and charging.* This policy outlines how internal pricing, cost transfers, or other chargeback processes work for supply cost allocation to floors and units, if any.

INVENTORY PLANNING

Planning and managing inventory are vital to effective inventory management, sales and operations planning, and collaborative planning forecasting and replenishment (both of which will be described later). The purpose of inventory is to buffer the variability inherent in both supply and demand environments. In a perfect world, where demand is constant and manufacturers or distributors supply the exact amounts in the plan, no inventory is necessary. However, in real life, this variability or fluctuation in the market is inevitable, and effective business processes have to be put in place to plan and manage accordingly.

The key aspects of inventory planning include:

1. Establishing safety and cycle inventory policy levels.

2. Obtaining the right amount of items just at the point of need or consumption.

3. Evaluating demand and planning inventory positioning accordingly.

4. Building effective replenishment processes based on collaborative demand plans and inventory policies.

The first of these, developing inventory policies, should be consistent with the ABC classification schemes for the key internal customers. ABC analysis assigns priorities based on volumes, margins, turnover, required service levels, or other relevant metric that shows relative importance compared to others across key dimensions. They should be statistically based (e.g., using previous forecasting errors and real demand forecasts) and should be continually updated with new assumptions, such as lead times. Finding an optimal safety stock level, for example, should not be taken lightly. In many companies, the safety stock levels are established by setting vague and general rules, such as "15 days on hand for all products." These types of policies have devastating results for firm economics. If an average hospital changes its blanket policy of 30 days on hand at all locations to a statistically based demand estimate, it could possibly reduce total inventories by nearly 25%—with no service impact on operations.

Additionally, hospitals must adopt some of the best practices for inventory management, such as:

- Continually updating business rules and assumptions.
- Using advanced statistical engines to calculate accurate inventory levels based on rough-cut demand-supply balances.

- Building safety policies around specific customer groups or product categories.
- Managing lead times, usage, and overall safety stocks held at each location.
- Using an ABC customer classification scheme to drive inventory business rules.
- Building and continually improving demand forecasts.
- Collaborating on schedules and changes in customer operations that might affect inventory (e.g., new operating room suite opening five additional beds).

One of the ways to improve inventory planning is to utilize vendor-managed inventory. **Vendor-managed inventory (VMI)** is a process whereby a supplier manages the inventory stock levels for its customers based on forecasted usage or demand. The largest healthcare distributors have VMI programs in place with many of their largest accounts. The process is designed to be proactive by the supplier, which controls the distribution plans and sends out orders with minimal involvement from the customer. VMI essentially places the control around inventory planning, and the risks of inventory levels, in the hands of the supplier, which can be very beneficial from a cost perspective.

INVENTORY AUDIT

Internal and external auditors routinely **audit** (i.e., examine, verify) inventories in most hospitals. The primary role of an audit function is twofold: financial and operational. Financial audits typically focus on ensuring four things:

1. The existence and completeness of inventory.
2. That valuations on the books are materially correct and use appropriate pricing methods.
3. That the presentation and disclosure of inventory balances on the published financial statements are accurate.
4. That ownership of all inventory has been established.

Operational audits tend to focus on whether hospitals are utilizing resources in the most appropriate manner; therefore, they focus on issues of effectiveness, efficiency, and compliance.

The following is a sample inventory audit program that may be similar to one used in a hospital. It is important that operational managers understand how they may be reviewed, so that appropriate policies, procedures, staffing, systems, and other management systems can be developed to ensure operational excellence.

A. Audit Overview, Purpose, and Scope

Audit guidelines exist to identify the specific financial controls and business procedures to be assessed as part of the inventory review and audit process. This includes existing cycle count procedures and controls over picking, packing, staging, and distribution of both inbound and outbound inventory. The objectives of this review are to:

- Confirm and test the accuracy of the ledger or subledger (i.e., book) to physical inventory balances in total and in all locations *(existence, completeness, ownership)*.

- Ensure that inventories are properly stated at the lower of cost or market determined by a specific method, such as FIFO *(valuation)*.

- Assess the effectiveness of these processes in ensuring, recording, and documenting the accuracy of the inventory balances *(presentation, disclosure)*.

- Assess the effectiveness of the area's inventory cycle count process in identifying shortages, shrinkage, and other errors in balance or counts *(effectiveness, compliance)*.

- Observe and document processes affecting inventory, such as shipping and receiving *(efficiency, accuracy)*.

B. Planning and Initial Review

During this phase of an audit, the auditors will:

1. Obtain and review prior working papers and historical audits, if any.

2. Send a copy of the prior audit cycle and periodic count programs, including documentation around ABC classifications or procedures, to the materials manager or inventory manager.

3. Discuss the scope of the audit and background information with management.

4. Request copies of any information required by warehouse or inventory location, including: current organizational chart, business procedures and inventory policies, cycle and periodic count procedures, and ratio analyses conducted year to date.

5. Request current book values or stock status (stock on hand) report for facility.

6. Request copies of reconciliations from general ledger balances against perpetual reconciliations, and for general ledger versus physical inventories (cycle counts).

7. Review custody chain and organizational structure. Meet management team, and get oriented to departmental layout and staff. Ensure existence and location of all inventory locations to be included in the count process.

C. Observation and Documentation

During this phase of the audit, operations managers can expect the auditors to do the following:

1. Follow up on results of last inventory audit and any solutions or action items that should have been implemented.

2. Discuss the organization. Specifically, identify the individuals responsible for the cycle count program, including those employees responsible for counting, reconciling, and reporting. Determine if there were any significant organizational changes (e.g., terminations, resignations) of warehouse or inventory staff recently, specifically, any management or senior-level changes. Document accordingly.

3. Inquire about any major systems changes at the facility or any major changes in the cycle count process since the last audit. Thoroughly review the documentation from the last audit, and document any changes.

4. Review the last audit of inventory counts. Review the ABC classification scheme for inventory. Select three of each item in each

classification for review. Count quantity on hand for each of these items, and document next to the stock status report from inventory or the ERP system. Document any reason for discrepancy or variance.

5. Review reported results for the year, including a focus on

   • Inventory turn ratios and loss calculations.

   • Adjustments that were conducted.

   • General ledger entries not related to receipts and issues.

6. Document the process for making, reviewing, and approving adjustments into the hospital resource planning system or the inventory system. Document cutoff times. Document if any adjustments were made for deleting inventory or changing entries once they were recorded. Document results of discrepancy.

7. Document any variances between the general ledger and inventory systems. Document if either system excludes quantities due to different status (e.g., consignment) or other locations (e.g., distributed par locations, patient rooms, etc.).

8. Observe the picking and packing process. Are there manual forms for tracking picking during the count process (so as not to affect book values)? Are there appropriate levels of documentation? How does the distribution manifest get into the ERP or inventory system? What happens to a product in the ERP or inventory system if a product is picked but not shipped or distributed? Do exception reports appear?

9. Inquire into the usage and status of systems. Are the ERP or inventory systems working properly? Do they appropriately decrement and increment inventory as materials are issued and received? Is there utilization of bar coding or other automated systems for tracking movements? Is there a data flow diagram available for the systems that shows information flows?

10. Observe the process of receiving inventory into the ERP or inventory system. Are purchase orders properly loaded? Compare system versus paperwork from manufacturer or distributor against system. Are receipts properly processed against the purchase order? Against the proper line number? Document the process for receiving goods. Select one receipt and observe processing into inventory.

11. Inquire into any expired products. Are they medical supplies or pharmaceuticals? If pharmaceuticals, were they controlled properly based on the control level of drug per the Drug Enforcement Agency? Were all adjustments out of inventory handled properly? Where do the items physically move to after inventory (e.g., donated to a distribution company that delivers them to countries in need, etc.)?

D. Reporting and Presentation

1. Summarize audit findings and discuss with local management on the last day of field work. Develop and agree to proposed solutions with local management. Draft audit report.

2. Submit draft audit report to inventory or materials managers for review and comments. Include these comments into final report. Finalize and distribute report.

INVENTORY MANAGEMENT EXPECTATIONS

Inventory ratios are metrics that gauge how well inventory is being utilized or managed over time. The expectation of materials managers is not only to continuously improve these metrics, but to also focus on inventory utilization, order fulfillment efficiency, revenue generation, and operational efficiency.

Inventory Utilization

This performance indicator measures how efficient the group is in delivering and managing overall inventories for the organization. The metric is defined as both the total inventory values, as well as the DIO, which is a better metric for measuring inventory when patient volumes are growing. Tracking current DIO, setting a targeted level, and then managing toward that goal improves inventory utilization.

Order Fulfillment Efficiency

This measures the efficiency of a department's picking, packing, and handling process. It should be measured as both the overall cycle time for fulfilling orders as well as number of items picked per hour, plus any number of other metrics available. Similarly, fill rates can be used.

Revenue Management

Inventory is responsible for maximizing revenue sources, such as for pharmaceutical items, medical supplies, or durable medical equipment. Capturing 100% of the potential revenues and minimizing the associated expenses is the goal. Tracking of the return on inventory, as calculated earlier, ensures that inventory is successfully generating revenues for the organization.

Operational Effectiveness

This metric measures the extent to which a department is effectively performing a variety of activities necessary to continually improve, including:

- Setting optimal inventory levels, including the creation of forecasts and plans with key vendors and distributors.
- Monitoring product mix and key item usage, including the development of ABC inventory classifications.
- Ensuring 100% customer service levels.
- Ensuring inventory accuracy through cycle counts and systematic tracking of issues and receipts.
- Continually improving staff productivity and eliminating redundancies.

Focusing inventory management efforts around each of these four areas, and developing the right set of metrics and ratios for inclusion in a scorecard, will improve the overall management and utilization of hospital inventories.

CHAPTER SUMMARY

Inventory represents supplies that have been purchased but not yet consumed or utilized. Inventory in health care is very disaggregated throughout hundreds of rooms, clinics, and storage areas. Managing and accounting for inventories represent a very complex subject that is common in the manufacturing or retail industries but not very well understood in health care, given its focus on managing COGS.

A number of important accounting entries need to be understood by the operations manager, since these entries form the basis for the financial statements. The uses of financial ratios are very important in providing internal controls over inventory because they allow analysts to understand typical inventory utilization behavior and look for exceptions and deviations. Other techniques and ratios use analytical techniques to minimize costs and continuously review asset utilization. Audits of inventory are focused on reducing risks of loss and maintaining adequate controls over these expensive resources. Incorporating audit concepts in daily inventory management improves operational effectiveness immensely.

KEY TERMS

audit; capitalize; case mix index; chargeable; consignment in; consignment out; cost of goods sold (COGS); cycle inventory; economic order quantity (EOQ); first in, first out (FIFO); first out (LIFO); generally accepted accounting principles (GAAP); inventory; last in, lower of cost or market (LCM); net realizable value; obsolete; periodic inventory; perpetual inventory; safety stock; shrinkage; timing; valuation; vendor-managed inventory (VMI); weighted average

DISCUSSION QUESTIONS

1. What is inventory?
2. What distinguishes inventory from a supply?
3. What are five benefits to having inventory in a healthcare supply chain?
4. What are two reasons not to hold inventory?
5. Why does GAAP help ensure accurate financial accounting of inventory?
6. Should consigned inventory be counted on the balance sheet for a hospital?
7. Does inventory normally have a debit or a credit balance?
8. Compare the basic differences among the LIFO, FIFO, and weighted average valuation methods.
9. Why is perpetual inventory so important?

10. What does DIO measure?

11. Describe vendor-managed inventory.

12. Define shrinkage and possible sources of loss.

13. Why is it important to understand the elements of an inventory audit?

EXERCISE PROBLEMS

1. A community hospital in Pennsylvania has a 15% supply expense ratio. If total operating expenses are $1,000,000 this month, what is the total annual cost of supplies? $(\$1 \text{ million})(12)(.15) = \$1.8 \text{ million}/\text{yr}.$

2. A hospital buys certain supplies for $50 each. The average markup is 100%. Additional selling costs are 25% of the total cost. What is the net realizable value? *ceiling price* $(\$50)(1+1)-(.25)(\$100) = \$75 \text{ (ceiling price)}$ *What is the 'floor price'?* ceiling – profit margin = $75 - 50 = 25$

3. Assume this same product has a current replacement cost of $40. What is the lower of cost or market?

Adjusted entry *spreadsheet entry would show additional $50,000 of expense* 4. An organization discovers in a physical inventory count that the actual inventory on hand is $50,000 less than the value on the books. Write the accounting entry to record this shrinkage transaction. *P. 291 total dollar value of avg. inventory on hand*

pp. 292–293 *$2 million* *($10 million/360 days) = 72 days* 5. Miami Trinity Healthcare has an average inventory balance of $2 million. The total annual supply expense is $10 million. Using a 360-day year, calculate the DIO. $\frac{COGS}{(p.289)}$ $10 \text{ million}/360 = \text{Avg. daily COGS}$ *DIO = 72 days.*

6. A product has total usage of 1,000 over the course of the year. Each item costs $20. The transactional order cost from procurement is $50 each transaction, and the annual carrying cost is 10% of the total annual cost. Calculate the EOQ.

DIO = days of inventory on hand or days of supply

REFERENCES

Bragg, Steven M. (2006). *Inventory Accounting: A Comprehensive Guide*. New York: John Wiley & Sons.

Healthcare Financial Management Association. (2005). *2005 Supply Chain Benchmarking Survey*. Washington, DC: HFMA.

Muller, Max. (2002). *Essentials of Inventory Management*. New York: American Management Association.

Classifying and Managing Products

Goals of This Chapter

1. Define items
2. Describe data classification and the United Nations Standard Products and Services Code (UNSPSC)
3. Understand the role of hospital resource systems
4. Understand the role of forecasting for new-item purchases

As discussed in previous chapters, a supply chain manages three key flows—information (data), finances (cash), and products (items). This chapter focuses on two of these: information and items. Specifically, the role of managing data quality and item structure is detailed because this is necessary to drive efficient procurement, replenishment, and inventory of goods. This chapter provides definitions of the term *item,* explains the rationale behind data classification schemes, describes the role that enterprise resource planning (ERP) and information systems play in managing item masters, and introduces a process for understanding the patterns in data that can help improve product forecasting and replenishment.

ITEMS AND ATTRIBUTES

Much of Part III has so far focused on the management of products, or goods, through a hospital's supply chain. These goods are also called *items*. For some, an item is inherently understood and needs no definition. For many others, an item is complex and needs further clarification.

An **item** is any physical good that is procured for ultimate use or consumption, whether in its current form or following some degree of processing or transformation. An item has physical characteristics—that is, it can be touched, weighed, moved, and stored—and it has quantitative characteristics. Quantitative characteristics include dimensions, such as size, weight, density, firmness, color, and the like. Contrary to services, such as healthcare service delivery that involves delivery of procedures or other qualitative characteristics, items are physical goods.

An item that is in its final form for consumption or utilization is called a **finished good**. A finished good will not be further processed, mixed, blended, processed, or otherwise transformed. Most of the goods purchased in hospital supply chains are finished goods. A finished item can be a syringe, a chair, or a loaf of bread.

Items that need further processing or transformation are called raw materials or **intermediate goods**. Intravenous injection, or IV bags, which might require additional processing with other injectable solutions, are intermediate goods. Hospital pharmacies that compound or mix their own drugs also manage intermediate goods. In pharmacies, the process of combining multiple fluids is called **admixture**, while the breakdown of tablets or solid substances is called **compounding**. These types of items are somewhat more complex, because they require understanding of bills of materials, or multiple items that comprise each finished goods item. A **bill of material** is a listing or recipe that defines the specific raw materials or components and the quantities required to create a finished good. For example, if 5% dextrose and 1% iodine are the two key components a pharmacy uses to blend with an IV bag, these two items are the raw materials on the bill of material.

Thus, items have quantitative and sometimes qualitative characteristics. These characteristics uniquely define each item and make it somewhat distinct. Walking down the bread aisle in the grocery store, you will see many loaves of bread, which can be described by their taste or weight attributes. For example, bread might be wheat, thinly sliced, honey flavored, one pound, oval shaped, artisan, or split-top.

Each of these defining characteristics of an item can therefore be called its **attributes**. Attributes are nothing more than the quantitative and qualitative characteristics that help to explain and define an item. These attributes are useful for three primary reasons:

1. They describe an item and allow categorization and classification to occur. Without classification, it would be impossible to purchase and manage thousands of items for a hospital's supply chain.

2. It facilitates electronic transaction processing among manufacturers, distributors, and hospitals, using common language, which expedites purchasing and logistical processes and streamlines commerce. Coding of each item, in a standardized system, can allow buyers and sellers to exchange data faster and more efficiently, which ultimately results in lower inventories and quicker response.

3. They allow sophisticated operations managers to analyze patterns and trends that otherwise would not be evident. By "slicing and dicing" data using attributes, and not just looking at discriminate analysis at the lowest levels, it is possible to find exceptions and patterns to improve overall results.

All of these are described in more detail later in this chapter.

DATA HIERARCHIES

A **hierarchy** is a classification system that organizes data around common attributes. These attributes as they are aggregated are called **categories** in supply chain and marketing terminology. A hierarchy helps analyze data from a different level and allows groupings to make sense of data more readily. For example, a hospital might use 2″ × 2″ bandages and then replace them with 1.5″ × 2″ bandages. The first bandage might be made and purchased from three vendors, and the second from two vendors. Therefore, at the lowest level for these items, there would be five distinct stock-keeping units. A **stock-keeping unit (SKU)** is a specific item at a specific unit of measure. SKUs represent the lowest level in an item hierarchy, as shown in **Figure 13–1**. Notice in this figure that one type of medical supply is a glove. A glove category can be decomposed by multiple attributes: latex versus nitrile, powder versus powder-free, a variety of different colors and scents, sterile and nonsterile, all sizes, and a variety of manufacturers. Exploding, or *decomposing,* each of these individual hierarchies shows different levels of details and attributes.

FIGURE 13–1 Item Hierarchy

In terms of an item or product hierarchy, products are classified according to a standard set of attributes, uses, and characteristics. An aggregation of items that share similar attributes creates different categories, and these categories roll up to others. Aggregating items up to higher levels allows decisions to be made that might not be evident if items were managed only at the lowest level of detail.

A non-healthcare example might make this clearer. When a consumer walks into a grocery store wanting to purchase toothpaste, he or she walks into that aisle and sees multiple brands, flavors, and sizes—each offering slightly different benefits. A specific tube of toothpaste is an individual SKU, but this can be aggregated up by brands: Crest, Colgate, Aquafresh, and so on. Each of these brands can then be aggregated based on other categories. If the grocery store wanted to decide which item was making the most profit so that they could market that item a little differently (e.g., position on an end-cap display, or to adjust pricing), it would be impossible given that an average large-scale store has more than 200 different toothpaste SKUs. But, if the store could slice that data differently among all 200 SKUs, they might find that a certain size, brand, or flavor dominated sales. What if the new strawberry mint toothpaste had 45% of sales in the last month, spread among 40 individual items? They never would have noticed the trend if they hadn't captured the attributes in the hierarchy.

In hospitals, the most commonly purchased items are in the general category called *medical supplies and equipment.* This category can further be described in multiple ways, depending on the hospital. The next lower level could be organized by specialty, such as surgical or cardiology, or by major type of use.

THE NEED FOR STANDARDS

Most hospitals create their own categories, which are usually quite limited and not very robust. It has been said that the average hospital has only about 25% of its items properly classified in a hierarchical categorical system. And, because healthcare distributors and manufacturers have not combined to create standards, each hospital has historically done its own thing.

Several companies and organizations have attempted to create a comprehensive standard for classifying items in health care. Unlike the retail and consumer goods industries, however, which are closely integrated and aligned, the healthcare supply chain is quite fragmented and segmented. In consumer goods, all manufacturers, distributors, and retailers use common coding and classification systems, and they share information routinely and often to help facilitate faster transactions and lower total costs. Organizations such as the Uniform Code Council and the Voluntary Interindustry Commerce Standards Association help promote commerce across the globe and across many industries. Health care, however, has been slow to adopt such standards and has not rapidly joined forces with overwhelming participation.

The healthcare industry lags behind other industries for the following reasons:

- *Late adopters.* Historically, hospitals and health care are always late adopters of new tools and technology when they relate to business operations instead of medical technology.
- *Fragmentation.* The healthcare supply chain is fragmented by groups that focus on nursing, medical, pharmacy, imaging, and

other specialties. Vendors tend to follow their specialty groups and not act as one with other vendors. Similarly, medical supply distributors are fragmented and highly competitive and have not historically collaborated well to create industrywide improvements. Neither have manufacturers, except for those that also serve retail chains with consumer-based medical supplies. Finally, hospitals are fragmented.

- *Lack of resources.* Hospitals especially are plagued by low hospital operating margins, which typically encourages operations management to allocate resources to pressing issues affecting them today, not those that can help improve their processes tomorrow.

- *Education.* In other industries, management is keenly aware of the gains that can be made from improving commerce flow among vendors. In hospitals, however, there is a lack of education about these types of issues; hospital management tends to be more concerned with patient and clinical issues and is simply not aware of the role standards can play in improving overall competitive advantage, reducing costs, and increasing productivity.

During the last decade, however, the healthcare industry has slowly started to work toward adoption of standards. Many healthcare organizations, such as the Healthcare Information and Management Systems Society and the American Hospital Association, are pushing for legislation, regulation, or other standards that unite the industry more comprehensively. This participation will not come easy, given the reasons listed earlier.

Three organizations are positioning themselves to help create standards in the industry: the Health Industry Business Communications Council (HIBCC), the Coalition for Healthcare eStandards (CheS), and the UNSPSC. The HIBCC has thus far focused on standards for communicating electronically using electronic data interchange. The HIBCC has advocated standards for unique hospital identification numbers, as well as standards for bar coding and universal product numbers. The HIBCC collaborative promises to be very beneficial to the industry in the long term (see Chapter 14 for a more detailed discussion). The CheS has also been pushing for standards around customer and product identification. For purposes of standards around items, the UNSPSC has been the lead organization for product classification and coding.

UNITED NATIONS STANDARDS PRODUCTS AND SERVICES CODE

The **United Nations Standard Products and Services Code (UNSPSC)** is a coding system that can be used across all industries, for all types of goods and services. It is a classification system that has evolved over many years, and it was originally developed by the United Nations Development Programme and Dun & Bradstreet Corporation in 1998 (UNSPSC. org, 2006).

UNSPSC classifies item level data into a hierarchy that is organized as follows:

Segment >> Family >> Class >> Commodity >> Business function

A segment is the highest level category, and the business function is the lowest. The code can be up to 10 digits long, with 2 digits representing each of the five levels of the hierarchy although the standard code is usually 8 digits long.

For example, look back to the gloves example in Figure 13–1. Gloves overall fit into the highest segment called "medical equipment, accessories, and supplies" in the UNSPSC schema. This is segment 42. Within segment 42, there are 20 different families, such as veterinary supplies, surgical products, nutrition, and many more. Gloves fit into family 13, "medical apparel and textiles." In this family, there are 3 classes—surgical textiles, housekeeping textiles, and medical gloves, which is class 22. At this point, the class can be broken down into another 5 commodities, including glove boxes, finger cots, and surgical gloves. Assuming that the gloves in the figure are medical, general-purpose gloves, they are categorized as commodity 03. The complete eight-digit code for these gloves would therefore be 42-13-22-03.

How can this code be useful? This code helps hospitals improve their overall operating efficiency. If the supply chain can standardize this coding, then, as hospitals purchase items from distributors, they can use this as a common code. Each party in the chain has its own fragmented system, so a distributor might code this same product 123, a manufacturer might code the product ABC, and the hospitals code the same product as XYZ. For hospitals to streamline their procedures, they need to use automated purchasing processes, sharing the right item numbers collaboratively among all parties. This code can then be shared with distributors during the ordering process automatically; with no manual intervention, then, the order can be filled and shipped.

Today, each party maintains a cross-reference table that links a hospital's item number against its own item master, or the party requires the hospital to disregard its own item numbers and use the vendor's. Either way, it takes multiple cross-references, duplicate entries, manual effort, and careful oversight for each item procured. This is a complex and lengthy process, which guarantees a high level of returns and lower productivity.

ITEM MASTERS IN THE ERP

Aligning the supply chain with a common product identification system will improve operational efficiencies, if adopted by the industry as a whole. In preparation, hospitals must ensure that the ERP, or other procurement and replenishment systems in use, have robust and complete item master data. An **item master** stores item-level data. These data include important attribute fields necessary for both transactional processing and analytical reporting. **Table 13–1** shows the optimal attributes for an item master in a hospital.

There are probably significantly more attributes that a hospital might want to manage if it used advanced analyses and planning, but those shown in Table 13–1 are some of the most significant ones for successful item master management. These attributes need to be maintained in database fields, which can be sorted and searched independently of the item. Many hospitals use one large comment field to capture free-form text and possibly significant attributes. This is a big mistake, though, because text fields are not searchable and therefore are of little value in terms of analysis, reporting, and managing items.

Thus, attributes are important because they allow users to separately sort them, report on different types of aggregation, and analyze patterns and trends. The term **slice and dice** is used to describe the process of breaking data down into component parts, using different angles or perspectives. If a hospital is negotiating a contract for sterile gloves, and all the information it has is at the lowest level, it loses significant bargaining power. If it walks into negotiations understanding all of the buying behavior, such as type, color, and size, as well as trends and forecasts for the future, its analysis will probably yield significant cost savings.

Table 13–1 Item Master Attributes

Attribute	Purpose
Item Number	Order fulfillment
UNSPSC	Electronic commerce
Segment	Spend analysis
Family	Spend analysis
Class	Spend analysis
Commodity	Spend analysis
Color	Spend analysis
Size	Spend analysis
Weight	Spend analysis
Unit of measure	Spend analysis
Manufacturer	Contract negotiation
Contract/GPO number	Contract negotiation
Cost	Spend analysis & contract negotiation
Chargeable flag	Revenue generation
Chargeable price	Revenue generation
ABC classification	Inventory management
Life-cycle stage	Forecasting

The concepts of rollup and drilldown are also important. A **rollup** is an aggregation in the hierarchy. Rolling up all gloves into higher-level families and segments provides useful reporting and analyses. Similarly, **drilldown** allows user to continuously explore data deeper by moving lower within the hierarchy, thus helping further refine, understand, and analyze data at more descriptive levels using narrowly defined attributes. Drilldowns are useful when the analyses need to move from general to more specific.

ENTERPRISE RESOURCE PLANNING SYSTEMS

In addition to storing item-level data, ERP systems are essential to integrate the activities of an organization, including financial, human resources, quality, procurement, and inventory management. In most industries, the **enterprise resource planning (ERP) system** is the primary "system of record" to track products or services provided, costs, customers, and cash associated with the entire operation. In health care, the ERP plays an important, but somewhat reduced role.

ERP systems originated in the manufacturing sector and evolved from the need to understand all aspects of goods manufactured—from the time they were procured until the time they were sold. ERPs were designed to integrate, or consolidate, all data and processes to eliminate redundant technology and business processes, to eliminate double-keying of information into multiple information systems, and to ensure a comprehensive view of the entire operation. Questions about the business—such as "What is the true cost of goods sold for a specific product" or "What is the real profit margin for a certain product line?"—could be addressed more accurately with one primary system.

Without integration of systems into a single ERP, manufacturing industries found that they did not have complete information and were often unable to make intelligent decisions (O'Brien, 1996). ERPs then became the repository for managing human resources and payrolls (because they play a critical cost and quality role in manufacturing goods), quality management (tracking returns, defects), production planning (which plant produces specific products at targeted production levels), procurement, inventory, general ledger and financial reporting, customer relationship management (tracking all details about customers, such as their locations, pricing, and usage patterns), and many other important activities. An ERP is very prevalent now in most industries. The primary roles of an ERP system are outlined in **Figure 13-2**.

In hospitals, ERPs play a somewhat reduced role. In Figure 13-2, those functions highlighted are hospital specific, while the others represent the range of functionality offered in other industries. The reduced functionality is primarily because hospitals are service intensive and don't have a manufacturing or finished goods conversion process. Management of service lines (e.g., radiology) often requires its own discrete specialized systems, like picture archiving and communication system, which are not part of a typical ERP.

The role of a hospital ERP tends to focus primarily on the financial, human resources, and supply chain components. If best practices are used—such as streamlining processes prior to the system implementation, eliminating paper-based reports, and validating organizational roles and responsibilities for the new processes—then hospital ERPs can make a significant contribution to a hospital's financial performance.

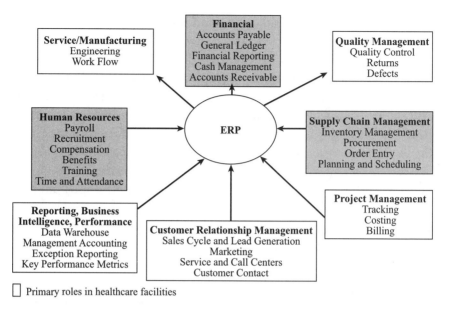

FIGURE 13–2 The Scope of ERP Systems

The largest ERP systems are offered by vendors such as SAP (www.sap.com) and Oracle (www.oracle.com), which offer solutions across multiple industries. For healthcare systems and hospitals, one of the larger ERP players is Lawson Software (www.lawson.com). There has been significant consolidation recently in enterprise systems, and many of the other large players, such as Peoplesoft, JD Edwards, and Baan, have all been acquired by one of these larger, more dominant vendors.

Advantages of an ERP

One of the primary advantages of an ERP is that it helps integrate all data and processes across the enterprise. For hospitals, if a stand-alone system is used for procurement and a separate system for inventory, then significant duplicate entry would be required to manage item masters, pricing, and product utilization. Similarly, if accounts payable doesn't leverage the same system as purchasing, then it would require extensive manual effort to confirm receipts of items purchased prior to payment. A single system helps integrate the business process, which helps improve overall internal business controls.

Another key advantage is that it helps eliminate redundant or duplicate systems. If each department or process used its own systems, there would literally be dozens or hundreds of small systems in existence. Each system requires specialized knowledge, training, and support, which is very expensive from an information technology investment perspective. ERP also helps eliminate paper; it provides formal electronic records for all aspects of a business process, thus eliminating the need for printing and filing each transaction (such as an order or invoice).

Most importantly, ERPs help provide full revenue cycle integration for patients—from point of invoice to point of cash receipt. If used properly in health care, it helps eliminate valuable cycle time and allows posting of charges on patients' bills at the time of administration, rather than batching hours or even days later.

THE ITEM LIFE CYCLE

As hospitals begin to use items, hierarchies, and item masters to improve the management of their data, it is important to understand the usage, or demand patterns for each item. In health care, innovation continuously brings new technologies, equipment, and supplies to market that help physicians and providers improve the quality of care. These new items replace older ones and have their own sets of attributes and economics. Behavioral and structural change in usage and demand determines the stage of the life cycle that the product occupies. For example, while a certain type of catheter might be on its way out, a new one is being introduced to replace it.

Therefore, all items move through a standard life cycle (Onkvisit & Shaw, 1989). This life cycle is comprised of six phases: pre-launch conceptual design, new-product introduction, growth, maturity, decline, and phase-out. A product that currently resides in a specific stage of the cycle has an entirely different demand pattern than a product in another stage (as discussed in the next section), and this demand pattern requires different ordering patterns and replenishment practices. The duration and magnitude of the pattern determine the overall shape of the demand pattern. **Figure 13–3** presents a standard, bell-shaped, product life-cycle curve highlighting each of these phases.

Although Figure 13–3 represents the life cycle as a bell-shaped curve, where a smooth predictable usage pattern exists in each phase, the actual

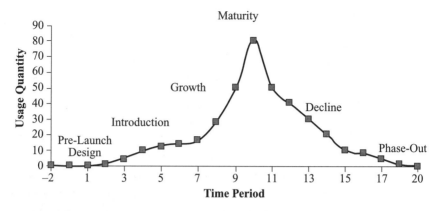

FIGURE 13–3 Life-Cycle Phases

shape of the curve is based on the specific item type, the competitive intensity of the manufacturers for that item, and the level of investment the industry is conducting for research and development. For instance, cardiology and oncology products are classic examples of industries in which items are continuously improving and evolving, while some other items, such as the syringe, have very few changes over time. As new items evolve, others must be phased out. Each of the phases is described in the rest of this section.

Pre-Launch Conceptual Design

Prior to any item ever generating usage or sales, it must be designed and launched. The pre-launch phase of the life cycle has no demand, but it is characterized by heavy investment in market and consumer research, pre-positioning of brands, test market deployment, product research and development, and extensive advertising. It is critical to focus on making planning decisions about retail outlets and channel positioning at this phase. Brand and product managers use their preliminary qualitative and quantitative figures to estimate potential demand for the product and to make a "go–no go" decision on whether to move forward with the product. Estimates of market share, prices, competitive maneuvers, and expected sales are all outcomes of this phase in the process. An estimate of the duration and magnitude of the life cycle is required. Additionally, time and speed are of the essence in this phase, because plans are continually revisited and adapted on an hour-by-hour basis.

New-Product Introduction

During the new-product introduction phase of the life cycle, demand can exhibit multiple patterns. In some cases, sales for well-known brand or product extensions can soar instantly, such as in high-tech industries or certain food lines. Other times, the pattern is less defined, and the slope of the demand curve is very gradual. At this point, demand is very uncertain, making planning more difficult. Margins can be high, depending on the specific industry—such as pharmaceuticals, which tends to start with premium pricing that declines over time. Management of demand should be based on either association of similar patterns experienced for other new products introduced historically or on market research estimates. Demand association involves taking a product that is being phased out and associating its demand with the new product to be introduced. For example, if a 25-gram hypodermic needle is being replaced with a 27-gram needle, the historical usage must be associated with the new item to ensure that future ordering plans, contracts, and inventory plans do not use zero history and usage as the baseline. Manufacturers' tendency to use promotions during this phase can distort the true demand picture, making planning even more complex as it moves to the next phase; from their perspective, however, it is essential to ensuring "mindshare" early to gain some successes. Decisions about inventory placement and location must be made during this phase. For innovative products, there is little competition, allowing for strong margins during the introduction phase.

Growth

As products reach this phase, demand becomes more stable and predictable. Supply chain and operational managers can use trends and statistics to accurately define the pattern and can use these figures to improve ordering patterns, as well as levels of inventories. Marketing promotions, such as manufacturers' rebates and pricing discounts, are still important, but play a lesser role in generating new business; it is more important to capture others' market share. Competition has escalated rapidly, forcing smaller margins at this stage.

Maturity

Usage and demand during the maturity phase are quite stable. Competition also tends to be quite intense because the industry's structural characteristics are well known, and most competitors have entered the market by this time. As a consequence, profit margins remain fairly low. During this phase, it is imperative to have new products introduced to begin balancing the portfolio and planning for the impending decline. Supply chains have to focus on cost minimization and maintaining high customer service levels during this phase because it is extremely important not to lose any customers at this stage.

Decline

If an item is having declining usage (e.g., down from 100 per month of a specific item to less than 10 per month), the item has entered the next phase of the product life cycle. If a hospital continues to order based on minimum thresholds that are not updated continuously, significant amounts of inventory will be built that will never be consumed, which is very costly and inefficient. However, predicting demand during the decline phase is often extremely difficult. The slope, intensity, and timing of the decline make it hard to understand the demand pattern. The best way to analyze the item's decline is to explore the company's historical product declines and associate a similar timing and intensity evidenced in other products and categories. During the decline phase, prices tend to be at historical lows, and no promotions are utilized, thus simplifying the planning process somewhat.

Phase-Out

At this phase, the product has been phased out. All demand that existed has either been transferred to a complimentary or replacement item or has been moved to another product. It is important that the transition to the replacement or extension items was handled smoothly to associate or chain this product demand to the replacement.

In summary, each phase of the life cycle results in changes to the demand pattern and likewise requires a different type of technique to analyze and manage supply and demand. Where the early stages rely on judgmental demand tools, such as market research, consumer profiling, test marketing, and demand association (or product chaining), the later stages rely heavily on trend analysis and statistical forecasting. The use of collaboration internally and externally within the supply chain is essential during all phases of the life cycle to achieve improved plans and forecasts (Campbell, 2000).

Example

Consider this example. A hospital purchases 500 central venous catheter trays per week of Model A. These trays cost approximately $25 each; the weekly cost, therefore, is $12,500. The usage patterns dictated an automated replenishment program: a once-weekly order is placed with the distributor for 500 trays, to be delivered on Monday mornings. At some point, Model B has been introduced by a manufacturer's sales representative, and a few physicians are starting to explore its efficacy. Model B was introduced to the hospital's material use evaluation committee and accepted. Materials management began to purchase a few of the new-model trays, based on initial requests of 10 each week, at a cost of $40 each, or $400 total. During week 3, all physicians began using Model B.

Model A just moved from maturity to phase-out; it skipped the decline phase entirely, which is quite probable. Meanwhile, materials management continues to use its heuristic rule of once-a-week ordering patterns and realizes—more than three weeks later—that more than 1,700 items have amassed in inventory, at a cost of $42,500. At the same time, after repeated service-level issues and physician complaints, materials management decided that it needed two weeks of safety stock inventory on hand for Model B to offset the problems it was encountering, so $40,000 of safety inventory was also being stored in central stores. The clinics, seeing their physicians continuously being without the proper supplies, have also horded Model B in various examination rooms and closets. In effect, then, a total of $75,000 of inventory has been stockpiled!

The distributor sees that the new product is taking off and simultaneously builds up inventories of Model B but, because it studies usage trends more proactively, has already realized a decline of Model A and holds only 50% of the normal cycle inventory.

What happens in this case?

1. The hospital has increased its inventories by 600%.

2. The distributor has also incurred additional stock and will have to find alternative ways to sell its products, or it will ultimately charge back the hospital through higher pricing later.

3. While volumes have now increased, because orders are being placed for both items, the real productivity of procurement and materials employees has declined significantly because they are all busy working on items that don't serve a purpose.

The mission of "right goods, right time, right location, right price, and the right condition" has obviously been neglected.

An item master that is robust and supports tracking of items by attributes and phases of the life cycle—where analysts continuously scrutinize the data looking for exceptions and outliers—could have prevented this from occurring.

PRODUCT USAGE PATTERNS

The stage that an item occupies in the product life cycle greatly affects the slope and shape of the usage and demand curve in the long run. However, in the short term, as planners focus on narrower time horizons, a variety of patterns can be seen. In general, there are nine types of usage or utilization patterns that products can exhibit. These include:

- Increasing trend
- Decreasing trend
- Seasonal demand
- Random patterns
- Intermittent or lumpy
- Cyclical
- Transient or irregular
- Horizontal, even, or constant
- Auto-correlated patterns

Because the goal of effective item management is to ensure optimal purchasing, replenishment, and inventory of the right products in the right quantities, understanding the key usage patterns is essential to predicting the right levels.

For example, if an item is showing signs of increasing trends, but the procurement department orders as if it were continuous usage, shortages or stockouts will occur. Similarly, if a item is declining, a purchasing strategy that adds 10% each week to historical usage patterns is not a good business practice. **Figure 13–4** shows some of the more common item usage patterns.

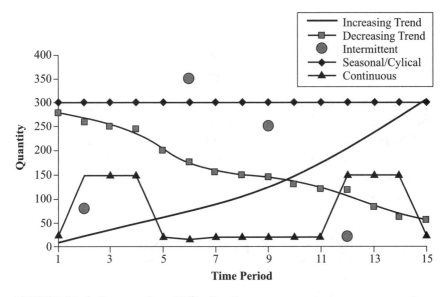

FIGURE 13–4 Common Item Utilization Patterns

The first two patterns are fairly straightforward: a product is exhibiting either **increasing** or **decreasing demand**. Increases or decreases can be detected if the **slope**, which is the tilt or angle of the rise or fall over the run, or the absolute value increases continuously over time. This change in usage is captured in most sophisticated ERP packages, or it can be extracted and calculated through spreadsheets. Mathematically, it can be calculated using the following basic formula:

$$Y = a + bx$$

where

Y = total usage
a = intercept or the point of the initial value
b = slope of the line
x = the time period

Consider this example. If an item has only two points of usage of 10 items in period 1 and 15 items used in period 2, the calculation of the slope represents a 50% increasing trend, calculated as follows:

$$Y = a + bx$$
$$Y = 10 + 5(1)$$
$$b = 50\% \text{ increase or slope}$$

This same formula can be used with additional data points to confirm trends, both increasing and decreasing, but it becomes significantly simpler to rely on advanced planning technologies or even spreadsheets.

Depending on the time frame analyzed, the increasing trend might indicate a product in the introductory or growth phase, while the decreasing trend might indicate the decline phase. A third pattern indicates strong **seasonal demand**—spikes in the Christmas months for toys, the sale of chocolate at Easter time, or even seasonal patterns when events are repetitive and periodic in nature (holidays, timing of specific promotions, and climate or weather). Another item usage pattern might be completely random, where no observed pattern can be found. This is especially evident when no systematic or constant patterns exist.

Another type of demand is called **intermittent** or lumpy **demand**. This is characterized by demand that is not dispersed evenly over time but tends to occur only at specific periods in batches or lumps. This might be caused by order batching (i.e., when customers tend to order in large lot sizes infrequently), by forward buying (i.e., when customers buy product earlier than is required for consumption purposes due to special pricing or to take advantage of financial reporting irregularities), or for some other reason entirely. As described earlier, **cyclical demand** can be seen when naturally occurring cycles tend to result in a predictable ebb and flow in the demand. Irregular or transient demand is one of the least predictable of all because it has no apparent pattern except that it just emerges for a specific period or two and then disappears.

The most predictable and regular of all demand patterns is the **continuous**, or horizontal **demand**, which refers to evenly dispersed usage throughout all time periods. Another demand pattern that exists (although it is not pictured in the graph) is the **auto-correlated demand** pattern, where the value of demand in one period is related to the demand for itself in previous periods. This type of demand pattern tends to be visible in areas in which trends and seasons are highly influential. Demand is a function influenced by many factors, such as trends, seasons, levels, causal factors, events, and other factors. The combination of any of these factors with the product's stage in the life cycle gives a very clear picture of the overall long-term behavior and pattern of the product.

CHAPTER SUMMARY

An item is any physical good that is procured for ultimate use or consumption. Items move through a chain—from manufacturers to vendors and on to customers. Understanding how items are being utilized (or "moving") is essential to being able to purchase an efficient quantity of items at the right time and avoid having either too much or too little inventory on hand. The UNSPSC is a highly structured categorization system that could be adopted by healthcare organizations to help understand the huge volumes of item data. Understanding the data requires an understanding of the phase of the product life cycle that the item currently occupies. Sophisticated purchasing managers can use both volume and pricing data to conduct a sourcing spend analysis to identify where value opportunities exist. The use of ERP systems helps support robust item masters, but ERPs also play a much larger role in supply chain and business management for health care. Forecasting item usage by quantitative techniques allows materials executives to become more efficient in the purchasing and replenishment processes. Tracking forecast accuracy and error rates is essential to understanding how forecasts compare with reality so that future adjustments can be made in both methodology and process.

KEY TERMS

admixture, attributes, auto-correlated demand, bill of material, categories, compounding, continuous demand, cyclical demand, decreasing demand, drilldown, enterprise resource planning (ERP) system, increasing demand, finished good, hierarchy, intermittent demand, intermediate good, item, item master, rollup, seasonal demand, slice and dice, slope, stock-keeping unit (SKU), United Nations Standard Products and Services Code (UNSPSC)

DISCUSSION QUESTIONS

1. How can attributes be used to improve the management of items?

2. What are the six steps of a product life cycle?

3. What is an item master, and what key attributes should it hold?

4. What is an ERP? What are three advantages to an ERP?

5. What are the reasons for the lack of standards in the medical supplies industry?

6. What role is the United Nations Development Programme playing in the creation of standards?

EXERCISE PROBLEMS

1. Assume the following time series data:

January	100
February	200
March	300
April	400

Is there a trend you can observe in the data? What is it called?

2. If a product has utilization of 50 in period 0 and has a slope of 10 each subsequent period, what is the expected forecasted value in period 2?

REFERENCES

Campbell, Mike. (2000). A Spirit of Collaboration Takes Over. *RetailTech Magazine:*23–24.

O'Brien, James A. (1996). *Management Information Systems*. 3rd ed. Chicago: Times Mirror.

Onkvisit, Sak, and John J. Shaw. (1989). *Product Life Cycles and Product Management*. Westport, CT: Greenwood Publishing Group.

UNSPSC. (2006). www.unspsc.org. Website of the United Nations Standard Products and Services Code.

CHAPTER 14

Supply Chain Collaboration

Goals of This Chapter
1. Define collaboration
2. Describe the role of sales and operations planning (S&OP) in health care
3. Understand how manufacturers and others use collaborative planning, forecasting, and replenishment (CPFR)

At its core, supply chain management (SCM) is highly collaborative in nature. **Collaboration**, defined as working jointly with others in an endeavor to accomplish similar goals, is fundamental to effective operations and SCM. Improving relationships, processes, and systems for key vendors and distributors is essential to SCM for pharmaceutical, medical, food, and other suppliers. There are two collaborative planning processes that have the potential to significantly improve distributor and manufacturer planning processes, and if used properly, they will help hospitals substantially achieve better results. These two processes are S&OP and CPFR.

Hospitals and providers do not use CPFR and S&OP today, but other components of the upstream supply chain definitely do. It is important for operations managers to know the processes involved in the rest of the chain to help reduce bullwhip effects and improve supply chain operations, and to understand the processes that their vendors utilize daily.

Although there are other business processes in existence that are also collaborative, such as quick response and efficient consumer response, they are variations on the two processes described in this chapter. In general, these processes are effective tools because they use demand to drive alignment through the supply chain, they promote the use of a single set of numbers to produce departmental and company plans, and they focus on improving results through streamlined business process management.

SALES AND OPERATIONS PLANNING

Sales and operations planning (S&OP) is a specific process that helps firms focus on one thing: making the best choices of where and how to fulfill demand. Distributors and manufacturers in health care widely use S&OP because of the huge array of SKUs in multiple distribution locations. Therefore, the demand side of the equation is difficult to predict and thoroughly understand. On the supply side, manufacturing plant capacities are often limited, and many constraints exist that complicate the ability to fulfill demand (such as distribution, lead time, manpower, and other resource constraints). Couple these constraints with the fact that the demand strategy for successful organizations is to serve demand with the highest customer economics first, and the process becomes even more complex.

The S&OP process is about matching demand with supply at aggregate levels. It involves managing these constraints to identify the demand that the firm seeks and fulfill this demand in the most responsive and efficient means possible. Balancing demand with supply to make profit-maximizing decisions (in all parts of the business) is the basic mission of S&OP.

Sales and operations planning is a collaborative process, and thus it is interconnected with other key business processes in the organization. The difference is that S&OP helps integrate the strategic aspects of the company (i.e., Where is the market heading?) with the tactical aspects (i.e., In which product families might we have supply problems?). Additionally, S&OP focuses on:

- A long-term view (e.g., next month or next quarter).
- Aggregated views at the higher product levels, such as categories or families.
- Fulfillment of key areas of market demand (e.g., satisfying the profitable demand).

- Finding key constraints in balancing demand and supply (e.g., such as targeting capacity issues and finding alternative sources of production).
- Achieving consensus among senior levels of management cross functionally.

OBJECTIVES OF S&OP

While the overarching purpose of S&OP is to provide aggregate demand and supply management, the objectives are clearly much more complicated. S&OP allows for the organization as a whole to collaborate around one of the most important business processes for the hospital. The collaborative S&OP process has four key objectives:

- *Provide a common base of information around the immediate market dynamics.* Driven by senior managers from the marketing/commercial side of the business, in conjunction with supply chain managers, the S&OP process helps all parties gain a common understanding of how the market is changing and the impact that this will have on demand and supply. A common understanding and implication of pricing, base demand, trends, competitive maneuvers, and market research findings all have an effect on the demand and supply chains. Therefore, the sales and operations process becomes extremely important in the overall planning process to drive alignment and share common assumptions about the future.
- *Manage the performance of the supply chain.* The S&OP process is the appropriate forum to discuss strategic aspects of the most recent supply and demand chain performance. This includes analyzing metrics such as target versus actual customer service levels, inventory days on hand (i.e., retailer inventory or similar measure), order fulfillment cycle time, as well as manufacturing yields versus plan. In addition, other relevant demand chain indicators, such as an analysis of promotion and assortment effectiveness, should also be explored.
- *Collaboratively manage product portfolios.* Plans for immediate or future development of new-product launches/introductions, product line extensions, product phase-outs, and other changes in product families can be jointly discussed in terms of impact on all areas of the extended hospital.

- *Create shared business plans and scenarios.* The end result of the S&OP meetings can be summarized with two words: better decisions and execution. S&OP processes help manufacturing, supply chains, demand chains, sales, marketing, and other departments make better decisions than they otherwise would have made. At the same time, each department can go out and execute against a plan that is shared by all other parties in the chain. Both better decisions and more effective execution are the two principal outputs in creating shared business plans and scenarios.

THE BASIC S&OP PROCESS

The basic S&OP process is a highly meticulous, collaborative process that occurs cross-functionally from senior management, supply chain, manufacturing, sales, marketing, and finance. The process can be broken down into five major phases:

Business planning >> Demand analysis >> Supply analysis >> Balancing >> Decisions

Each of these steps has many more activities and subprocesses. These steps will be defined at a high level in the rest of this section.

Business Planning

The purpose of *business planning* is to define the key strategic aspects of the business. This includes an analysis of sales, market share, profits, and expected return on investment. At this stage, the sales and marketing groups are responsible for providing general direction to the hospital in terms of managing the product portfolio. This business plan should guide decisions on manufacturing capacities, logistics requirements, and retail distribution strategies.

The next few steps have to be undertaken within the context of optimizing the primary business goals for the firm, such as improving the profit and loss position and increasing market share by market segment and category.

Demand Analysis

In the *demand analysis* phase, companies must focus on obtaining a collaborative unconstrained plan that can be expressed quantitatively by a single forecast for demand by product category. It is more accurate and productive to plan a chain around a single forecast, than a range of expectations, so the focus should be to center around a single view of the future. Specifically, this includes the following tasks or subprocesses:

3) • Run statistical forecasts on historical demand (based on combinations of historical sales, confirmed or booked orders, and committed customer schedules).
 • Share these preliminary forecast figures.
4) • Obtain collaborative business intelligence on volume sales plans, retailer or supplier promotions, and planned price increases.
 • Gain collaborative input on other key events that might occur during the period.
2) • Perform sensitivity or simulation analysis.
1) • Secure a common demand scenario.
 • Publish the final unconstrained demand plan.

Note

In addition, during this phase it is important to look at demand not only for current products in the portfolio, but also for product line extensions, new display or bonus packs, and completely new items as well. Every product must undergo a thorough demand analysis to identify and validate its phase of the product life cycle to finalize the demand plans. New items to be introduced or utilized should be a part of this process.

In general, it is the primary role of the sales and marketing team to obtain field input on all demand factors to establish the most accurate demand plan. It is important to remember the following equation for a good demand plan:

$$\text{Demand plan} = \text{Statistical forecast} + \text{Business intelligence} + \text{Collaboration} + \text{Action}$$

The output of the demand analysis phase is typically a report or system view that outlines at the product family level the following information: sales history analysis, target inventory levels (based on the cycle inventory policy), customer service levels (e.g., order backlogs, out of stocks, fill rates), and all demand assumptions taken.

Supply Analysis

During the *supply analysis* phase, the key inputs are the reports prepared during the demand analysis phase that define demand for each product family. The supply planners use this information to review and refine the operations plan to determine if sufficient supply exists to meet expected demand. The available supply equation is fairly easy to define:

$$\text{Supply} = (\text{Capacity} \times \text{Utilization}) + \text{Inventory on hand} + \text{Goods purchased for resale}$$

Given this, the supply planners need to explore the assumptions taken during the planning period (i.e., next month or quarter) and analyze if capacity additions have occurred (e.g., new plants coming on line), if capacity reductions have occurred (e.g., plants have been transitioned to other families or have been closed entirely), if plant utilization or yield rates have changed (e.g., due to maintenance), or if any other supply factors have a bearing on supply. For example, obtaining adequate supply of components or raw materials in certain industries, such as the chip fabrication sector, often creates frustrations for planners in their attempt to balance supply with demand.

The end result of this phase is a rough-cut capacity plan that details the planned available inventory levels and supply positions at the family level, as well as listing issues that are the source of the supply constraints (such as manufacturing line bottlenecks, resource limitations, and upstream supply chain or vendor-related problems). Following this rough-cut capacity analysis, summary reports should be distributed to key members of the full sales and operations planning team to begin their analysis.

Balancing

At this point, the key input is the combined demand/supply rough-cut planning report. This report details the potential problem areas for the company so that the group can focus on attacking the exceptions (those areas where demand and supply are seriously misaligned). The balancing process typically takes place in two parts: an informal pre-S&OP discussion and a formal S&OP meeting. The pre-S&OP discussions are with the key members of the team to begin making some recommendations on how to balance demand and supply, including many demand or supply management decisions. For example, if demand exceeds supply, such actions might include:

- Increasing prices temporarily to reduce demand.
- Allocating available supply to only key retail or downstream locations.
- Adding new capacity or resources, such as people, shifts, equipment, or plants.
- Purchasing product for resale from other collaborating companies.
- Establishing customer priorities (based on customer service level expectations, customer value added, and ABC rankings) to determine which demand will not be immediately fulfilled.

If supply exceeds demand, some appropriate actions that might be recommended include:

- Decreasing prices temporarily (i.e., **temporary price reductions**), to generate additional demand.
- Adding additional promotions, such as premiums or rebates.
- Scaling back on the production plans, which might result in labor and resource savings short term.
- Building or "loading" inventory, especially if demand is increasing and the cost of shutting down production is greater than the cost of capital attached to finished goods inventory.
- Adjusting other constraints that might affect the balance.

In the process of deciding on these demand and supply strategies for balancing, there should be an aggregated view of all product families in the business units to roll up the financial or top-line business impact of all decisions and assumptions. Once completed, the planning process is ready for senior-level decisions.

Decisions

The high-level view of the plans at this point should be summarized and presented in the monthly, formal sales and operations meeting. This meeting should summarize and review the key elements of the business plan, the current financial climate, the supply chain performance metrics, the family-level rough-cut plans, and the summary of the key decisions that need to be taken to balance demand and supply. At this point, the S&OP process must be focused on aligning the business (i.e., manufacturing, logistics, extended supply chain) around a core S&OP business scenario, so decisions have to be made quickly and must be fully supported. Consensus in the multifunctional meetings must be found, because the goal of S&OP is to create a common, collaborative scenario for how to best manage the combined hospital.

In summary, S&OP is an effective collaborative business process for managing demand and supply activities in large distribution and manufacturing organizations. While hospitals and providers are historically less involved, an understanding of this process helps drive alignment with the upstream supply chain. Benefits from the S&OP process include better cross-functional alignment, gap analysis, more efficient resource planning, and more effective use of promotional resources. This process is essential to synchronizing the demand and supply chains with shared scenarios that can streamline operations, reduce demand variability, and create consistent actions and strategies for all parts of the extended hospital.

COLLABORATIVE PLANNING, FORECASTING, AND REPLENISHMENT

Collaborative planning, forecasting, and replenishment (CPFR) is the name for the process that seeks to improve the relationship or partnership between retailers and suppliers. The intent of the process is to achieve full collaboration and improve the sharing of information around consumer point-of-sales data through the retail supply chain to improve overall chain performance.

OBJECTIVES OF CPFR

While the primary objective of CPFR is to improve the relationships within the other parties in the supply chain, there are many other objectives:

- Alignment of the chain around a common process, common formats for data exchange, common systems, and common performance metrics.
- Sharing of one common forecast and demand plan, based on downstream sales and usage data, which ensures that suppliers, manufacturers, distributors, and hospitals all share common business and supply chain plans.

- Communication of issues around meeting demand, prioritizing demand, and managing supply allocations within a collaborative framework.
- Advanced notification of pricing or promotions to more adequately plan future months without experiencing the bullwhip effect.
- Better visibility of demand, inventory, and shipment data through the supply chain by sharing common technology and messaging formats among parties in the chain.

Each of these objectives translates into maximizing collaboration in the planning process to streamline operations and maximize the effectiveness of the entire chain—not just components within the chain.

CPFR GUIDELINES

Fifteen years ago, the **Voluntary Interindustry Commerce Standards (VICS) Association** was created by industry executives who got together to brainstorm how to collectively improve the supply chain coordination in the retail industry among retailers, manufacturers, and suppliers. The overall objective of the VICS Association at the time was to use better demand information to drive alignment through the supply chain by focusing on creating voluntary standards within the industry that all parties would use to share data in consistent manners (Schenck, 1998). As VICS states, the committee's objective is as follows:

> The Association's overall global objective is to improve product availability to the consumer by providing leadership and encouragement in the identification, development, and implementation of volunteer standards, protocols, guidelines, and other mechanisms, that when properly utilized are expected to lead to better anticipation of, and reaction to, changes in consumer demand for these products with the subsequent optimization of production and carrying costs (VICS, 2006).

The VICS committee has been the driving force behind the creation of a CPFR process and standards within the consumer packaged goods and retail industries. VICS has not yet had much influence on the healthcare industry, although many of the manufacturers that sell through retail chains are currently participating such as Johnson and Johnson and GlaxoSmithKline. It has been a very slow process; however, it has been well received by the world's leading firms, such as Procter & Gamble,

Hewlett-Packard, Wal-Mart, Nabisco, and JC Penney. Other firms, while interested in the concept and excited about the opportunities, have been slow to embrace the actual CPFR standards.

The guidelines for CPFR allow for the creation of a common trading framework. Specifically, this means common language, common process models, and common data standards (Cross, 2000; Hoque, 2000). Of these, the most important is obviously to share a common philosophy or paradigm with all parties in the CPFR framework. This shared philosophy is carried out with the use of common vocabulary and language within the process. Both business and technology terminologies and definitions must be designed to support a common base of understanding among all participants. Achieving this common base is essential for multiple retailers and suppliers to interact and improve relationships.

Second, the business process used has to be very well defined and detailed. In successful firms using CPFR, the process models describe exactly which elements of the relationship need to be documented, which key aspects of the combined business plan must be shared, which categories will be emphasized and which strategies will be used, which steps will be used to provide a sales forecast, how to handle exceptions in the process, and how to evaluate performance. The use of a very detailed process model enables maximum returns.

Third, these process models and common terminologies must be translated into specific and common data standards. In fast, flexible supply chains, the CPFR process has to allow for quick and accurate exchange of data among parties. As such, the data sets must be standardized across all parties to ensure that the parties are translating and interpreting the data the same way. Specifically, this translates into information technology standards for data structures, data interfaces, data integrity, and security.

PERFORMANCE METRICS IN CPFR

The outcomes of CPFR processes should focus on the creation of systemwide performance improvements through completely collaborative business processes. Hospitals and health systems, as downstream members of the chain, need to focus on critical metrics that impact the reliability and cost of the goods and services they procure. The performance metrics that CPFR seeks to affect include an improvement in forecasting accuracy, improvements in customer service levels or fill rates to providers, increased product line availability, reduction of inventory levels, and generally better financial cash flows.

CHAPTER SUMMARY

The healthcare industry has an extended supply chain that spans manufacturers, distributors, providers, and patients. This chain is very fragmented, and there is a need for significantly greater collaboration among the parties. Two of the most common collaborative business processes are S&OP and CPFR. While hospitals and providers do not today have much of a role in these processes, it is important to understand them and to use them to promote improved communication and collaboration and to begin utilizing similar processes in health care to improve relationships and to build better supply chains.

Both processes attempt to link systems, business plans, and processes to achieve a tighter integration of information and products among parties in the chain. Aligning patient and provider demand all the way upstream to manufacturers in a CPFR environment will be useful when the industry is ready. The goal of improved collaboration within the extended supply chain focuses on reducing inventories and improving overall cycle time and responsiveness. The use of highly collaborative planning processes between multiple parties internally and externally will help drive improved overall supply chain economics.

KEY TERMS

collaboration; collaborative planning, forecasting, and replenishment (CPFR); sales and operations planning (S&OP); temporary price reduction; Voluntary Interindustry Commerce Standards (VICS) Association

DISCUSSION QUESTIONS

1. In what specific ways can hospitals improve their collaboration with key vendors, such as the large distributors in food services, pharmacy, and medical supplies? What type of data could be shared that would help improve the overall supply chain?

2. Has VICS had much of an impact on health care? On which part of the chain?

3. Sales and operations planning is a process adapted from industrial and manufacturing settings. How can it be applied to hospitals?

REFERENCES

Cross, G. (2000). How e-Business Is Transforming Supply Chain Management. *Journal of Business Strategy*, March–April:36–39.

Hoque, Faisal. (2000). *e-Hospital: Business Models, Architectures, and Components.* Cambridge, UK: Cambridge University Press.

Schenck, J. (1998). CPFR: Stitching Together the Partnership. *Apparel Industry Magazine*, 59(8):72–73.

Voluntary Interindustry Commerce Standards Association Web Site. (2006). (www.vics.org).

CHAPTER 15

Pharmaceutical Operations Management

Goals of This Chapter
1. Define a pharmacy
2. Describe the role it plays in both clinical and operations management
3. Understand the national drug codes
4. Describe key trends affecting pharmacy administration

There are many departments and functions throughout the hospital that are primarily operational management in nature. Besides materials management, departments such as pharmacy, operating room, laundry and linen, food services, admissions, asset management, housekeeping, and many more are all business support services that rely on operations management to convert resources efficiently into outputs. Because of the significance of the pharmacy in terms of both resources consumed and revenue generated, a separate discussion of operational management for the pharmacy department will be provided in this chapter.

THE MODERN PHARMACY

The **pharmacy** is often one of the largest and most profitable departments in a hospital. A pharmacy is a facility that exists to fill and dispense drugs and medications that are prescribed by physicians or other caregivers. Pharmacists and pharmacies are active participants in the health delivery process (along with physicians and nurses) and are often structurally organized within the clinical care or clinical support services divisions (Griffith, 1992). They play a partnership role with physicians and other providers in evaluating the overall efficacy, safety, and quality of medications on patient outcomes.

The purpose of this chapter is to describe the modern pharmacy from an operational perspective, so any discussion on the clinical role in patient healing and health has been purposely omitted here. There are a number of characteristics about pharmacies that make it primarily operational and logistical in structure. In many respects, pharmacy management is quite similar to operating a retail establishment. For example, pharmacies actively "sell" goods, whose cost can represent 50% to 90% of the total expenses of the department. There are typically two components of expense, similar to retail: labor (for filling, dispensing, and compounding orders and drugs) and cost of goods sold. Lastly, pharmacies also provide service to customers or patients and are responsible for ordering, replenishing, storing, and providing controls over drugs.

A **drug** is a substance or article that is "intended for use in the diagnosis, cure, mitigation, treatment, or prevention of disease in man or other animals" and "intended to affect the structure or any function of the body of man or other animals" (Food and Drug Administration, 2004). Drugs are formally recognized through the U.S. Food and Drug Administration (FDA) and the National Formulary or the U.S. Pharmacopoeia.

Pharmacies can be quite complex in their operations. They are required to be staffed and managed primarily by pharmacists because state and national boards require all dispensing of drugs and medications to be performed by registered pharmacists licensed in that state. There are a number of laws and regulations, such as those set in place by the U.S. Drug Enforcement Agency (DEA), the FDA, the National Association of State Boards of Pharmacy, and many others. Pharmacies must maintain strict management controls over certain drugs, such as those classified as narcotics or other controlled substances.

Controlled drugs (also known as **scheduled drugs**) are those that are tightly monitored around usage and distribution, because of potential for misuse and abuse. The DEA, through the Controlled Substances Act (Title 21, Chapter 13, Drug Abuse Prevention and Control) has outlined specific guidelines for safe registration, handling, and documentation requirements for drugs that have high potentials for abuse. These drugs are placed in a schedule, which is organized C-I through C-V. C-I (or Schedule I) represents those drugs with the highest risks and potential for abuse, such as heroin or marijuana, with very little medical value. The others are organized by descending risk levels (C-II through C-V) and are all drugs that typical hospital pharmacies might dispense. Accordingly, there is a need for stricter controls around all business processes for pharmacy inventory management than in other areas in the hospital—for both inbound and outbound flows of product. **Figure 15–1** depicts the hierarchy of items, from those that require a degree of control similar to other medical-surgical supplies to those that require very strict management processes.

Information systems, business policies and procedures, and the level of documentation and internal controls must be directly related to the item type managed in a pharmacy. For example, although a pneumatic tubing system might be used to quickly send certain products to a floor, it can't be used for any scheduled drugs because the chain of custody can't be directly established and the drug could end up being administered to the wrong patient. **Chain of custody** refers to the handling audit trail, which details who handled specific items and when and where the transfers of physical products occurred. This is necessary to maintain integrity in the process and to ensure comprehensive management of the life cycle of an item, from initial acquisition to final disposition.

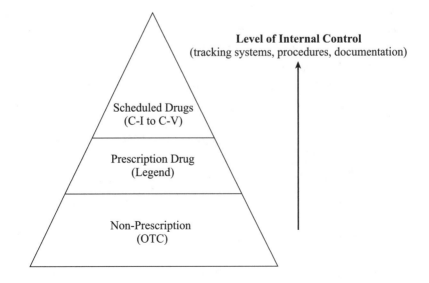

Level of Internal Control
(tracking systems, procedures, documentation)

Scheduled Drugs
(C-I to C-V)

Prescription Drug
(Legend)

Non-Prescription
(OTC)

FIGURE 15–1 Pharmaceutical Goods Control Hierarchy

THE PHARMACEUTICAL SUPPLY CHAIN

In smaller hospitals, a pharmacy might be defined as one finite, centralized geographic facility. In these environments, the pharmacy has higher intrinsic control because direct oversight takes place in one location, where drugs are both received and dispensed. In more complex and larger hospitals, however, a pharmacy department might have dozens or even hundreds of distributed locations. In the most complex pharmacies, there are both inpatient and retail pharmacies. Within each of these categories, there could be multiple locations and technologies and literally hundreds of employees.

Most of the largest pharmacy manufacturers don't deal directly with hospital or retail pharmacies, primarily because of the highly fragmented competitive nature in the manufacturing industry. Hundreds of pharmaceutical suppliers might have to contract with thousands of hospitals, so an intermediary or middleman role has developed to help procure, transport, store, and replenish in a much simpler manner. Firms such as Amerisource Bergen, McKesson, and Cardinal Health distribute products from thousands of suppliers to thousands of providers, simplifying the network significantly. These large **distributors** have also taken on other roles to help provide value and extend their competitive influence in the chain, such as offering systems and technology to providers, providing outsourced labor and services, and even manufacturing generic supplies.

The pharmaceutical supply chain tends to move through several phases, beginning with a concept for a biologic or chemical reaction that has potential; to eventual manufacture and commercialization; to full-scale production, distribution, and sale through either a retail or hospital pharmacy. **Figure 15–2** shows the healthcare value chain, describing both the new-product development chain and the operational supply chain.

The pharmaceutical manufacturer, or a biotechnology firm, is responsible for new-product development. This process is expensive, is time consuming, and requires extensive testing and trials over multiple years and phases. It has high risks, usually has multiple failures that requires restarting or changes to medications, and has high levels of regulation from the FDA and others. As such, the highest level of risk and investment is performed early in the supply chain, significantly prior to the commercialization and full-scale production and distribution.

As this happens, there is a constant struggle for power and for financial value in the pharmaceutical network. Hospitals typically lose this struggle.

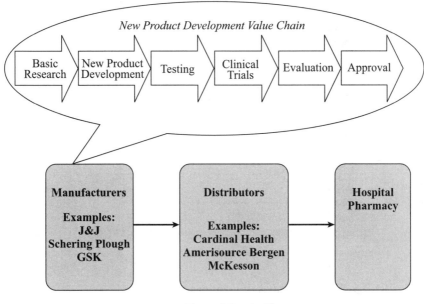

FIGURE 15–2 Pharmaceutical Value Chain

Manufacturers are dominated by some very large firms, including Johnson & Johnson, Pfizer, Merck, Schering Plough, GlaxoSmithKline, and Eli Lilly, although there are hundreds of smaller pharmaceutical and biotechnology firms located throughout the world.

The major pharmaceutical manufacturers in 2005 earned an average profit of about 15%. The largest pharmaceutical distributors averaged less than 2%, while leading retail pharmacy chains (such as Walgreen's and CVS) averaged around 3%. Meanwhile, hospitals averaged only about 4% profit margin (see **Figure 15–3**).

MANAGING ITEMS USING THE NATIONAL DRUG CODE

Pharmacies represent multiple operations management challenges, including inventory, personnel management, technology and automation, management controls, location analysis and selection, procurement, and network distribution. The most difficult is that of managing the move-

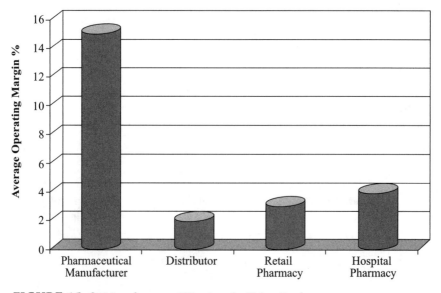

FIGURE 15–3 Manufacturers Winning the Value Battle

ment of these drugs, which accounts for the largest percentage of expenses for hospital pharmacies.

The primary purpose of a pharmacy is to dispense medications; thus, pharmacies ultimately are "physical" supply chains, managing the physical flow of goods both inbound and outbound. The management of drugs acquired for replenishment to each physical location requires careful control over stock-keeping units and item categories, much the same way as materials management departments manage general-purpose medical supplies. Pharmacies are somewhat different, in that most items are stamped or coded with a proprietary pharmacy-industry coding system called a national drug code. The **national drug code (NDC)** is an industry identifier created in 1969 by the FDA to provide a comprehensive listing of all approved drugs. The NDC is a 10-digit identification number assigned by the FDA to all commercialized products, which helps uniquely identify the manufacturer or labeler of the product, the specific product, and the packaging type.

The first segment of the NDC (the labeler) is either a 4- or a 5-digit number that identifies the firm that manufactured, packaged, or labeled the product. For example, the GlaxoSmithKline labeler identifier is 00173, and Merck has been assigned 61258.

The second segment of the 10-digit code is the product identifier. This can either be a 3- or a 4-digit number, which uniquely identifies the specific product. For example, Vytorin product in tablet form is 0311.

The third segment of the code is the packaging type. This is either a 1- or a 2-digit code that defines the base unit of measure and specific packaging size (i.e., vial, bottle, cartridge). **Figure 15–4** shows the NDC coding structure for Merck's Vytorin medication in a bottle with 30 tablets.

There are some exceptions and issues to the NDC coding system. In any of these NDC numbers, 0's can cause problems because they can be scanned by bar-coding technology or information systems as either null values (i.e., no entries or blanks) or actual zeros. In some cases, asterisks (*) are used to identify digits. In addition, many government agencies use an 11-digit NDC identifier, which creates comparison problems for the same unique drugs. All labelers, products, and packaging types can be queried on the Internet at the FDA Web site at this address: http://www. fda.gov/cder/ndc/database/default.htm.

With the NDC number, a bar code can be applied, which allows tracking of items into the hospital and then through the dispensing and administration process. A bar code has also been called a "license plate," but it is basically a label that is placed on a product to provide visual representation through a set of identifiers that contain useful information about the product. When you walk into a grocery store, the common label used in retail is the universal product number (UPN) code. In health care, although there are many standards, the most common are the national health-related items code, the UPN, and several more (see Chapter 13 for a more complete discussion).

Using NDC and bar code technology, it then becomes possible to monitor the physical movements of drugs, ensure proper internal controls

FIGURE 15–4 Example of Pharmacy National Drug Codes

around the inventory, and ensure proper charging of the medications to patients using bedside scanning at the time of administration of the drug by the provider.

PROCESS WORKFLOW AND AUTOMATION IN THE PHARMACY

The process of providing drugs and medications to patients requires a licensed healthcare provider to provide a written script or prescription. A **prescription** is a doctor's written order for medication or other course of treatment. This script then has to be filled, which is the primary role of pharmacies. In large, modern hospitals, this script might be entered directly into a computerized physician order entry (CPOE) system. A CPOE allows the physician to enter the treatment and medication information for patients directly into an information system, which captures that information, routes it to the appropriate person in the workflow process (i.e., pharmacies for filling orders, nursing for delivering other services), applies any number of business rules to further promote patient safety, and ensures that the right patient receives the right medications. While this process can be very manual and labor-intensive, technology is being deployed quite extensively in pharmacies that automate much of the process. In less sophisticated hospitals, these prescriptions are given to nursing, and that department then either faxes or manually transports these forms to the nearest pharmacy location, which might be located in a nearby nursing supply room or pod or on a centralized floor somewhere else. Typically, these orders are scanned into an imaging system and routed to a pharmacy technician for entry into the pharmacy order entry system. There are a large number of information systems that exist to enter and fill pharmacy orders, from vendors such as Siemens, General Electric Healthcare, McKesson, and many others.

Once entered into a system, the items have to be picked, packed, and distributed back to the point of care. Items are picked manually off shelves by automated pickers, often with **robots** and **carousels**. This equiment uses technology and large mechanized systems to help select single- and small-dose packages, label them, and store them in the right location. Robots and carousels work together with other ordering and dispensing systems to automate the storage and retrieval process of goods. Automation helps reduce manual labor, reduces error rates, minimizes patient waiting times, and generally increases the number of orders filled with the same staffing level—all key goals of operations management. Several specialized pharmacy technologists, including ScriptPro, McKesson, and Swisslog (three of the largest competitors in this arena), offer this technology.

Oftentimes, the use of forward positioning of inventory is used in pharmacies. **Forward positioning** refers to the placement of medications near the point of use, prior to their actual usage, based on forecasted needs. For example, if three doses of a specific drug are needed today at 5 P.M., instead of the pharmacy waiting for the order to appear; entering it; and then picking, packing, and dispensing the order, the drug could be staged in a forward position nearer the unit or floor on which it will be used.

The use of automated dispensing solutions, from vendors such as Pyxis, Omnicell, and McKesson, allow forward positioning. These medication-dispensing systems are very similar in concept to vending machines, which require a form of consideration (e.g., cash) that, when supplied, renders appropriate products (e.g., soft drinks). In pharmacies, however, the consideration is a secure identification (through badge, employee identification entry, or biometric means) that appropriately identifies the person as an authorized user who should be granted access to the appropriate medications and drugs. **Biometric methods** are newer security systems, which use physiological characteristic, such as fingerprints or retinal scans, to uniquely identify an individual. Dispensing systems use these various types of security measures to ensure that the right provider enters the right product information to be dispensed to the right patient, thus providing controls and safety for the patient.

Medication-dispensing systems allow for much tighter controls over inventory, especially where required for scheduled or controlled drugs. If a nurse scans her badge, enters the patient medical record number, and selects a product, and if all three entries meet established controls and security, then a drawer or cabinet is opened that grants access. Simultaneously, inventory controls are checked as nurses are prompted for a count of remaining items in the bin.

Finally, once dispensed, the drugs are taken to a patient's room for administration. The administration phase should be the trigger for charging patients, because this is the point of true consumption. The provider should record the administration in the medical record (whether paper or electronic), and this information becomes the formal written record of consumption.

KEY OPERATIONS MANAGEMENT TRENDS FOR PHARMACIES

Some of the key trends in pharmacy management toward achieving operational excellence include the following: perpetual inventory, strategic pricing analysis, systems integration, and location and network optimization.

Perpetual Inventory

Many large hospital pharmacies are now pursuing perpetual inventory. As the dollar value of most large pharmacy inventories continues to climb into the multi-million-dollar range, there is a much stronger need for higher levels of internal controls over these resources, as well as being able to monitor for theft, shrinkage, and other forms of loss. **Perpetual inventory** denotes the expansion of the use of information systems to ensure real-time, continuous tracking of inventory through the purchasing, receiving, distribution, dispensing, and medication administration workflow. *Perpetual* refers to the ability to know, at all points in time, actual balances through continuous tracking of receipts and issues.

Strategic Pricing Analysis

Strategic pricing analysis refers to the application of differential pricing markups to each drug based on its potential for reimbursement, usage, the item's history and life cycle, payer mix, and other factors. Strategic pricing suggests that some drugs will have higher margins than others, but the net impact will be larger net revenues for the pharmacy as a whole. As pharmacies closely monitor the usage of medications, and the associated reimbursement levels from payers, continuous analysis of price points must be conducted.

System Integration

Most pharmacies have dozens of systems: robots that pick, cabinets that dispense, procurement systems that order, carousels that store, pricing systems, retail charging systems, and many more. Integrating all of these pharmacy systems, from the point of order through administration, including synchronization of other major systems, from CPOE to electronic medical records to patient billing, is required to ensure that all information flows quickly and accurately between systems. Such **system integration** also ensures higher levels of internal controls because there are reduced opportunities for manual error or abuse.

Location and Network Optimization

One of the biggest elements of large-hospital pharmacy strategy centers around the dichotomy of distributed versus central (often called bulk) pharmacies. Larger hospitals tend to have multiple pharmacy locations distributed throughout hospital floors, units, and clinics, in addition to dispensing cabinets positioned in dozens of locations. In other hospitals, a centralized pharmacy is used to buy and store items, and a greater number of pharmacy technicians are employed to provide frequent distribution and replenishment of orders as they come in from providers on each of the floors. The strategy with optimal economic results typically is one or the other; however, most hospitals utilize a mixed strategy, which seems like it offers many positives, but in reality guarantees higher inventories and more personnel providing distribution services, both of which create excessive cost infrastructures.

Careful analysis of strategy and locations ensures efficient operations. These analyses should be based on profitability of existing transportation, stocking, and other process costs—in order to ensure that the right network of pharmacies exists. In general, more locations translate into higher numbers of items held and greater investment in inventory. Similarly, more locations suggest higher service levels. Finding the right trade-off, or optimization point, is essential. To illustrate this point, consider the square root law of consolidation. The **square root law of inventory** suggests that the total costs will increase dramatically as the number of stocking points increases. This can be written as the following equation:

$$I_t = I_i \sqrt{n}$$

where

I_t = amount of inventory at one location
I_i = amount of inventory at each of n locations
n = number of stocking points

Consider the following example. A pharmacy has three physical locations on different floors. Each location has \$200,000 worth of inventory, so the total inventory is currently $600,000. If this hospital were to consolidate from three locations down to one central location, the result would be a 30% reduction in inventory, calculated as follows: The square root of 3 is 1.732051, multiplied by the average inventory in each location ($200,000) is $346,410. So, if all three locations were collapsed into one, then a savings of nearly $154,000 in inventory investment would be reduced. This is equivalent to a 30% reduction in inventory levels:

$$\sqrt{3} \times \$200,000 = \$346,410$$

$$\$500,000 - \$346,000 = \$154,000$$

$$\$154,000 \div \$500,000 = 30\%$$

As this shows, even ignoring the costs of staffing and replenishing, there is a large benefit to be gained from closely monitoring the number and location of pharmacy locations.

EFFECT ON PHARMACY PERFORMANCE

Hospital administrators evaluate a pharmacy's performance in several ways: these can be clinical (impact on patient safety and effectiveness), organizational (collaboration with other healthcare providers), operational (ability to satisfy demand at high quality and service), and financial (ability to earn reasonable returns on drug expenditures). Strategic effectiveness ensures that pharmacies cover all four of these dimensions, which can be summarized as "providing clinical efficacy through high quality medications, with minimal error rates, in a patient-centered service environment, while still delivering financial value". If compounding or mixing is occurring, the outcomes of these medications must be monitored to ensure that the pharmacy augments the clinical care process.

In addition, most pharmacies have financial expectations and are considered "profit centers." **Profit centers** are organizational units that generate revenues, and they are required to earn reasonable returns on those revenues, after considering all costs of operation. Achievement of expected operating margins for pharmacy is another strategic performance indicator.

From an operations management perspective, however, there are many more key performance indicators that are critical:

- *Cycle time,* from order request through order fulfillment. Cycle time represents the service level given to both providers and patients and is expected to continuously decrease.
- *Cost per dose or order filled.* This figure should be tracked continuously to ensure that the operational labor costs decrease over time.
- *Percent of inaccurate orders or doses.* This metric, which is defined as the number of errors (wrong dose, wrong location) over the total number of orders filled, represents a quality metric for pharmacies. A similar metric, *percent of items returned,* measures how many items are being sent back to the central or bulk pharmacy locations for any reason.
- *Total days of inventory on hand.* Calculated as the average inventory balance divided by the average daily pharmacy operating expense, this metric describes how efficient the pharmacy is, the level of safety inventory being held, and how quickly items are being turned. Average figures for hospital pharmacies are 10 to 12 turns per year, or 30 days of inventory on hand.

Together, these metrics help continuously improve the operations of a pharmacy.

Spotlight on McKesson

One of the largest healthcare technology and distribution firms is McKesson. McKesson operates as the largest pharmaceutical distributor, but the scope and vision of the company portfolio is much larger than just drug distribution. As a *Fortune* 15 firm with more than $80 billion in revenues, McKesson operates three business units focused on a number of complex healthcare problems, including the largest healthcare technology business in the United States.

In a recent interview, I had an opportunity to discuss McKesson's strategy and the healthcare industry with one of its top executives—Marc Owen. Owen is the executive vice president of corporate strategy and business development, and he is responsible for corporate strategy, new initiatives, mergers and acquisition, and international markets. Owen has many years of strategy and technology experience, following an extensive consulting background with McKinsey Consulting.

McKesson's business strategy is to "attack $300 billion in operational administrative inefficiencies" in the healthcare system, coupled with interrelated safety and quality issues. These challenges are complex and unique to this industry, and McKesson is uniquely situated to help address these issues for all aspects of the healthcare value chain, from providers to payers. McKesson's strategy combines four critical success factors that differentiate the service offerings: deep clinical expertise, process knowledge, technology capabilities, and scale. In fact, more than 10% of McKesson's company is clinically trained, and the solutions reach more than 50% of U.S. hospitals today.

According to Owen, "Some hospitals have a stronger process mindset than others, but most attack processes one at a time." He sees a "cause for hope" in that certain hospitals are achieving dramatic results in some areas, like an 80% to 90% drop in medical error rates or a double-digit improvement in revenue cycle metrics. McKesson's focus on pharmacy distribution, pharmacy automation, and healthcare decision support and technology allows the key challenges in all major areas of the healthcare business to be addressed.

Interestingly, Owen points out that one of the primary reasons health care lags behind other industries in technology is because of the focus on mobile computing. "Health care involves mobility of people and resources, which are not stationary as in other industries. Mobile technologies, such as Wi-Fi, RFID, and mobile computing, are relatively new technologies." He sees these technologies receiving a lot of interest and being adopted fairly quickly.

Finally, Owen offers some very prudent advice to healthcare professionals. "Start slowly on process improvement, and continue to improve and build on it. It is not necessary to have revolutionary or breakthrough change all at once."

Sources: Interview with Marc Owen, 2006; *Fortune April 17, 2006.*

CHAPTER SUMMARY

The pharmacy is essential for hospitals and health care. Modern hospital pharmacies play a key role in providing clinical care as well as improving operational efficiencies. Understanding the pharmacy's business challenges, from use of standardized NDC codes to automation of the prescription order process, is necessary for operations managers. Multiple key performance metrics can be established and monitored to ensure continuous improvement in this area. The role of technology, including the use of robots, carousels, and other automation, helps make the pharmacy much more operationally efficient than other parts of the hospital.

KEY TERMS

bar code prescription, biometric method, carousel, controlled drug, chain of custody, distributor, drug, forward positioning, national drug code (NDC), pharmacy, perpetual inventory, profit center, robot, scheduled drug, square root law of inventory, strategic pricing analysis, system integration

DISCUSSION QUESTIONS

1. What role does a pharmacy play in operations management?
2. Should controlled drugs be given the same level of oversight as prescription drugs?
3. How are systems and technology streamlining pharmacy operations?

REFERENCES

Food and Drug Administration. (2004). *Federal Food, Drug, and Cosmetic Act.* Chapter II, Section 201. United States Code Title 21, Chapter 9.

Fortune. (2006). *Fortune 500 Rankings.* April 17 issue.

Griffith, John R. (1992). *The Well-Managed Community Hospital.* 2nd ed. Ann Arbor, MI: AUPHA/Health Administration Press.

Owen, Marc. (2006). Personal interview conducted via telephone by Jim Langabeer on December 18, 2006.

PART IV

Summary

This final part provides some final thoughts on how operations and logistics management can guide hospitals toward achieving significantly differential results. It summarizes best practices and provides a launching point for deploying improved management within individual facilities.

CHAPTER 16

The Future of Operations Management

Goals of This Chapter

1. Explore future trends and opportunities in healthcare operations management
2. Understand initial steps to get started in applying operations management successfully

---

Hospitals and healthcare systems have been showing signs of improved profitability. This reverses a trend of declining and predominantly negative margins that have saddled the industry for much of the past decade. This will not continue for long, however. Economics dictate that the long-term profitability of all industries will continue to diminish until normal profits approximate zero and that pricing, competition, and industry structure will evolve to make this happen. We have seen many signs of this happening recently.

As the industry searches for payer reimbursement mechanisms that shift the burden of health care off the government and toward consumers and businesses, the drive toward this evolution gains speed. Other policy issues, such as incentives, pay for performance (i.e., aligning reimbursement levels with outcomes), changing access mechanisms, and other macro political issues continue to evolve, focused on long-term cost reductions but felt by healthcare organizations in terms of reduced profit margins.

Management must continue to evolve, innovate, and differentiate if it expects profits or returns that are greater than the normal, long-run expectations for the industry. This chapter discusses the future of operations management in health care and summarizes the trends discussed in this text.

EVOLVING TRENDS

There are a number of key trends evolving that have been discussed in this text. Many of these have been discussed in their respective chapters, such as procurement or pharmacy. This chapter focuses on the macro-level changes that are affecting operations management as a whole. There are eight broad trends in operations management, as shown in **Figure 16–1**.

Strategy Focused on Agility, Speed, and Visibility

One of the biggest challenges in large hospitals and systems is the inability to know where patients and expensive resources are at all times, which effectively reduces capacity and causes excessive amounts of resources to be deployed. Imagine, however, the following scenario. A new patient is finalizing registration in admissions; subsequently, an order is given to housekeeping to make the room ready; a request also is made to materials management to order the typical procedural supplies required for the patient's stay and to si-

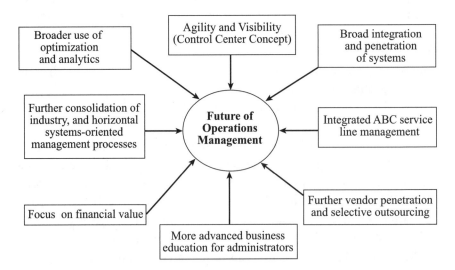

FIGURE 16–1 The Future of Healthcare Operations Management

multaneously update the census, electronic medical records (EMRs), and other key systems. If this same hospital tracks the flow and movements of all wheelchairs, infusion pumps, medications, crash carts, and other key resources as well, there would be higher utilization and throughput with reduced level of investments. All of the manual bed boards, tracking sheets, and paper processes could be discontinued, and in its place would be real-time visibility shared by all clinical and support services.

Healthcare business strategy is moving toward greater agility and speed in business processes in an effort to improve throughputs and service simultaneously. These strategic capabilities will drive decision-making processes and will ultimately result in greater operational excellence.

In the long run, hospitals will evolve over time much the same way that other low-margin, operationally focused industries have, such as telecommunications, retail, and energy. The technology and processes in these industries have evolved to where a continuous, real-time monitoring environment is used to manage the key aspects of the business. In health care, the use of scorecards (or dashboards) is primarily retrospective, in that it looks back over the previous day or month for metrics and results. As health care improves its operational focus, a control center concept using tracking technologies supports:

- Radio frequency identification (RFID) tags for use on key resources.
- Visibility of patients from admit to discharge—and all departments that are visited in between.
- Movement of expensive drugs and supplies to reduce the risk of theft or loss.

Health care is in the early phases of this evolution. Organizations are selectively putting tracking technologies such as patient bar coding and RFID on equipment and are simultaneously implementing real-time clinical systems in place to improve processes such as discharge planning. These systems will prove useful, will have a limited return on investment (ROI), but will eventually dictate the need for further system integration (discussed later) to achieve greater benefits throughout the entire organization. This will eventually lead to the need for a new, integrated department that can monitor and control the flow and throughput of resources throughout the entire system. A control center concept—staffed by professionals focused on operational efficiencies and driven by new metrics of speed, agility, and acuity—will be implemented that can significantly decrease the organizational barriers and process inefficiencies. **Figure 16–2** shows a conceptual control center concept, where multiple systems and technologies are utilized to manage key resources.

Integration and Penetration of Technology

Technology plays a vital role in integrating disparate processes and automating manual ones. As operations management begins to understand and influence the infrastructure to produce better costs and outcomes, technology will become even more pervasive. Much of this technology will be focused less on clinical needs than on business needs.

Most large hospitals have hundreds of enterprise and stand-alone systems, many of which are quite interdependent. Health care in the future will have much broader integration of these key systems and technology to allow for sharing and linking of data so that applications can operate as one large system. This is called **interoperability**, and extensive work is currently underway to define integration standards, middleware, and platforms on which this can occur. Interoperability ensures that all key systems—such as EMRs, a picture archiving and communication system, medication administration, enterprise resource planning, charge descrip-

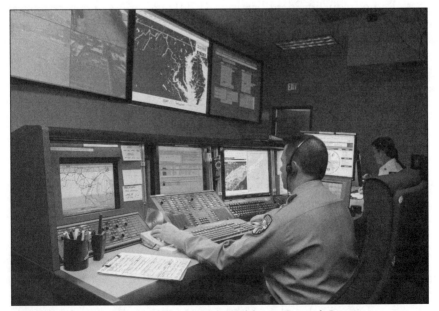

FIGURE 16–2 Visibility and Tracking in Healthcare Control Centers

tion master, and many more—work together seamlessly. This interoperability will allow the first trend (strategy) to be fully realized.

Integrated Service Delivery with Activity-Based Costing

Healthcare organizations are moving away from vertical, stand-alone, silo-based business units, where patients are treated differently at each department or clinic. More streamlined business processes will result in an integrated, or horizontal, service delivery. The current redundancy that exists—where each unit captures similar patient data, creates its own schedules, and manages separate systems—will be replaced by a more holistic and integrated service line approach.

This new approach will help drive improved throughput and patient flow, but it will do little to reduce costs if it is not paired with an activity-based costing approach. **Activity-based costing (ABC)** defines total costs at a detailed level, where activity drivers and resource consumers are used. Understanding the costs at an activity level is necessary because, in most health care organizations, there has been very little work done to understand what drives costs and where the true costs lie. Many of the hidden or fixed costs that are dormant in vertical processes are more easily exposed in a horizontal cross-functional approach, which is why ABC should be used in conjunction with integrated service delivery.

Greater Vendor and Payer Collaboration

There are opportunities in the healthcare value chain for significantly higher levels of collaboration with both vendors and payers. Interactions with both today are still highly manual and don't involve electronic commerce and collaborative processes. Collaboration can take the form of automated reconciliations of charges and patients, shared business plans, and collocation of employees.

In many large facilities, limited outsourcing is already in use for support services such as gift shops and cafeterias. As health care continues to focus on operational efficiencies, many organizations will discover that their **core competency** (or expertise that underlies their reason for existing and the source of the competitive advantage) doesn't involve operating all aspects of a business process directly. A shift toward more selective outsourcing, in both clinical and business areas, will be significantly greater in the future than what currently exists.

Vendors will also control much more of the supply chain in many areas. Vendors possess more specialized knowledge and technology, which will penetrate deeper into many organizations, and complicated mechanisms will be used to better align incentives between vendors and providers—much different than the cost-plus arrangement that is common today. The large healthcare distributors will have an expanded role. Incentive payments for improved bottom-line performance in key metrics will be used, and vendors will offer more attractive solutions that are comprised of labor, technology, and process.

Different managerial skills are required to manage vendor arrangements such as these, and operational managers must also include business acumen such as contract administration, performance management, and vendor collaboration.

More Advanced Business Education

Many administrators can benefit from improved management and business education. There are nearly 75 accredited graduate-level programs in healthcare administration, yet far too many programs focus predominantly on public and social policy and not enough on management, financial, and business issues. While most healthcare degree programs focus on the healthcare enterprise as a governmental organization, this will change as programs evolve to teach a broader curriculum focusing on operations, finance, and technology. In those facilities governed by physicians, the pursuit of the MBA degrees has risen steadily: an estimated 22% of physician executives in large medical centers have dual MD-MBA degrees (Westfall, 2005). Yet, far too many physicians are relatively inexperienced in business practices that will help improve financial and operational performance.

As the healthcare industry continues to change into a more dynamic one, where financial pressures force administrators to act as true business managers, there will be a much higher need for well-rounded graduates with advanced business skills. Being able to use accounting and financial data to help drive improved decision making and processes currently relies on skills that are better developed outside of health care. Having and using these skills, though, is necessary if hospitals are to manage increasing scale, horizontal integration, and effective operations.

Financial Value

Clinical and support services need to continuously measure and improve the financial value offered. As health care becomes more sophisticated, organizations will be managed much more like a financial portfolio, where departments and units that offer the greatest value at the lowest risk are cultivated, while those that destroy value (i.e., where total costs of operations are greater than the returns provided) are mitigated or eliminated. As healthcare organizations continue to measure performance more holistically, the emphasis on tracking ROI and value creation will force differential management of service lines. This emphasis on financial value will ultimately help each unit deliver better and more competitive services.

Consolidation and Horizontal Management Processes

The healthcare industry will most likely continue to consolidate, as it has over the past few decades. Horizontal integration—through mergers, acquisitions, and joint ventures—will probably be used (much more than vertical integration) to create integrated delivery networks, as organizations attempt to use their current skills to manage similar operations in other geographic areas.

This consolidation will create the need for a systems approach that can manage the interrelated facilities to achieve better results. Standardization, aggregation, and alignment are all necessary if hospitals are to achieve any synergistic effects from integration. Operational management, therefore, has to evolve from a narrow perspective to a much larger network view that can take disparate operations and connect them to achieve better results. This will require better leadership skills and the ability to manage and align processes that are expansive and currently decentralized.

Deployment of Analytical and Optimization Techniques

Health care has significantly greater potential for utilization of optimization and analytical techniques. As discussed in this text, all of the key operational processes in most healthcare organizations have developed over time using trial and error and do not deliver optimal results. The use of game theory, process engineering, Six Sigma, and other techniques will help augment the deployment of analytical techniques. Use of linear programming, simulation modeling, and other mathematical tools will become much more widespread in hospitals of the future than they are today. The use of analytics and optimization in the future will support a broad range of processes, including labor scheduling, patient routing, wait line and service delivery, and department or resource location analysis, to name just a few.

ACHIEVING SUCCESS IN OPERATIONS MANAGEMENT

With the concepts and tools learned from this text, there should be a number of opportunities for improvement that can quickly be addressed. Here are some final thoughts on how operations managers can get started in the process of improvement and change by applying their knowledge to achieve better results quickly.

1. *Learn as much as possible about the organization,* and develop a list of the high-priority problems that it faces. Create a list or a plan of the processes that need the most improvement. Chart those initiatives that have the highest value and that can be achieved with minimal risks and faster timelines. This will allow for some "quick hits" or initial success to build an improvement program, one process at a time.

2. *Innovate and challenge the status quo.* To a large extent, healthcare organizations are governed by the people who are the most averse to change or who don't understand the financial or business reasons that make change necessary. Many clinicians and administrators won't see the need for continuously improving processes, managing performance on a routine basis, and identifying opportunities for breaking down barriers to increased throughput and operational efficiencies. Challenging this behavior and thought process is required if health care is to improve cost and quality simultaneously. Operations managers must be change agents.

3. *Comprehensively analyze and improve everything, using a MECE approach.* In quality and continuous improvement projects, it is important to encourage team-based decision processes that are **mutually exclusive and collectively exhaustive (MECE)**. MECE

is a systems-oriented approach to decision making whereby each idea is distinct and can stand on its own; it also completely covers the range of possibilities for that issue (Rasiel, 1999). The MECE approach ensures that managers fully explore all issues yet are clear and separate in their thought processes, ensuring comprehensive coverage. MECE should be used in all process engineering and project management methodologies to develop the broadest and clearest depiction of the relative topics.

4. *Always look for analytical or quantitative approaches to problems.* Operations managers should not settle for outdated **heuristics** (i.e., rules of thumb) or other biased methods for making decisions. Quantitative techniques, wherever possible, should be used to model processes, productivity, and performance and to substantially improve decision-making processes. Quantitative data form the basis for many operations techniques, such as forecasting demand and capacity and then aligning healthcare operations strategies accordingly.

5. *Measure everything important, graphically, in scorecards.* Relying on text reports and tables makes trends and changes over time very difficult to identify and measure. Whether looking at statistical control charts of clinical procedures or financial outcomes, viewing data graphically in a scorecard puts things in perspective. All key processes and business units should have scorecards developed, so that pre- and post-project performance can be measured and planned results can be achieved. Comparison of trends to published benchmarks or targets helps instantly focus management on opportunity areas.

Of course, these are just some of the things that must be done if operations management is to be successful in transforming healthcare organizations. Remember, there are always new tools and techniques that can be adopted to improve outcomes. Good luck on the journey!

CHAPTER SUMMARY

Operations management in health care will continue to evolve over time. Eight key trends are identified that will further drive operational excellence: increased visibility of patients and resources; expansive system integration; integrated service delivery; greater collaboration with payers and vendors; additional business education for administrators; strategic focus on achieving financial value in all parts of the organization; consolidation of competition and the need for improved horizontal management processes; and broader use of optimization and analytics. It is important that operations managers, at all points in their careers, develop a comprehensive plan for identifying and improving operations. Lastly, several suggestions for how to comprehensively begin incorporating operations management into the daily practice are provided.

KEY TERMS

activity-based costing (ABC), core competency, heuristics, interoperability, mutually exclusive and collectively exhaustive (MECE)

DISCUSSION QUESTIONS

1. What are some of the key trends that are evolving in healthcare operations management?

2. Discuss the rationale behind systems interoperability.

3. How might an operational control center work in health care?

4. Why should administrators and medical executives continue developing business skills?

5. What are five initial steps that can be taken to begin the operations management process?

REFERENCES

Rasiel, Ethan M. (1999). *The McKinsey Way*. New York: McGraw-Hill.
Westfall, Carol. (2005). 2005 Compensation Survey. *The Physician Executive*. November–December:32–37.

Major Teaching Hospitals

Source: Association of American Medical Colleges.
Reprinted with Permission.

Alabama
1. Birmingham Veterans Affairs Medical Center
2. Carraway Methodist Health Systems
3. UAB Health System, University of Alabama at Birmingham
4. University of Alabama Hospitals
5. University of South Alabama Medical Center

Arizona
1. Banner Good Samaritan Medical Center
2. Bannerhealth
3. Department of Veterans Affairs, Veterans Integrated Service Network, VISN 18
4. Maricopa Medical Center
5. St. Joseph's Hospital & Medical Center CHW Arizona–Nevada
6. Southern Arizona Veterans Affairs Health Care System
7. University Medical Center

Arkansas
1. Arkansas Children's Hospital
2 Central Arkansas Veterans Healthcare System
3. University of Arkansas for Medical Sciences

California

1. California Pacific Medical Center
2. Catholic Healthcare West
3. City of Hope National Medical Center
4. Cedars-Sinai Medical Center
5. Community Health Network
6. Department of Veterans Affairs, Veterans Integrated Service Network, VISN 22
7. Jerry L. Pettis Memorial Veterans Affairs Medical Center
8. Harbor–UCLA Medical Center
9. Huntington Memorial Hospital
10. Kern Medical Center
11. Loma Linda University Medical Center
12. Long Beach Memorial Medical Center
13. Los Angeles County/USC Medical Center
14. San Francisco General Hospital and Medical Center
15. Santa Clara Valley Health and Hospital Systems
16. Scripps Green Hospital
17. Scripps Health
18. Stanford Hospital and Clinics
19. Tenet Healthcare Corporation
20. UCLA Healthcare
21. UCLA Medical Center
22. UCSD Healthcare
23. UCSF Medical Center
24. USC University Hospital
25. University of California, Irvine, Medical Center
26. University of California, Davis, Health System
27. University of California, San Diego, Medical Center
28. University Medical Center
29. Veterans Affairs, Greater Los Angeles Health Care System

30. VA Sierra Pacific Network (10N21), Department of Veterans Affairs, VISN 21

31. Veterans Affairs, Long Beach Healthcare System

32. Veterans Affairs, Northern California Health Care System

33. Veterans Affairs, Palo Alto Health Care System

34. Veterans Affairs, San Diego Healthcare System

Colorado

1. Children's Hospital

2. Department of Veterans Affairs, Veterans Integrated Service Network, VISN 19

3. National Jewish Medical and Research Center

4. University of Colorado Hospital

5. Veterans Affairs, Eastern Colorado Health Care System

Connecticut

1. Bridgeport Hospital

2. Central Connecticut Health Alliance Inc.

3. Danbury Hospital

4. Greenwich Hospital

5. Hartford Hospital

6. Hospital of St. Raphael

7. John Dempsey Hospital, University of Connecticut Health Center

8. Norwalk Hospital

9. Saint Francis Care

10. Saint Francis Hospital and Medical Center

11. Stamford Health System

12. Stamford Hospital

13. Veterans Affairs, Connecticut Health Care System

14. Yale–New Haven Health System

15. Yale–New Haven Hospital

Delaware
1. Christiana Care Health System
2. Veterans Affairs, Medical and Regional Office Center

District of Columbia
1. Children's National Medical Center
2. George Washington University Hospital
3. Georgetown University Hospital
4. Howard University Hospital
5. Universal Health Services Inc., George Washington University Hospital
6. Washington DC Veterans Affairs Medical Center
7. Washington Hospital Center

Florida
1. All Children's Hospital
2. Department of Veterans Affairs, Veterans Integrated Service Network, VISN 8
3. H. Lee Moffitt Cancer Center and Research Institute
4. Jackson Memorial Hospital
5. North Florida/South Georgia Veterans Health Care System– Malcolm Randall VA Medical Center
6. Miami Veterans Affairs Medical Center
7. Mount Sinai Medical Center
8. Orlando Regional Healthcare System
9. Shands Healthcare
10. Shands Jacksonville Medical Center
11. St. Luke's Hospital
12. Tampa General Hospital
13. Veterans Affairs, Medical Center, James A. Haley Veterans Hospital

Georgia
1. Atlanta Medical Center

2. Augusta Veterans Affairs Medical Center

3. Central Georgia Health Systems

4. Children's Healthcare of Atlanta

5. Children's Healthcare of Atlanta (Includes Egleston and Scottish Rite)

6. Crawford Long Hospital of Emory University

7. Department of Veterans Affairs, Veterans Integrated Service Network, VISN 7

8. Emory Healthcare

9. Emory University Hospital

10. Grady Memorial Hospital–Atlanta, GA

11. MCG Health, Inc.

12. Medical College of Georgia Hospital and Clinics

13. Veterans Affairs Medical Center (Atlanta)

14. Medical Center of Central Georgia

15. Memorial Health University Medical Center

16. Memorial Health Inc.

Hawaii

1. Queen's Medical Center

Idaho

1. Boise Veterans Affairs Medical Center

Illinois

1. Advocate Christ Medical Center

2. Advocate Health Care

3. Advocate Illinois Masonic Medical Center

4. Advocate Lutheran General Hospital

5. Children's Memorial Hospital

6. Department of Veterans Affairs, Veterans Integrated Service Network, VISN 12

7. Edward Hines Jr. Hospital, Department of Veterans Affairs

8. Evanston Northwestern Healthcare

9. Hospital Sisters Health System

10. John H. Stroger Jr. Hospital of Cook County

11. Loyola University Health System

12. Loyola University Medical Center

13. MacNeal Hospital

14. Memorial Health System

15. Memorial Medical Center

16. Mount Sinai Hospital

17. Northwestern Memorial Hospital

18. OSF Saint Francis Medical Center

19. Rehabilitation Institute of Chicago

20. Rush System for Health

21. Rush University Medical Center

22. St. John's Hospital

23. University of Chicago Hospitals

24. University of Chicago Hospitals and Health System

25. University of Illinois at Chicago Medical Center

26. Veterans Affairs, Chicago Health Care System

Indiana

1. Ball Memorial Hospital Inc.

2. Cardinal Health System Inc.

3. Clarian Health Partners Inc.

4. Richard L. Roudebush Veterans Affairs Medical Center

5. St. Vincent Hospitals and Health Services Inc.

6. Wishard Health Services

Iowa

1. Iowa Health–Des Moines

2. Iowa City Veterans Affairs Medical Center

3. University of Iowa Hospitals and Clinics

Kansas

1. University of Kansas Hospital

Kentucky

1. Jewish Hospital

2. Jewish Hospital Healthcare Services

3. Lexington Veterans Affairs Medical Center

4. Louisville Veterans Affairs Medical Center

5. University of Kentucky Hospital

6. U of L Health Care University Hospital

Louisiana

1. Baton Rouge General Medical Center

2. General Health System

3. Kenner Regional Medical Center

4. Lindy Boggs Medical Center, Inc. Tenet Louisiana

5. Medical Center of Louisiana at New Orleans

6. Ochsner Clinic Foundation

7. Overton Brooks Veterans Affairs Medical Center

8. Touro Infirmary

9. Tulane University Hospital & Clinic

10. Veterans Affairs Medical Center of New Orleans

Maine

1. Maine Medical Center

Maryland

1. Department of Veterans Affairs, Veterans Integrated Service Network, VISN 5

2. Franklin Square Hospital

3. Greater Baltimore Medical Center

4. Holy Cross Hospital

5. Johns Hopkins Bayview Medical Center

6. Johns Hopkins Health System

7. Johns Hopkins Hospital

8. LifeBridge Health, Inc.

9. MedStar Health

10. Mercy Medical Center

11. Sinai Hospital of Baltimore Inc.

12. The National Institutes of Health (NIH) Clinical Center

13. University of Maryland Medical Center

14. University of Maryland Medical System

15. Veterans Affairs, Maryland Health Care System

Massachusetts

1. Baystate Health System

2. Baystate Medical Center

3. Berkshire Medical Center

4. Beth Israel Deaconess Medical Center

5. Boston Medical Center

6. Brigham and Women's Hospital

7. Cambridge Health Alliance

8. CareGroup Inc.

9. Caritas Christi Health Care System

10. Caritas St. Elizabeth's Medical Center of Boston

11. Children's Hospital

12. Dana-Farber Cancer Institute

13. Department of Veterans Affairs, Veterans Integrated Service Network, VISN 1

14. Faulkner Hospital

15. Lahey Clinic Medical Center

16. Massachusetts General Hospital

17. Mount Auburn Hospital

18. Partners HealthCare System Inc.

19. St. Vincent Hospital Worcester Medical Center

20. Tufts–New England Medical Center

21. University of Massachusetts Memorial Health Care

22. Veterans Affairs, Boston Healthcare System

23. Veterans Affairs Medical Center (West Roxbury/Brockton)

Michigan

1. Bronson Methodist Hospital

2. Department of Veterans Affairs, Veterans Integrated Service Network, VISN 11

3. Detroit Medical Center

4. Henry Ford Hospital

5. Hurley Medical Center

6. Ingham Regional Medical Center

7. John D. Dingell VA Medical Center

8. McLaren Regional Healthcare Corporation

9. McLaren Regional Medical Center

10. Michigan State University Kalamazoo Center for Medical Studies

11. Oakwood Healthcare System

12. Oakwood Hospital and Medical Center

13. Sinai-Grace Hospital

14. Spectrum Health

15. St. Joseph Mercy Hospital

16. St. John Hospital and Medical Center

17. Trinity Health

18. University of Michigan Health System

19. University of Michigan Medical Center

20. Veterans Affairs, Ann Arbor Healthcare System

21. William Beaumont Hospital

22. William Beaumont Hospital System

Minnesota
1. Abbott Northwestern Hospital

2. Allina Hospitals and Clinics

3. Department of Veterans Affairs, Veterans Integrated Service Network, VISN 23

4. Fairview Health Services

5. HealthPartners Inc.

6. Hennepin County Medical Center

7. Mayo Medical Center

8. Minneapolis Veterans Affairs Medical Center

9. Regions Hospital

10. Saint Mary's Hospital

11. University of Minnesota Medical Center, Fairview

Mississippi
1. Department of Veterans Affairs, Veterans Integrated Service Network, VISN 16

2. Methodist Rehabilitation Center

3. University Hospitals and Clinics/ University of Mississippi Medical Center

Missouri
1. Barnes-Jewish Hospital

2. BJC HealthCare

3. Children's Mercy Hospital

4. Department of Veterans Affairs, Veterans Integrated Service Network, VISN 15

5. Saint Louis University Hospital

6. St. John's Mercy Medical Center

7. St. Louis Children's Hospital

8. Saint Luke's Hospital of Kansas City

9. Saint Luke's Shawnee Mission Health System

10. St. Mary's Health Center

11. Truman Medical Center Hospital Hill

12. University of Missouri Health Care

Nebraska

1. Department of Veterans Affairs, Veterans Integrated Service Network, VISN 14

2. Saint Joseph Hospital

3. The Nebraska Medical Center

4. VA Nebraska–Western Iowa Health Care System–Omaha Division

New Hampshire

1. Dartmouth Hitchcock Alliance

2. Dartmouth–Hitchcock Medical Center

New Jersey

1. Atlantic Health System

2. Cooper University Hospital

3. Department of Veterans Affairs, New Jersey Health Care System

4. Hackensack University Medical Center

5. Jersey Shore University Medical Center

6. Monmouth Medical Center

7. Morristown Memorial Hospital

8. Meridian Health System

9. Newark Beth Israel Medical Center

10. Robert Wood Johnson Health System

11. Robert Wood Johnson University Hospital

12. Saint Barnabas Health Care System

13. Saint Barnabas Medical Center

14. Saint Peter's University Hospital

15. University of Medicine and Dentistry of New Jersey–University Hospital

16. University Medical Center at Princeton

New Mexico

1. New Mexico Veterans Affairs Health Care System

2. University of New Mexico Hospital

New York

1. Albany Medical Center Hospital

2. Albany Veterans Affairs Medical Center

3. Bellevue Hospital Center

4. Beth Israel Medical Center

5. Brooklyn Hospital Center

6. Bronx Lebanon Hospital Center

7. Bronx Veterans Affairs Medical Center

8. Coney Island Hospital

9. Continuum Health Partners Inc.

10. Department of Veterans Affairs, Veterans Integrated Service Network, VISN 2

11. Department of Veterans Affairs, Veterans Integrated Service Network, VISN 3

12. Elmhurst Hospital Center

13. Harlem Hospital Center

14. Hospital for Joint Diseases Orthopedic Institute

15. Hospital for Special Surgery

16. Jacobi Medical Center

17. Kaleida Health

18. Kaleida Health/Buffalo General Hospital

19. Kings County Hospital Center

20. Lenox Hill Healthcare Network

21. Lenox Hill Hospital

22. Long Island College Hospital
23. Long Island Jewish Medical Center
24. Lincoln Medical and Mental Health Center
25. Montefiore Medical Center
26. North Central Bronx
27. Maimonides Medical Center
28. Mary Imogene Bassett Hospital
29. MediSys
30. Memorial Sloan-Kettering Cancer Center
31. Metropolitan Hospital Center
32. Mount Sinai Hospital
33. NYC Health and Hospitals Corporation
34. NYU Hospitals Center
35. NYU Medical Center
36. New York–Presbyterian Healthcare System
37. New York–Presbyterian Hospital, The University Hospital of Columbia and Cornell
38. New York Methodist Hospital
39. North Shore–Long Island Jewish Health System
40. Northport Veterans Affairs Medical Center
41. North Shore University Hospital
42. Our Lady of Mercy Healthcare System
43. Our Lady of Mercy Medical Center
44. Queens Hospital Center
45. Roswell Park Cancer Institute
46. Saint Vincent's Catholic Medical Centers of New York
47. St. Luke's–Roosevelt Hospital Center
48. Sound Shore Health System
49. Sound Shore Medical Center of Westchester
50. Strong Health System

51. Strong Memorial Hospital

52. Staten Island University Hospital

53. Syracuse Veterans Affairs Medical Center

54. University Hospital, SUNY Health Science Center, Stony Brook

55. University Hospital, SUNY Upstate Medical University

56. University Hospital of Brooklyn, SUNY Health Science Center

57. United Health Services Hospitals

58. Veterans Affairs New York, Harbor Health Care System–Brooklyn Campus

59. Veterans Affairs New York, Harbor Health Care System–New York Campus

60. Veterans Affairs, Western New York Healthcare System

61. ViaHealth

62. Westchester Medical Center

63. Winthrop South Nassau University Health System Inc.

64. Winthrop–University Hospital

65. Woodhull Medical & Mental Health Center

North Carolina

1. Carolinas HealthCare System

2. Carolinas Medical Center

3. Department of Veterans Affairs, Veterans Integrated Service Network, VISN 6

4. Duke University Health System

5. Duke University Hospital

6. Durham Veterans Affairs Medical Center

7. North Carolina Baptist Hospital

8. Pitt County Memorial Hospital

9. University Health System of Eastern Carolina, Inc.

10. University of North Carolina Hospitals

11. UNC Health Care System

North Dakota
1. MeritCare Hospital

Ohio
1. Akron General Medical Center
2. Arthur G. James Cancer Hospital and Richard J. Solove Research Institute
3. Aultman Hospital
4. Children's Hospital Medical Center of Akron
5. Children's Medical Center
6. Cincinnati Children's Hospital Medical Center
7. Cincinnati Veterans Affairs Medical Center
8. Cleveland Clinic Foundation
9. Cleveland Clinic Health System
10. Columbus Children's Hospital
11. Dayton Veterans Affairs Medical Center
12. Department of Veterans Affairs, Veterans Integrated Service Network, VISN 10
13. Forum Health
14. Forum Health–Western Reserve Care System
15. Good Samaritan Hospital
16. Grant–Riverside Methodist Hospitals, Grant Medical Center Campus
17. Grant–Riverside Methodist Hospitals, Riverside Campus
18. Health Alliance of Greater Cincinnati
19. Kettering Medical Center
20. Louis Stokes Veterans Affairs Medical Center
21. MetroHealth System
22. Miami Valley Hospital
23. Ohio State University Health System
24. Ohio State University Hospitals

25. OhioHealth
26. St. Elizabeth Health Center
27. Summa Health System Hospitals
28. University Hospital
29. University Medical Center
30. University Hospitals Health System
31. University Hospitals of Cleveland

Oklahoma
1. OU Medical Center
2. Oklahoma City Veterans Affairs Medical Center

Oregon
1. Oregon Health & Science University
2. Portland Veterans Affairs Medical Center

Pennsylvania
1. Albert Einstein Medical Center (Albert Einstein Healthcare Network)
2. Allegheny General Hospital
3. Children's Hospital of Philadelphia
4. Crozer–Keystone Health System
5. Crozer–Chester Medical Center
6. Department of Veterans Affairs, Veterans Integrated Service Network, VISN 4
7. Geisinger Health System
8. Fox Chase Cancer Center
9. Frankford Hospital of the City of Philadelphia
10. Hamot Medical Center
11. Hospital of the University of Pennsylvania
12. Jefferson Health System
13. Lehigh Valley Hospital
14. Lankenau Hospital

15. Magee–Women's Hospital

16. Mercy Hospital of Pittsburgh

17. Philadelphia Veterans Affairs Medical Center

18. Pittsburgh Mercy Health System, Inc.

19. St. Christopher's Hospital for Children

20. St. Luke's Hospital

21. The Milton S. Hershey Medical Center

22. Temple University Health System

23. Temple University Hospital

24. Tenet Health System, Graduate Hospital

25. Tenet Health System, Hahnemann University Hospital

26. Thomas Jefferson University Hospital

27. University of Pennsylvania Health System

28. University of Pittsburgh Medical Center (UPMC)

29. UPMC Presbyterian Shadyside

30. Veterans Affairs Pittsburgh Healthcare System

31. West Penn Allegheny Health System

32. Western Pennsylvania Hospital

33. Wellspan Health

34. York Hospital

Puerto Rico
1. San Juan Veterans Affairs Medical Center

Rhode Island
1. Care New England Health System

2. Lifespan Inc.

3. Memorial Hospital of Rhode Island

4. Miriam Hospital

5. Rhode Island Hospital

6. Roger Williams Hospital

7. Women and Infants Hospital of Rhode Island

South Carolina

1. Greenville Hospital System
2. Medical University of South Carolina Medical Center
3. Palmetto Health
4. Palmetto Health Alliance
5. Ralph H. Johnson Veterans Affairs Medical Center

South Dakota

1. Avera McKennan Hospital and University
2. Sioux Valley Hospital USD Medical Center
3. Sioux Valley Hospitals and Health System

Tennessee

1. Department of Veterans Affairs, Veterans Integrated Service Network, VISN 9
2. James H. Quillen Veterans Affairs Medical Center
3. Johnson City Medical Center Hospital Inc.
4. Methodist Healthcare–University Hospital
5. Mountain States Health Alliance
6. Regional Medical Center at Memphis
7. Saint Thomas Hospital
8. Vanderbilt University Hospital
9. Vanguard Health System
10. Veterans Affairs Tennessee Valley Health Care System
11. Veterans Affairs Medical Center of Memphis

Texas

1. Baylor University Medical Center
2. Central Texas Veterans Health Care System
3. Children's Medical Center of Dallas
4. Dallas County Hospital District, Parkland Health & Hospital System
5. Department of Veterans Affairs, Veterans Integrated Service Network, VISN 17

6. Harris County Hospital District

7. Medical Center Hospital

8. Memorial Hermann Healthcare System

9. Methodist Health Care System

10. Methodist Health System

11. Methodist Hospital

12. Michael E. DeBakey Veterans Affairs Medical Center

13. Scott and White Memorial Hospital

14. St. Luke's Episcopal Health System

15. St. Luke's Episcopal Hospital

16. Texas Children's Hospital

17. University Health System

18. University Medical Center

19. University Medical Center Health System

20. University of Texas M. D. Anderson Cancer Center

21. University of Texas Health Center at Tyler

22. University of Texas Medical Branch Hospitals at Galveston

23. University of Texas Southwestern Medical Center

24. Veterans Affairs, North Texas Health Care System

25. Veterans Affairs, South Texas Health Care System

Utah

1. University of Utah Health System

2. University of Utah Hospital

Vermont

1. Fletcher Allen Health Care

2. Veterans Affairs Medical and Regional Office Center

Virginia

1. Carilion Medical Center

2. INOVA Fairfax Hospital

3. INOVA Health System

4. Hunter Holmes McGuire Veterans Affairs Medical Center

5. Medical College of Virginia Hospitals

6. Salem Veterans Affairs Medical Center

7. Sentara Norfolk General Hospitals

8. University of Virginia Medical Center

Washington

1. Children's Hospital and Regional Medical Center

2. Department of Veterans Affairs, Veterans Integrated Service Network, VISN 20

3. Harborview Medical Center University of Washington Hospitals

4. University of Washington Academic Medical Center

5. University of Washington Medical Center

6. Veterans Affairs Puget Sound Health Care System

West Virginia

1. Cabell Huntington Hospital

2. CAMC Health System

3. Charleston Area Medical Center

4. West Virginia United Health System

5. West Virginia University Hospitals Inc.

Wisconsin

1. Aurora Health Care

2. Children's Hospital of Wisconsin

3. Froedtert Hospital and Health System

4. Gundersen Lutheran Health Care System

5. Lutheran Hospital–LaCrosse

6. Sinai Samaritan Medical Center

7. St. Luke's Medical Center

8. University of Wisconsin Hospital and Clinic

Answers to Selected Chapter Exercise Problems

CHAPTER 1

1. Some questions to consider include the following.

   - What is the current level of productivity in terms of packages per hour?

   - What is the cost of the new software? How long is its useful life? What is the amortized cost?

   - What is the expected level of productivity post-implementation?

   - Does the delta in productivity metrics justify the cost?

CHAPTER 3

1. Average deduction rate is 52%.

2. 30 days of working capital.

3. 3.6% return on capital.

CHAPTER 5

1a. 5-day moving average forecast is 28.2.

1b. 3-day moving average forecast is 29.3.

2. Using the calculation of $W = \dfrac{L}{\lambda}$ average wait time is 15 minutes (10/40). Note that this is not the same as the total wait in the system (W_q).

CHAPTER 6

1. Single-factor productivity rate is 12.2.

2. Productivity has decreased by 6.9% from the previous month.

3. Yes, total annual cost would be $20,000 and total savings would be $23,787.50. Therefore total benefit would be $3,787.50.

CHAPTER 7

1. PERT calculation is 26.3 days.

2. PERT is higher by 1.3 days.

CHAPTER 8

1. The program would break even at 1,000 procedures.

2. The new breakeven point is 857 procedures.

3. The second option should be chosen.

CHAPTER 9

1. NPV is $1,243. Yes, the project should be accepted since it is greater than $0.

2. 2.85 years.

CHAPTER 12

1. $1,800,000 (15% × $1 million × 12)

2. Net realizable value is $87.50 ($100 sales price – $12.50 cost to sell).

3. Current replacement cost falls between the ceiling and the floor, so $40 is the lower of cost or market.

4. Debit COGS, credit inventory

5. Days of inventory on hand is 72 days.

6. Economic order quantity is 7.07.

CHAPTER 13

1. Yes, this is definitely an increasing trend.

2. This is calculated using $Y = a + bx$, with a slope equal to 10, an intercept of 50, so the forecast for period 2 is 70.

Glossary of Terms

activity-based costing (ABC)

A classification scheme in which inventories or supplies are grouped according to usage or sales volumes, typically in terms of quantities or dollar volumes. "A" items tend to be the highest usage or highest dollar items and typically represent about 80% of the usage but only 20% of the items.

academic medicine

Clinical patient care that occurs in a teaching hospital or one of its facilities. Care delivered by the faculty, residents, fellows, or students of an affiliated medical school as part of a formal training program.

acquisition

A type of growth strategy in which one organization acquires another organization. Examples include a hospital purchasing a physician practice or a large, investor-owned hospital purchasing a small, rural independent hospital.

acute care

A specific episode or event requiring care.

adjusted patient day

A calculation that measures hospital volumes in which both inpatient and outpatient volumes are incorporated. Calculated as total gross revenue divided by total inpatient revenue, multiplied by the number of inpatient days.

admixture
: The pharmaceutical process of combining multiple fluids.

allowances
: Deductions or discounts from gross patient revenues that reduce the amount of charges to be collected. Typically these are contractually negotiated (for managed care) or regulated (for government payers).

as-is process
: Process map that depicts the actual, current process in place prior to any process engineering.

asset
: Anything the hospital owns that has immediate or long-term monetary value. Examples of assets are cash, marketable securities and investments, prepaid expenses, accounts receivable, inventories, fixed assets (also called plant, property, and equipment), and other assets.

attributes
: Characteristics that describe an item.

audit
: An examination or verification of finances, compliance, and/or operations. Most common audits are financial in nature, ensuring adherence to generally accepted accounting principles (GAAP), which ensure that the organization's finances are materially correct and that internal controls are adequate.

average length of stay (ALOS)
: The average number of days a patient stays, from admission to discharge. An inpatient metric, which is calculated as the number of patient days during a period divided by the number of discharges.

balance sheet
: One of the three most common financial statements; shows the financial position of a hospital at a specific point in time. Key elements focus on the accounting equation of Assets = Liabilities + Net assets.

bar code
: Single- or two-dimension machine-readable code that contains a number of key pieces of information. Also called a "license plate" and is visually represented either by an array of bars linearly or a matrix diagram of dots.

bar code reader	Scanning devices that can be used to scan, de-code, and interpret bar codes.
benchmarking	Comparison of a key performance measurement relative to the competition or other leading organizations. The process of seeking best practices among better performing organizations, with intentions of applying those internally.
benefit	A gain or positive change in an outcome.
bill of material	Listing or recipe that defines the specific raw materials or components in a finished good.
biometric methods	Newer security systems that use physiological characteristics, such as fingerprints or retinal scans, to uniquely identify an individual.
bottleneck	A choke point, or a point in a process where capacity is limited, that effectively reduces the number of outputs due to physical or logical constraints.
brand equity	The combination of assets and liabilities unique to each teaching hospital that determines its overall image or perception in the marketplace.
breakeven analysis	Analytical technique that studies cost structures and volumes to identify at what point total returns equals total costs.
budget	A quantitative plan that represents management's financial expectations; typically converts patient activities into associated revenues, costs, and margins.
bulk replenishment	A method of replenishment of resources where items are simply augmented to the existing cart or location.
bullwhip effect	A phenomenon whereby demand varies or fluctuates significantly as the demand is viewed or interpreted further upstream. Although the actual consumer demand might be fairly constant, the impact of promotions, nonsystematic ordering, and other factors tends to cause the upstream supply chain to interpret downstream demand as highly variable. Caused by lack of visibility into actual consumer demand, among other factors.

business plan	The written, detailed plan for an existing or proposed program, facility, service line, or other operation. Typically used to assess the financial practicality, plus detail key strategies.
business strategy	The managerial process responsible for formulating dynamic decisions about critical elements of the business that establishes hospital direction, creates a significantly differentiated competitive game plan, and results in a competitive advantage. Also called *competitive strategy* or simply *strategy*.
buy-in	Similar to partnering, where sponsors and managers craft a story or vision for their change, and then obtain support from others to ensure that no organizational obstacles prevent the project's advancement.
cannibalize	To draw demand away from another product. For example, when a cellular phone manufacturer introduces a new model, this new model cannibalizes or diminishes sales for existing models.
capacity	The amount of resources or assets that exist to serve demand.
capacity planning	The process of aligning capacity with demand.
capital	A factor of production that represents investments in assets to offset labor, or assets used to produce even more assets.
capital substitution	A term used to describe the role that technology or capital can play in displacing labor.
capitalize	The accounting process of recognizing assets on the balance sheet and spreading or depreciating the costs over the time periods in which the benefits will be realized.
capitation	Method of physician or provider reimbursement that transfers financial risk of care to physicians and away from health plans or insurers. Standard primary care capitation in health plans reimburses the provider on a per member per month basis, such that a flat payment is made per capita to a defined population over a certain period of time.

carousel	Pharmacy equipment that automates the picking, packing, and dispensing of drugs.
case mix index (CMI)	A measurement that shows the complexity of a procedure. Used to normalize data so that comparisons can be made relative to other procedures and to perform benchmarking against competitive hospitals. Adjusting supply expenses by case mix index is one common use.
cash inflow	Cash that is generated or returned from a project, and represents sources of funds.
cash outflow	Cash that is expended or otherwise utilized, and represents uses of funds.
categories	In data hierarchies, a grouping of attributes for analysis purposes.
causal factor	A data series that is used to help improve product forecasts because it has a suspected strong relationship with the item. For example, "new building starts" is often used to help improve the prediction of demand for "lumber" because quantity of lumber consumed has a strong tie to the number of houses or buildings being built.
chain of custody	Refers to the handling audit trail, which details how and who has handled specific items, when and where the transfers of physical products occurred.
channel	A type of outlet for selling hospital services, or a specific set of processes and parties that gets products from source of supply to end consumer. Hospital channels include clinics, hospitals, mobile clinics, and even in-store retail locations. A type of facility where patient care is provided.
Charge Description Master	A hospital's master list of prices for all procedures, services, and supplies provided to patients.
chargeable	An item or service that will be charged back, directly or indirectly (through room or procedure rates) to patients.

collaboration	Open, participative process and environment where internal and extended supply chain partners work together to share common information (such as point-of-service data), formats, languages, and processes to achieve a common goal (increase profitability and improve demand).
collaborative planning, forecasting, and replenishment (CPFR)	A process deployed in consumer industries in which the entire extended supply chain network uses a specific collaborative planning and forecasting framework to improve inventory and sales plans. A partnership for sharing information about consumer point of sales data between suppliers and retailers.
community hospital	Term used to describe facilities that are available for use by the entire community. Represents the majority of hospitals in the United States and includes all nonfederal, short-term hospitals of either for-profit or nonprofit status.
competition	A term used to describe the existence of substitute providers of a product or service. In most industries, the greater the intensity of the competition, the greater the need for business strategy because heightened competition leads to reduced margins over time.
competitive advantage	Differential outcome or differential performance achieved by an organization relative to the competition. A result of the activities and processes that are performed significantly better than the competition.
competitive bidding	Formalized sourcing process; ensures that multiple vendors are contacted and encouraged to respond to solicitations (such as requests for proposals or information) to ensure a competitive marketplace, which improves economics and typically lowers the total cost of ownership.
competitiveness	Management's ability to respond to environmental changes, as well as competitors' actions, to protect and enhance overall financial outcomes.

compounding | Pharmaceutical process of breaking down tablets or solid substances.

concentration | A term used to describe the existence of competition, in terms of size and distribution, in a market. Typically expressed in a ratio format from 0 to 1, where a number closer to 0 indicates an extremely fragmented and competitive market, while a number closer to 1 indicates a near-monopoly environment.

consignment in | A type of inventory that is being held or stored on the hospital's facility at no charge until sold, and is owned by a vendor or distributor.

consignment out | Inventory that is owned by the organization and is placed elsewhere until it sells.

continuous improvement | A constant focus on achieving better outcomes.

control chart | Chart that shows process data values over time, relative to both a mean and standard deviations.

controlled drug | Drugs that are tightly controlled around usage and distribution by the U.S. Drug Enforcement Agency because of potential for misuse and abuse.

core competency | Expertise that underlies an organization's reason for existing and is the source of its competitive advantage.

cost of capital | The weighted average cost of all funding sources for a hospital, including both debt and equity, typically expressed as a percentage.

cost of goods sold (COGS) | The total cost of the inventory sold in a specific period.

cost-quality continuum | A theoretical tradeoff or dichotomy where a focus on one side of the equation leads to diminishing returns on the other.

cost report | An institutional report that details the financial and operational transaction summary for a hospital, such as revenues and expenses by key services, as well as balance sheet and activity information.

Council of Teaching Hospitals (COTH)
: A group of major hospitals that play a significant role in educating future medical providers and providing basic and advanced research, in addition to providing patient care. An organization of the Association of American Medical Colleges with restricted membership to only those hospitals with primary missions in academic health care.

critical path method
: A technique that helps to identify the longest path in a project, which therefore makes it the most critical, because a delay in this path will negatively impact the entire project.

current asset
: An asset (something producing a future benefit) that is expected to be converted to cash through sales or consumption in the next 12 months, or the next operating cycle, whichever is longer. Cash, accounts receivable, and inventory are current assets.

current liability
: A liability (obligations owed to another party) that is expected to become due or be paid in the next 12 months. Accounts payable is a current liability.

current procedural terminology (CPT)
: The code that describes the types of services provided by hospitals. Often used interchangeably with *healthcare common procedural codes*.

current ratio
: The relationship found by dividing current assets by current liabilities.

customer
: Within health care, a customer is a potential, current, or previous user, consumer, or other interested party involved in the exchange of healthcare services. The primary customer is the patient (i.e., the individual receiving care), but many secondary customers of hospitals exist, such as payers, community, patients' families, government, or other key stakeholders in the healthcare transaction.

customer service
: The means by which a provider attempts to keep customers happy and loyal, while differentiating themselves from others.

cycle inventory
: The inventory that accrues over time due to supply chain production or procurement process that is

tied to inflexible lot sizes. For example, if demand in period A was 10,000 units, but the retailer can only purchase from their supplier in a 20,000-unit lot size, the difference between the two over time becomes the average cycle inventory.

cyclical demand
A demand pattern where cycles tend to result in a predictable ebb and flow in business or demand.

de-bottleneck
To eliminate constraints or obstacles that limit capacity or throughput.

deductions
Similar to *allowances.* Adjustments—whether for contractual, regulatory, or charitable care provided—that reduce gross patient revenues.

deliverable
The tangible outcome that results from the project.

demand
The need for a specific product at a specific time. In a perfect world, demand would equal sales, but in reality they can be significantly different. As an example, if sales were 500 in period X but two manufacturing plants were down and thus the firm had no inventory to sell, the lost demand plus actual sales would equal demand.

demand association
A process that allows planners to estimate the demand for new products, or to estimate demand for current products at new selling locations, by associating the historical demand of one product with another. This process brings a degree of analytical validation to otherwise judgmental means for estimating demand, especially for new-product introductions. Also called *product chaining* or *demand chaining.*

demand chain
As opposed to a supply chain, demand chain is a relatively new term that focuses on the more complex set of business processes and activities that help firms understand, manage, and ultimately create consumer demand. Tends to focus more on generating demand than fulfilling supply.

demand forecast
A collaborative process that estimates the quantity of items that will be used or required over a specific

time period. Projection of demand by item, location, and time dimensions.

depreciation
: A decline in value over time, or an allocation of the original cost of an asset during the total productive or useful life of that asset.

design capacity
: Maximum stated or theoretical output for a resource.

diagnosis
: Physician or medical provider's explanation for the cause or source of the problem or symptoms.

diagnosis-related group (DRG)
: A classification system for illnesses that comprise 495 groups of medical conditions, each of which has a different reimbursement schedule for Medicare payments. Used by the Centers for Medicare and Medicaid Services to standardize payments and promote more efficient patient care.

distributor
: Brokers, intermediaries, or other middlemen that aggregate supply, store inventory, and serve to connect the manufacturer with retailers and consumers.

downstream
: Refers to positioning closer toward the consumers or users of goods and services.

drilldown
: Allows users to continuously explore data deeper by moving finer and lower in the hierarchy, thus helping to further understand and analyze data at more descriptive levels using narrowly defined attributes.

drug
: Substance that is intended for use in the diagnosis, cure, mitigation, treatment, and prevention of disease.

durable medical equipment (DME)
: Equipment used in the delivery of patient care that meets several criteria: it is used repeatedly for multiple patients, it is used for a medical necessity, it is appropriate for use outside of the hospital, and it is no longer beneficial to patients once they resume normal health.

economic order quantity
: A basic calculation that approximates the optimal quantity of items to procure at one time.

economic performance
: The financial viability and outcomes measured over the long term. Often measured by multiple metrics,

such as return on capital. Typically refers to true cash operating position after the costs of the capital employed have been extracted.

economies of scale
Synergies or reductions in total costs due to purchase and usage of larger, bulk quantities.

effective capacity
An adjustment of the design capacity, which is calculated by multiplying average expected utilization rates.

efficiency
One of the primary goals of operations management. Measures the degree of resource and costs consumed per unit of output.

electronic data interchange (EDI)
The standardization of specific, common data through common message formats, such as invoices, point-of-service data, and shipping notices, that helps simplify exchanges and electronic transfer between different components of the supply chain. EDI is used to enable tracking of point-of-service demand to synchronize the supply chain, thus reducing overall inventories, reducing planning response cycle times, and improving overall collaboration.

enterprise resource planning (ERP)
The primary "system of record" to track products or services provided, their costs, customers, and cash associated with the entire operation.

evidenced-based medicine
Medicine that follows the scientific method to medical practice and seeks to quantify the true outcomes associated with certain medical practices by applying statistical and research methods.

exchange cart
A replenishment system where an entire fixture (or cart) is swapped entirely with all new items.

exclusions
Services for which an insurer or payer will not provide reimbursement.

extended SCM
Term used to describe the internal hospital supply chain plus channel partners external to the firm. Also referred to as the *supply chain network,* this can include manufacturers, wholesalers, distributors, bro-

kers, retailers, dealers, third-party logistics providers, transportation carriers, and public warehouses.

external environment
Includes all forces external to the industry that potentially influence business strategy, such as competition, industry, legal, and other aspects outside of the organization.

fee-for-service
An approach in which a hospital charges additionally for each service provided. Becoming less common as managed care and indemnity providers contractually negotiate bundled services for fixed fees in efforts to reduce overall costs.

finished good
An item that is in its final form for consumption or utilization.

first in, first out (FIFO)
An accounting method for inventory in which the first item purchased and received is the first item used, and therefore ending inventory is comprised of the most recently purchased items.

fiscal year
An accounting period of one year, used for financial reporting and budgeting purposes. May be the same as a calendar year, but could be any 12-month period.

fixed costs
All expenses that are necessary to delivery services and do not vary with total services provided. Used in breakeven analysis and financial ratio analysis.

forecast
A projection or estimate of future demand. Can be created using a variety of qualitative and quantitative methods.

forward positioning
The placement of medications (or other inventory) near the point of use, prior to their actual usage, based on forecasted needs.

future value
The value of money in the future, taking into account the time value of money and interest.

GAAP
Generally accepted accounting principles. Required for use by public companies, but used by many private and not-for-profit organizations, to accurately record expenses and inventory values in a standard fashion.

game theory	Economic technique where the organization can attempt to estimate how the competition will respond to its strategies and what will be the impact on performance.
Gantt chart	A type of chart that shows activities as blocks or bars over time, named for its founder Henry Gantt.
group physician practice	An organized group of physicians that comes together to leverage economies of scale in administrative and facility infrastructures. Typically involves management of all back-office and financial functions so that physicians can focus on providing care and not the daily aspects of business management.
group purchasing organization (GPO)	A collaborative arrangement in which multiple parties (buyers) unite for purposes of increasing their collective bargaining power with vendors (sellers).
Hawthorne effect	Phenomenon whereby individuals perform differently when they are given attention or being observed than they would in normal situations.
healthcare common procedural code (HCPC)	A code, often used interchangeably with *current procedural terminology* code, that describes the types of services provided by a hospital.
healthcare operations management	A discipline of management that integrates scientific or quantitative principles to determine the most efficient and optimal methods to support patient care delivery. The quantitative management of the supporting business systems and processes that transform resources (or inputs) into healthcare services (outputs).
health maintenance organization (HMO)	A health plan that represents managed-care alternative delivery systems. Offers enrollees unlimited access to care from a qualified, select list of providers.
Herfindahl-Hirschman index (HHI)	Measures market concentration. It is used primarily by the Department of Justice and the Federal Trade Commission to assess the impact of a merger on that market's competitive dynamics. Calculated by

a sum of the squares of the individual market shares for each of the hospitals in the market. The higher the number, the closer the healthcare market is to being a monopoly. Alternatively, the lower the concentration, the more competitive the market.

heuristic
A rule of thumb or general guideline.

hierarchy
A classification system that organizes data around common attributes. Used here to refer to information systems, but can also apply to organizations and other management systems.

horizontal integration
Refers to consolidation, mergers, acquisition, or alliances among several competitive or cooperative hospitals that have resulted in multi-hospital health systems.

hospital
An organization devoted to delivering patient care; provides services centered on observation, diagnosis, and treatment.

hurdle rate
The minimum rate of return that an organization's management requires before they accept or approve projects.

improve
To make something better.

innovation
The continuous process of doing new things, or just doing current things better. Often a driver of industry economics.

input
All resources to be used or consumed in a process, such as labor hours, staff, supplies, space or facilities, information systems, and any other resources.

integrated delivery network
Any combination or integration between a hospital and other providers or partners in the healthcare industry that work together collaboratively across a spectrum of care to provide more competitive and comprehensive services.

interest
Payment received by those who hold money to forgo current consumption.

intermediate good
Items that require additional processing before they can be sold. Used here from a drug compounding perspective.

intermittent demand	Utilization behavior that is not dispersed evenly over time, but tends to occur only at specific periods in batches or lumps.
internal rate of return (IRR)	Computation of project outcomes where the net present value of a project is equal to zero.
interoperability	Integration of technology to allow for sharing and linking of data so that applications behave as one large system.
inventory	Materials that are available for sale and therefore represent future benefits for an organization. Requires special financial accounting treatment to determine proper valuation. Buffer against demand variability.
item	Any physical good that is procured for ultimate use or consumption, whether in its current form, or following some degree of processing or transformation.
item master	A system that stores item-level data. These data include important attribute fields, necessary for both transactional processing and analytical reporting.
joint venture	A type of growth strategy in which two or more organizations combine financial and operating resources to create a new jointly owned entity for a specific project or purpose.
just in time (JIT)	The process of moving goods (either finished, semifinished, or materials) to the next stage of the supply chain at the exact point in time that they are required for use in the process or for consumption by customer. The goals of JIT programs typically are to reduce or eliminate inventory levels, minimize process cycle times, and increase the level of responsiveness and flexibility in the manufacturing and logistics processes. The opposite of *supply to stock*.
key performance indicator (KPI)	A limited number of performance metrics that quantify operating results in critical areas, typically focused around strategic outcomes or productivity.

last in, first out (LIFO)
: An inventory accounting method that states that the oldest items purchased and received are the last to be sold, or that newer items purchased are the first ones sold.

laundry management
: The process of collecting, processing, transporting, and replenishing linens during the linen life cycle, from acquisition to final disposition.

lean process
: Process focused on quality improvements that increase speed, improve flexibility, reduce lot sizes, increase customization, and reduce waste.

liability
: A financial obligation in the future that must be settled by transfer of cash or other assets, and is recorded on the balance sheet as either current or long-term in nature.

linear programming
: An optimization technique that seeks to either maximize or minimize an objective function, given a set of variables and constraints.

linens
: Fabrics used for healthcare purposes, including scrubs, pillows, cases, sheets, blankets, towels, lab coats, rags, protective gear, and gowns.

logistics
: The efficient coordination and control of the flow of all operations, including patients, personnel, and resources.

loss leader
: An item that is sold by a vendor at a loss to attract customers to buy other premium items. Loss leaders are usually either very early or late stage, have poor growth prospects under normal conditions, or might not otherwise sell well.

lower of cost or market (LCM)
: Concept used in inventory accounting that states that inventory must be capitalized at whichever price is lower—cost or market.

lowest unit of measure (LUM)
: Term to describe a practice where items are purchased and stored in the unit in which they will ultimately be consumed.

managed care
: Organized efforts to achieve cost containment in health care. Typically, managed care has two key

characteristics: (1) structurally integrated alternative delivery systems, such as health maintenance or preferred provider organizations, and (2) different reimbursement mechanisms and financial incentives that change provider and patient behaviors toward less utilization and less expensive treatments.

managed care organization (MCO)
An organization that is designed to capture the benefits of managed care. A generic term that includes health maintenance and preferred provider organizations.

managed competition
The application of managed-care principles within a competitive environment.

management
The process of planning, organizing, leading, and controlling that helps steer an organization and achieve the mission and objectives.

manufacturers
Companies that produce goods or transform raw materials and components into useable finished products.

markup
The difference between the invoice cost and the price charged to patients, typically expressed as a percentage. Used to generate reasonable returns or margins.

materials management
The department in a hospital typically responsible for supply chain management, including the business processes associated with acquiring, storing, distributing, and replenishing supplies and other resources.

mean absolute deviation (MAD)
A calculation of the amount of error in a forecast. Calculated as the sum of the absolute difference between the average of the actual values and the forecasted values, divided by the number of observations.

measurable
A state or condition where inputs and outputs can be readily observed and calculated.

Medicaid
A health insurance program for low-income persons who are elderly, blind, disabled, or are members of families with dependent children. Medicaid is funded and controlled primarily by individual states,

although the U.S. government does share in providing resources.

medical record
The formal, auditable account and history of a patient's encounter in the hospital, including description of illnesses, procedures performed, supplies provided, notes, and discharge procedures. When in electronic form, it is also referred to as electronic medical record or electronic health record.

Medicare
Federally funded national health insurance program for persons aged 65 and older, and for disabled persons, regardless of income or age.

milestone
The key date by which a major project deliverable should be achieved.

multivariate
A forecasting approach that relies on multiple data series to predict future demand.

mutually exclusive and collectively exhaustive (MECE)
A systems-oriented approach to decision making where each idea is distinct and stands on its own, and also completely covers the range of possibilities for that issue.

national drug code (NDC)
A 10-digit pharmaceutical industry code that uniquely identifies each drug.

net patient revenue
The difference between gross patient revenues less discounts and deductions. Also called *operating revenue.*

net present value (NPV)
The present value of all cash inflows less expected cash outflows. A measure of the relative profitability of a project over the long term, after full consideration of the time value of money.

net realizable value
An accounting term used in valuation of inventory, equal to the sales price less all cost of sales.

network
A group of providers—including doctors, clinics, academic medical centers, and hospitals—that is contractually organized, either loosely or formally, to provide a full range of integrated healthcare services to enrolled members and patients.

observation
Involves analyzing or studying patients, running tests and checks, all of which will ultimately lead to a diagnosis.

obsolete	Implies that the useful life of a product has expired.
operating margin	The difference between net patient revenue and total operating expense. Reflects the profits cleared in the course of normal business operations. As a percentage, it is calculated by dividing profit margin by net revenues.
operational effectiveness	A measure of how well an organization is managed.
operational excellence	A term used to describe an organization that continuously seeks to improve its productivity, business processes, and overall effectiveness.
operations management	Quantitative management of the supporting business systems and processes that transform resources (or inputs) into healthcare services (outputs). Discipline of management that integrates scientific principles to determine the most efficient and optimal methods to support patient care delivery.
optimization	A mathematical approach to solving a problem, where an optimal (or best) solution can be reached given the constraints and parameters defined.
output	The level of production or yield (of goods and services) that results from a conversion process. Outputs are the result of the work conducted through business processes and automation.
outsourcing	Contracting of an outside firm to perform services that were once handled internally.
par	Inventory location that holds a specific product mix with minimum quantities that will cover the location for a predetermined number of hours or days. Used for supplies, pharmaceuticals, and for linens.
Pareto chart	Graphical representation of the vital few issues that exist. Based on the 80–20 concept, which states that 80% of the cumulative percentage of problems are caused by 20% of the issues.
partnering	Establishing mutually beneficial and cooperative relationships with others, where trust and teamwork help to create synergies.

payback	The number of periods required to complete the return of the original investment. Calculated by dividing the initial investment by the average expected cash flow each period.
payer	A party to a hospital transaction that provides financial reimbursement through specific mechanisms and protocols, typically based on negotiated or settled pricing.
payer mix	The relative percentages of volumes and revenues that is generated by each payer group (e.g., Medicare, commercial, self).
payoff	Payback or return on decisions or investments.
penetration	Term used in procurement to represent the percentage of usage or purchases against a specific contract.
per diem	A method of reimbursement where payers will compensate hospitals a flat reimbursement amount each day, regardless of actual services performed or resources consumed.
performance scorecard	A tool to visualize measurements of key performance indicators for an organization relative to time, targets, or other baselines.
periodic inventory	A method of accounting for inventory where inventory balances are physically counted and adjusted at established intervals, rather than being perpetual.
perpetual inventory	Ability to know, at all points in time, actual balances due to continuous tracking of inventory receipts and issues.
pharmacy	A facility that exists to fill and dispense drugs and medications that are prescribed by physicians or other caregivers. In hospitals, they are often one of the largest revenue generators and resource consumers.
physician preferences	A situation where a provider selects established vendors and known products based on existing comfort level and possibly reluctance to change.

pilot	An initial test of a proposed new process, under limited conditions, to help gauge issues and success in achieving the desired goals.
point of service	A type of managed care plan that offers a network of preferred providers, like the health maintenance organizations, but also allow members the flexibility to seek care outside of the network, albeit at a higher cost and with higher out of pocket expenses.
point of use	The position in the chain where drugs, supplies, or other resources are actually being administered for use by the patient. Also refers to a type of technology that allows for distributed resources to be managed more efficiently.
portfolio	A collection of investments (could be systems or other assets) grouped by different categories, which are selected to help ensure a balanced and systematic approach to improve overall outcomes.
postponement	A supply chain concept in which goods are procured at the latest point in the process; helps reduce inventory levels and encourage rapid response on the part of vendors.
preferred provider organization	A health plan that contracts with a limited panel of independent providers. Patient care services are offered with little or no out-of-pocket expenses for enrollees when all patient care has been performed by members of this network of preferred providers.
prescription	A doctor's written order for medication or other course of treatment.
present value	The value today of a future payment.
price elasticity	The responsiveness of the market to changes in prices. The relationship between pricing variability and demand variability.
process	Set of activities and tasks that are performed in sequence to achieve a specific outcome.

process engineering The careful scrutiny of a current-state process to identify value creation opportunities, such as eliminating hand-offs or steps in the process.

process flowchart Diagram depicting the flows or activities in a process.

product life cycle A process and an indicator that define the major phases involved in the development of a product. The major phases of the life cycle include prelaunch, introduction, growth, maturity, decline, and retirement (or death).

productivity The ratio of outputs to inputs for a specific process. One of the primary goals in operations management is to increase this ratio on a continuous basis.

profit center Organizational units that generate revenues and are expected to earn reasonable returns on those revenues, after considering all costs of operations.

profit margin The excess of revenues less expenses, which represents the residual value of a hospital that is available for funding future operations.

program evaluation and review technique (PERT) A project management technique that builds timelines and project plans based on estimates of three cases: a best case, worst case, and most likely case.

project An organized effort involving a sequence of activities that are temporarily being performed to achieve a desired outcome.

project management The application of knowledge, skills, tools, and techniques to a project to achieve project success.

project manager The individual who leads the planning and daily activities to achieve the project deliverables.

prospective payment A generic term for a payment methodology in which fee schedules are calculated based on treatment type or illness classifications and are paid prospectively (i.e., in advance of the treatment) without regard to actual costs incurred.

quality A condition where goods and services uphold high standards for safety, reliability, and excellence, and exceed customers' expectations.

quality management | The application of quantitative and qualitative methods to ensure that healthcare services and products possess the characteristics necessary to completely satisfy the needs that they are designed to serve.

quantitative | Suggests that data and numbers are used for measurement purposes. The application of mathematical rigor and analysis into managerial processes.

quick response | A process in which lead times are minimized, rapid processing of orders occurs, and changes in demand and business requirements are instantly communicated over the supply chain via collaborative information systems.

radar diagram | Graphical analyses that show target versus actual performance in the key internal areas helps to identify issues that potentially exist.

radio frequency identification (RFID) | Technology that uses small radio transponders to read and transmit data over existing wireless standards and frequencies.

rapid prototyping | A concept where ideas and solutions can be targeted toward a very small sample, to see if the solution improves results prior to wide-scale implementation.

realization | A condition where assets or benefits are actually received.

reliable | Stable and uniform results over time, used in measuring data and performance.

receipt | Physical documentation of actual quantities of goods that were delivered. Receiving documents are often called *proof of delivery*. Receipts must be matched against orders prior to payment.

requisition | A request for an item from a user or consumer of goods and services. The first step in the purchasing process.

return on investment (ROI) | A ratio calculated as total amount of profits earned from a project or investment, divided by the total cost of that investment. Typically looks at profits and expenses over a specific time period, such as three or five years, to capture the time value of money.

reverse logistics
: The process and methods by which hospitals reverse the physical flow of goods, returning them back internally to the originating department or all the way back the chain to distributors and suppliers.

risk
: The factors that jeopardize project success or might cause potential impairment or delay.

robot
: Automation technology that assists in picking and packing pharmaceuticals.

rollup
: An aggregation in a hierarchy.

root cause analysis
: Process for identifying and correcting the major issues causing problems.

safety stock
: Inventory carried in excess of forecasted demand to help manage unexpected variability or uncertainty in demand behavior. Also referred to as *inventory buffer* or *reserve stock*.

sales and operations planning (S&OP)
: The process used in many industrial, process, and manufacturing industries that helps plan production around demand estimates derived collaboratively by multiple internal departments, such as sales, marketing, and logistics.

scheduled drug
: Medications that are classified by the U.S. Drug Enforcement Agency as narcotics or other controlled substances.

scorecard
: A quantitative evaluation tool that lists the key attributes or decision criteria and forces weighted scoring across a number of areas. Typically used for either evaluating vendors or projects.

sensitivity analysis
: A simulation tool that allows a user to change key variables and assumptions, using known mathematical relationships, to estimate the impact on a dependent variable.

service level agreement (SLA)
: Formal agreement that clearly communicates the types of services to be offered, performance expec-

tations, hours services are to be provided, inputs or resources to be committed, and payments if any.

service line

A discrete group of closely related product items. In health care, a service line is equivalent to the number of medical offerings available in the portfolio. Also referred to as *healthcare services* or *product lines*.

shrinkage

Loss, due to theft, mishandling, or other cause.

Six Sigma

Methodology focused on improving processes and quality by eliminating defects and reducing variability or volatility of outcomes.

slice and dice

Term used in information technology to describe the process of breaking data down into component parts, using different perspectives and dimensions to view data.

slope

The tilt or angle of the rise (or fall) over the run.

software maintenance

Support payments due to vendors to cover upgrades and enhancements.

soiled

Dirty or used. Commonly used in laundry and linens.

spectrum analysis

An analysis of the electromagnetic spectrum to assess waves, ensure that there will be no interference from other equipment or devices, and ensure that channels and frequencies are clear. Used prior to implementation of *radio frequency identification* technology.

spend analysis

An in-depth comprehensive analysis of a hospital's expenditures, primarily routine operating expenses, focused on what, how, and with whom an organization spends dollars.

square root law of inventory

Theory of inventory management that suggests that total costs will increase dramatically as the number of stocking points increase.

standard deviation

A statistical measure of the degree of fluctuation or dispersion around the mean.

standardization

Common goal in logistics and supply chain processes to use consistent procedures, resources, items, and services to achieve consistent results across multiple departments.

statement of cash flows
: One of the three key financial statements. Represents all of the cash inflows a hospital receives from its ongoing business activities and investments, as well as its cash outflows for expenditures, labor, and other activities.

statement of financial position
: One of the three key financial statements that details assets, liabilities, and equities or net assets. Also known as the balance sheet.

stock-keeping unit (SKU)
: The combination of the specific end item sold in a particular location. Typically the lowest level in the product hierarchy of a planning system.

stockout
: A shortage of a specific product in inventory, resulting from lack of adequate understanding of demand. Results if an order arrives and no product is available. Also called a *sellout* in certain industries.

strategic alliance
: An often ambiguous term used to imply any number of working relationships between two or more organizations. Often results in a joint venture or merger.

strategic management
: The process for orchestrating organizational resources toward the development of an alignment between business strategies and the environment to improve financial performance. Involves the behavior of complex organizations in responding to turbulent environments, and aligning hospitals' services with the needs of the market.

strategic planning
: The process of formulating competitive strategies that determine a hospital's overall direction and approach.

supply chain
: The activities, people, facilities, and processes involved in moving products through a network to procure, assemble, manufacture, distribute, and sell products to consumers.

supply chain management (SCM)
: The management of all activities involved in sourcing and procurement, conversion, and logistics.

supply to stock (STS)	Philosophy where larger quantities of materials are purchased and placed into an inventory location for storage and distribution. The opposite of *just in time*.
SWOT analysis	A type of analysis used in strategic planning that identifies an organization's strengths, weaknesses, opportunities, and threats.
system integration	The ability to connect or combine two or more systems.
teaching hospital	A major healthcare organization offering observation, diagnosis, and treatment through the practice of academic medicine, via a variety of distribution channels. A limited number of large, complex hospitals that have a major commitment to the missions of academic medicine, including graduate medical education, medical research, and patient care. These organizations are the primary training grounds for future medical doctors, as well as nurses and other allied health professionals.
third-party payer	A payer that is neither the patient or the provider.
three-way match	A method of ensuring strong internal controls, by reconciling purchase orders against receipts and invoices prior to payment.
throughput	The rate or velocity at which services are performed or goods are delivered. Refers to the amount of output that a process can deliver over a specific time period; used in both productivity analysis and process engineering.
time and motion study	Analysis of the details of a process; identifies the total amount of time and effort required to perform a procedure.
time series	Set of values or observations at successive points in time.
time value of money	The financial concept where money received in the present is worth more than the same amount if it were received in the future.

to-be process	A version of a *process map* that depicts the future state or the state following design and process engineering.
tracking system	Tools that monitor the position, flow, and movement of resources. Both *radio frequency identification* and *bar coding* systems fall within this category.
United Nations Standard Products and Services Code (UNSPSC)	Worldwide classification system used to describe item-level data. Supports standardization among vendors and providers about items.
univariate	Refers to dependence on a single variable, where demand forecasts are based on only one historical data series.
upstream	Refers to positioning closer toward manufacturers.
utilization	Usage.
valuation	An assessment of the financial value of an asset.
value chain	The collection of activities that define how work is accomplished in an organization, from inputs to final outputs. In the healthcare industry, the value chain is comprised of the parties and activities involved in delivering patient care. This involves the procurement of materials from suppliers, the delivery of care by physicians and nurses, the financing of care by third-party payers, and the receipt of care by patients.
variable cost	Costs that vary directly with production.
variation	Inconsistency or dispersion of results. Variability in process outcomes is the major source of operational inefficiency and should be minimized as much as possible. Measured by standard deviation.
vendor	A party in the supply chain that sells goods to others, irrespective of ownership of assets. Typically either a manufacturer or a distributor.
vendor-managed inventory (VMI)	A process whereby a supplier manages the inventory stock levels for its customers based on forecasted demand. The process is designed to be proactive by

the supplier, which controls the distribution plans and sends out orders with minimal involvement from the customer.

vertical integration
A type of growth strategy in which one organization acquires another organization—usually a key supplier or a buyer. An example is if a teaching hospital purchased a health insurance plan.

Voluntary Interindustry Commerce Standards (VICS) Association
An organization that helps to promote commerce across the globe and across many industries. Provides standards for CPFR and for collaborative planning.

wait time
Time interval during which there is a temporary cessation of service.

weighted average
A calculation method that uses relativity and means. A type of inventory valuation method.

work breakdown structure (WBS)
Decomposes project activities into more detailed components to allow for better planning. Use of a hierarchy effect to organize tasks, where the top level is the highest level, and each subsequent level below that provides more detail for that task.

working capital
A valuation metric that defines the excess of current assets (comprised of cash, accounts receivable, and inventories) less current liabilities (primarily trade and other payables). It measures liquidity and the ability to cover short-term debt.

About the Author

Dr. James R. Langabeer II is an Associate Professor of Management at the University of Texas School of Public Health at Houston. He has also served as a senior-level manager at two world-renowned academic medical centers, where he had responsibilities over a variety of functions, including management engineering, budgeting and planning, supply chain operations, financial management, and business analysis. He was the executive vice president for one of the fastest growing consulting and technology firms in the United States, where he consulted in more than 30 countries globally for the world's leading *Fortune* 500 firms across the healthcare, retail, and manufacturing industries. Earlier in his career, he was a senior operations manager for a *Fortune* 300 manufacturing firm, where he led the integration and transition processes for multiple mergers and acquisitions. He holds a bachelor's of business administration from the University of Texas at San Antonio; a master's of business administration from Baylor University; and a doctorate in leadership and administration from the University of Houston, where his research focused on economic performance and strategic management of large teaching hospitals. Dr. Langabeer is also a Fellow in the Healthcare Information and Management Systems Society and is a Certified Management Accountant.

Previously, Dr. Langabeer served on the graduate management faculty at Boston University in the department of Administrative Sciences and also at the University of Houston–Downtown. He is the author of three other books: *Creating Demand Driven Supply Chains* (2003), *Competitive Business Strategy for Teaching Hospitals* (2000), and *The Market Driven Enterprise* (1994). He extensively researches healthcare financial and management issues and has been published in more than 35 leading journals, including the *Journal of Healthcare Finance*, *Academic Medicine*, *Supply Chain Management Review*, the *Journal of Healthcare Management*, and the *Journal of Healthcare Information Management*.

INDEX